MESCALINE

Mike Jay has written extensively on scientific and medical history. His books on the history of drugs include *High Society: Mind-Altering Drugs in History and Culture* (Thames and Hudson, 2010) and *The Atmosphere of Heaven: The Unnatural Experiments of Dr Beddoes and His Sons of Genius* (Yale, 2009).

Further praise for *Mescaline*:

'Outstanding. Jay tells a fascinating story with style. He handles a large cast of often-eccentric and difficult individuals with sensitivity and deals expertly with the varied cultural, anthropological, racial and legal issues.' William Bynum, author of *The History of Medicine*

'Jay's excellent book . . . combines joy and gravitas and adds up to a comprehensive history of a still-enigmatic substance . . . Jay's great achievement here is his integration of the two halves of the mescaline story, the Western and the indigenous, rooting it in its proper context and rescuing it from the kitsch that has gathered around psychedelics since the 1960s. The result is a fascinating look into the varieties and potential of human consciousness.' Phil Baker, *Literary Review*

'A highly readable and erudite history, which is also amply and elegantly illustrated. Alongside its obvious appeal to drug historians, it also should offer a valuable primer for any general readership interested in Native American rituals and ceremonies, radical psychiatry or the counterculture of the 1960s.' Peder Clark, *Social History of Medicine*

'Jay is our foremost cultural historian of psychotropic substances and this is a fascinating and brilliantly researched account. Mescaline emerges out of the generic haze of "psychedelics" as a particular substance with its own particular history.' Marcus Boon, author of *The Road of Excess*

'*Mescaline* manages to balance the challenges of a global outlook with the intricacies of personal experience . . . Jay, as with his many other works, expertly places the 'important details in these larger trends, and the result is a wonderfully engaging narrative; informative and entertaining. It will no doubt prove to be an important go-to text for researchers, academics, and trippers alike.' Robert Dickins, *Psychedelic Press*

'An engaging, sensitive history of human interest and interaction with the psychoactive alkaloid mescaline. Jay skilfully weaves insights gained from a range of academic disciplines as well as from popular culture – and provides dramatic evidence that not all of Nature's treasures readily transfer to the contexts of modern society.' Daniel C. Swan, author of *Peyote Religious Art*

'Jay's history of mescaline use is a bit of a mind-altering experience itself, both rollicking and intellectually rigorous . . . he takes seriously mescaline's ability to produce such visual and emotional revelations. But he also wants to demystify the heroic accounts of some of its evangelists.' *The Economist*

'Highly readable . . . the mescaline alkaloid has a long and storied history, and has attracted the attention of some remarkable individuals along the way.' Philip Smith, *AlterNet*

'A must read for understanding the fascinating tension between indigenous traditions and Western clinical modernity that is emblematic of the psychedelic ethos'. Erika Dyck, author of *Psychedelic Psychiatry*

'Very readable and fascinating . . . certainly the most detailed and comprehensive social and medical history of mescaline.' Peter Carpenter, *British Society for the History of Medicine*

'Mike Jay is one of the most wise, well-informed, clever and funny voices on drugs in the world. Everyone should read everything he writes – it is consistently brilliant.' Johann Hari, author of *Chasing the Scream and Lost Connections*

'Engrossing . . . a pioneering attempt to grapple with the different uses and knowledge of this substance.' David Robertson, *Synapsis*

'An undeniably rich and fascinating history that is intimately linked to the story of indigenous culture, Western colonialism and Western medicine over the past several centuries.' Zoe Hackett, *Chemistry World*

'Mike Jay is the Neil Armstrong of today's psychonauts. In *Mescaline* an incredible amount of scholarly and personal research is beautifully presented and ordered in a sensible chronology that really works to channel potentially disruptive and mad matter into a fascinating cultural history. I just loved the last chapter which brought everything back to its proper place in a careful Native American ritual. It made the most emotionally satisfying ending to an extraordinary trip . . .' Nicholas Rankin, author of *Telegram from Guernica*

'Mike Jay's book carefully describes those who came before Huxley: North, South and Central American Indians, Victorian scientists, pioneering physicians and modern aesthetes.' Kate Womersley, *TLS*

'Illuminating . . . richly informative about the many connections between mescaline and visual experience, both the making and the viewing of art . . . *Mescaline* suggests a connection among consciousness, self and seeing.' Philip Alcabes, *Los Angeles Review of Books*

'Jay deftly sets down the cultural and scientific history of mescaline in its heyday: a curious chronicle that deserves not to be forgotten.' Alison Abbott, *Nature*

'Jay tracks the emergence of peyote and its derivative mescaline, bringing incredible and previously untold nuance to the complicated story of peyote's role in the collision between Native Americans and white colonisers. Channeling the major players, including the meeting of Comanche chief Quanah Parker and Euro-American ethnologist James Mooney, the heart of Jay's book is both gripping narrative and often tragic culture-wide cautionary tale.' Jesse Jarnow, *Aquarium Drunkard*

'Jay forces readers to think about the cultural and biomedical elements of the cactus-derived drug. And he wonders why historians and others have given mescaline so little attention.' *Psychology Today*

'Beautifully written, deeply researched, and wonderfully captivating . . . this is a study that the general reader will enjoy and that the drug scholar will be compelled to read and re-read.' James Pugh, *The Social History of Alcohol and Drugs*

MIKE JAY

MESCALINE

A Global History of
the First Psychedelic

YALE UNIVERSITY PRESS
NEW HAVEN AND LONDON

For information about this and other Yale University Press publications, please contact:
U.S. Office: sales.press@yale.edu   yalebooks.com
Europe Office: sales@yaleup.co.uk   yalebooks.co.uk

Set in Adobe Garamond Pro by IDSUK (DataConnection) Ltd
Printed and bound by CPI Group (UK) Ltd, Croydon, CR0 4YY

Library of Congress Control Number: 2019933930

ISBN 978-0-300-23107-6 (hbk)
ISBN 978-0-300-25750-2 (pbk)

A catalogue record for this book is available from the British Library.

10 9 8 7 6 5 4 3 2 1

CONTENTS

List of Illustrations   ix

Acknowledgements   xii

PROLOGUE **ONE BRIGHT MAY MORNING**   1
3 May 1953: Hollywood Hills

1 **CACTUS MYSTERIES**   13
2000 BCE–present: Andean South America

2 **THE DEVIL'S ROOT**   31
1519–present: Mexico

3 **MAKING MEDICINE**   51
1880–93: Oklahoma, Texas, Detroit, Berlin

4 **BRILLIANT VISIONS**   77
1895–98: Washington DC, Philadelphia, Leipzig,
London

5 **HIGHER POWERS**   101
1899–1918: London, Missouri, New York, Taos,
Oklahoma

6 **DER MESKALINRAUSCH**   129
1919–28: Vienna, Heidelberg, Chicago,
Côte d'Azur

7   **PROFANE ILLUMINATIONS**   147
1929–36: Warsaw, Bucharest, Paris, Berlin, Mexico

8   **M-SUBSTANCE**   169
1936–52: Oklahoma, Taos, London, Hamburg,
Basel, Saskatchewan

9   **THE DOORS BLOWN OPEN**   199
1953–59: California, Wisconsin, Mexico, Paris,
Atlantic City, Oxford

10   **TRIPPING WITH MESCALITO**   225
1960–2014: New York, California, Texas, Arizona,
Las Vegas

EPILOGUE   **UNDER A COMANCHE MOON**   247
7–8 October 2017: Oklahoma

Endnotes   257
Bibliography   275
Index   288

ILLUSTRATIONS

CHAPTER FRONTISPIECES

Prologue: The mescaline molecule.

Chapter 1: A bas relief, Chavín circular plaza, *c.* 1200 BCE. Drawing by Pauline Stringfellow for Richard L. Burger, *Chavín and the Origins of Andean Civilization*, Thames & Hudson, 1992.

Chapter 2: *Anhalonium williamsii* by Paul Christoph Hennings, 1888. Courtesy of https://sacredcacti.com/blog/lewinii/

Chapter 3: Peyote ceremony, ritual objects. From Weston La Barre, *The Peyote Cult*, 1938, with the kind permission of Crescent Moon Publishing.

Chapter 4: Silas Weir Mitchell in his study. Printed in the *Topeka State Journal*, 28 October 1902.

Chapter 5: *The Peyote Ritual* by Monroe Tsa Toke, 1957. © Leslie Van Ness Denman.

Chapter 6: Merck Pharmaceutical Co.'s 'Mescalinium-sulfat' solution in a bottle.

Chapter 7: *Portrait of Nena Stachurska* by Stanisław Ignacy Witkiewicz (with peyote and alcohol, after three days without smoking), 1929, pastel on paper. Courtesy of National Museum, Poznań.

Chapter 8: *Stage II (Mescaline Drawing with Cones)* by Julian Trevelyan, 1936. Courtesy of Bethlem Museum of the Mind.

Chapter 9: A photograph of Aldous Huxley, 1952. Keystone Pictures USA / Alamy Stock Photo.

Chapter 10: 'Mescalito', tattoo art. © 2016 Marek Kaot.

Epilogue: 'Arrangement of Interior of Tipi for Peyote Meeting'. From Weston La Barre, *The Peyote Cult*, 1938, with the kind permission of Crescent Moon Publishing.

PLATES

1. San Pedro cacti growing at Chavín de Huantar, 2003. Photo © Aliya Saleem.

2. *Stirrup-Spout Vessel with Feline and Cactus*, 900/200 BCE, north coast of Peru. The Art Institute of Chicago.

3. A hand-coloured lithograph after an original drawing by Walter Hood Fitch, *Curtis' Botanical Magazine*, Vol. 73, 1847, plate 4296. © The Board of Trustees of the Royal Botanic Gardens, Kew.

4. *Le peyotl: la plante qui fait les yeux émerveillés* by Alexandre Rouhier, 1926.

5. A Huichol *mara'akame* collecting peyote. Hemis / Alamy Stock Photo.

6. *The Rite Begins* by Alejandro Lopez Torres, 1997, coloured yarn on board. From the collection of Wade Davis, courtesy of the October Gallery, London.

7. A photograph of James Mooney. Courtesy of the National Anthropological Archives, Smithsonian Institution.

8. A photograph of Quanah Parker of the Kwahadi Comanche, standing in front of a tipi.

9. *Peyote Ceremony* by James Mooney, 1893. Courtesy of the National Anthropological Archives, Smithsonian Institution (gelatin glass negative BAE GN 01778a 06305400).

10. *Peyote Medicine Man* by James Auchiah, 1973, tempera on paper. Courtesy of the Arthur and Shifra Silberman Collection, National Cowboy & Western Heritage Museum, 1996.027.0014.

11. *Portrait of Nena Stachurska, Merck Mescaline + C* by Stanisław Ignacy Witkiewicz, 1929, pastel on paper. From the Teodor Białynicki-Birula collection, Museum of Middle Pomerania, Słupsk, Poland.

12. *Mescaline Painting – Red and Blue Abstract* by an anonymous artist, 1936. Courtesy of Bethlem Museum of the Mind.

13. *Green Abstract* by Basil Beaumont (Basil Ivan Rakoczi), 1936. Courtesy of Bethlem Museum of the Mind, with the kind permission of Christopher Rakoczi.

14. *The Doors of Perception* by Aldous Huxley. Cover art by John Woodcock, Chatto & Windus, 1954.

15. 'In the Magic Land of Mescaline', cover illustration for a feature by Claude William Chamberlain, *Fate*, January 1956.

ACKNOWLEDGEMENTS

At an early stage of writing Toni Melechi and Alan Piper were both very generous in pointing me towards primary sources they had uncovered in their previous researches. Thanks also to Toni for reading an early draft of the manuscript. I owe a great debt to Keeper Trout for sharing his prodigious knowledge of the botany and history of peyote and San Pedro, and for giving me detailed feedback on the manuscript. Trout works together with Martin Terry and Ted Herrero at the Cactus Conservation Institute (cactusconservation.org), an essential resource for the preservation of peyote's natural habitat; it was a great pleasure to meet Martin and Ted in Oklahoma and I thank them for their insights into peyote's current status. I owe my education in the traditional use of San Pedro (*huachuma*) in the Andes to Anthony Henman (Peru), and Roberto Calzadilla and Maria Yana (Bolivia). I greatly appreciated Andrew Lees' expertise in biochemistry and the neurosciences, as well as his fine literary judgement. Jesse Jarnow responded enthusiastically to my queries about the early years of psychedelic counterculture. Erik Davis made several invaluable connections on my behalf. Thanks also to Peter Moore for many enjoyable conversations and his stimulating feedback on the manuscript. And, as always, very special thanks to Louise, the perfect companion in these researches.

In Oklahoma: my deep gratitude to William Voelker Wahathuweeka and Troy (The Last Captive) Kwihnai Mahquuitsoi Okweettuni of Sia, the Comanche Nation Ethno-Ornithological Initiative and Piah Pha Kahni (Mother Church) of the Numunuh (Comanche) Native American Church, for their wonderful food and hospitality, their great generosity in sharing with me the history of their people and their precious life items, and for hosting the meeting that I describe in the epilogue. Udah! Warmest appreciation to Charlie Haag, President of the Native American Church of Oklahoma, for sharing with me the stories of his grandfather Mack and the founding of the Native American Church, and for making tracks with James Mooney around Calumet and Concho. Many thanks to Daniel Swan, curator of the Sam Noble Museum of Natural History in Norman, OK, for sharing his deep knowledge of the NAC and its artistic traditions, and for his generous introductions. Thanks also to Amie Tah-Bone at the Kiowa Cultural Centre in Carnegie, and Diana Cox at the Gilcrease Museum in Tulsa.

In New Mexico: special thanks to Mark Hoffman and the Bad Shaman for their hospitality in Taos and their insights into local history and ethnobotany. Thanks also to Carol at the Mabel Dodge Luhan house for her welcome and guided tour. In Gallup, many thanks to Donovan Ferrari at Silver Dust Trading and to Rick and Kathy at Shi'ma Traders for sharing their knowledge of the contemporary NAC scene.

Among many other people to whom I'm indebted for conversations, pointers and other assistance are: Ian Baker; Michael Bird; Jacob Blandy; Paul Bloom; Joseph Calabrese; Ru Callender; Anthony Day and Ross Macfarlane at the Wellcome Library; Rob Dickins; Patrick Everett; Colin Gale and Amy Moffat at the Bethlem Art and History Collections Trust; Richard Grant; Kathelin Gray and Chili Hawes at the October Gallery; Adam Green; Ivo Gurschler; Tim Harvey, editor of the Cactus and Succulent Journal (USA); Rhodri Hayward; Matei Iagher; Gary Lachman; Brian Leese; Rachael Lonsdale; Dave Luke and Anna Hope; Stella Luna; John Marks; Jelena Martinovic; Michael Neve; Jerry Patchen; Mark Pilkington; John Robertson of the Poison Garden, Alnwick; Sonu Shamdasani; John Smythies; Michael Somple of the Munson William Proctor Art Institute; and Beata Zgodzińska at the Museum of Central Pomerania.

Many thanks for all their support and encouragement to my literary agent, Caroline Montgomery, and to my editor Julian Loose, whose early suggestions steered the book towards its eventual form.

ONE BRIGHT MAY MORNING

3 MAY 1953

HOLLYWOOD HILLS

Mescaline molecule.

'One bright May morning' in 1953, at his home in the Hollywood Hills, Aldous Huxley swallowed 400mg of mescaline sulphate crystals dissolved in water. The book that resulted, *The Doors of Perception*, made mescaline world famous.[1] Huxley first described the experience in a letter to his editor at Chatto and Windus as 'without any question the most extraordinary and significant experience available to human beings this side of the Beatific Vision'.[2] To his readers it became 'what Adam had seen on the morning of his creation – the miracle, moment by moment, of naked existence'.[3] It went far beyond words and Huxley and Humphry Osmond, the psychiatrist who had supplied the vial of mescaline and witnessed the experiment, exchanged letters in which they tossed around suggestions for a new term to encompass mescaline's action and that of its recently discovered chemical cousin LSD. Huxley consulted Liddell and Scott's dictionary for Ancient Greek roots that captured the sense of 'to make visible or manifest' the psyche; he suggested 'phaneropsychic', 'psychophans' or 'phanerothymes'. Osmond responded with 'psyche-delic'.[4] Huxley maintained the correct spelling should be 'psychodelic' and persisted with it, to little avail.

Reading it today, Huxley's book seems an improbable springboard for the psychedelic revolution. The sixties counterculture rarely recalled the high seriousness of its aesthetic canon (Bernini, Watteau, Vermeer) or its profusely capitalised metaphysical abstractions ('Mind-at-Large', '*Istigkeit*', 'the Dharma-Body', 'the Void', 'the Nature of Things'). Most fondly remembered in the decade to come was the author's rapt scrutiny of the folds in his grey flannel trousers. At the time of its publication in 1954, however, *The Doors of Perception* compelled attention with two grand claims: one about mescaline's future and one about its past. The first was of a scientific breakthrough, the 'new and perhaps highly significant fact'[5] that mescaline might reveal the cause of schizophrenia and potentially its cure. The second was Huxley's claim that the dimensions of mind opened up by mescaline were virtually unexplored: 'How many philosophers, how many theologians, how many professional educators have had the curiosity to open this Door in the Wall? The answer, for all practical purposes, is, None.'[6]

By the time *The Doors of Perception* was published, mescaline was already a hot topic in biomedical and psychiatric research. During 1953 and 1954 readers of *Time* and *Newsweek* had learned about the schizophrenia hypothesis proposed by Humphry Osmond and John Smythies on which Huxley's first claim was based. But Huxley promoted the drug to the status of popular sensation. The *New Yorker* gave over a dozen pages to a narrative of the healing powers and Native American ceremonies involving the peyote cactus, from which mescaline had originally been extracted. Simultaneously with Huxley's essays, articles and broadcasts about the prospect of a society in which psychedelic drugs were used for spiritual illumination, the French artist and poet Henri Michaux was publishing the first of his gruelling investigations into the effects of mescaline on consciousness and creativity; the anthropologist James Sydney Slotkin produced his acclaimed ethnography of Native American peyote use; and the pioneers of the drug culture to come, William Burroughs and Allen Ginsberg among them, were adding peyote to their diets of marijuana, heroin and Benzedrine. Suddenly mescaline was everywhere.

In addition to mescaline and LSD, in 1957 a *LIFE* magazine cover splash announced the discovery of a new psychedelic drug. The investment banker and amateur ethnobotanist Gordon Wasson had tracked down a tribal community in Mexico which still used vision-giving mushrooms according to ancient tradition, and in 1958 Albert Hofmann, the discoverer of LSD, isolated the mushrooms' active chemical and named it psilocybin. The issue of *LIFE* following Gordon Wasson's feature 'Seeking the Magic Mushroom' demonstrated that intrepid members of the public were already undertaking their own adventures. It included a letter from one Jane Ross advising that Wasson's journey to the mountains of Oaxaca had been unnecessary: 'I've been having hallucinatory visions accompanied by space suspension and time destruction in my New York City apartment for the past three years.' She had been alerted to mescaline by *The Doors of Perception* and acquired it in its natural form, the dried top of the peyote cactus, from a Texas mail order supplier for $8 per hundred 'buttons'. 'It usually takes about four "buttons" for one person to have visions,' she wrote.[7] William Burroughs had already sniffed out the same supplier, and within three years peyote would be on open sale in the bohemian haunts of lower Manhattan.

Laboratory-grade mescaline was also available to the determined seeker: in practice, anyone who could claim a PhD or rustle up a plausible-looking business letterhead. My uncle Peter had neither, but after reading *The Doors of Perception* he visited the office of Aldrich, the research chemical supplier, outside London and casually requested some. The assistant informed him that 'we've been told to be careful about who we supply it to', and asked if he was a doctor. 'Well, I am a physicist,' Peter offered (he was working for Kodak at the time). He was sold half a kilo, over a thousand doses, which kept the beatnik vanguard of Soho and the Sussex coast supplied for some time.

These early adopters were few and scattered, but their traces give a flavour of the diverse interests that would soon be subsumed within the new category of 'psychedelic'. In 1952 Osmond's collaborator John Smythies, who had first been drawn to mescaline by his interest in mystical and paranormal experiences, supplied some to the British psychic researcher Rosalind Heywood. Heywood had a very different experience from Huxley: 'for him the outer world was transfigured, whereas for me it became extremely drab and boring. My consciousness fled away into a stupendous inner world.'[8] She advertised in the *Manchester Guardian* for artists to participate in mescaline visualisations, an offer accepted eagerly by Bryan Wynter, a graduate of the Slade art school who already knew *The Doors of Perception* virtually by heart. Wynter went on to pursue his own experiments at his remote cottage in the far west of Cornwall, where from 1956 onwards mescaline inspired his 'new consciousness' turn, in which he sought to catch through seething abstract canvasses 'the moment at which the eye looks out at the world it has not yet recognised'.[9]

    ✦   ✦   ✦

As the sixties unfolded, Huxley's bright May morning came to stand alongside Albert Hofmann's first LSD-fuelled bicycle ride in 1943 as the founding experience of the psychedelic era. Yet the two grand claims with which he had announced mescaline to the world had already receded from view. The theory that schizophrenia was caused by a neurotoxin related to mescaline was, like many of the scientific theories in Huxley's late writings, quickly forgotten.[10] Over the next few years it was overwritten by the dopamine hypothesis that emerged from studying the action of new drugs such as chlorpromazine. Discovering a chemical cause for schizophrenia, let alone finding a chemical cure, seems no closer today than it did in 1954.

Huxley's second claim, that the states of consciousness opened up by mescaline were all but unexplored, must have seemed odd even at the time to the attentive reader. Huxley had clearly made careful study of an extensive literature on the subject. The very first page of *The Doors of Perception* cites a series of pharmacological, medical and literary descriptions of mescaline's effects dating back over fifty years, including Louis Lewin's nineteenth-century pharmacological writings[11] and the pioneering self-experiments of the neurologist Silas Weir Mitchell and the *fin-de-siècle* psychologist Havelock Ellis. It goes on to outline a written history of mescaline's indigenous use spanning five centuries, from pre-Hispanic Mexico to the contemporary Native American Church in the United States.

Havelock Ellis in particular seems to have been a direct inspiration. Ellis's 1898 report opens, like Huxley's half a century later, with a genealogy dating back to ancient Mexico and a crisp scene-setting gambit that, like Huxley's, fuses scientific detachment with confessional intimacy: 'On Good Friday I found myself entirely alone in the quiet rooms in the Temple which I occupy when in London, and judged the occasion a fitting one for a personal experiment.'[12] The core of Ellis's essay, like that of Huxley's, is a dazzling aesthetic performance in which he compares the effects of peyote (from which mescaline was at that moment being isolated) to everything from Maori architecture to the painting of Claude Monet. His conclusion, like Huxley's, is a manifesto for the drug's transformational possibilities, both for the individual and for society at large. Ellis predicts that 'the favourite poet of the mescal drinker will certainly be Wordsworth', whose work precisely captures the drug's power to enchant even the humblest object.[13] Huxley cites Wordsworth twice as an exemplar of how to perceive, in nothing more remarkable than a hedge or a table, 'the gift, beyond price, of a new direct insight into the very Nature of Things'.[14]

Mescaline launched the psychedelic era but would play little part in its future. By 1954 it was already being superseded in scientific research by LSD, which produced similar effects on the mind at less than a thousandth of the dose and with fewer physical side effects. By the time Timothy Leary had his psychedelic awakening on psilocybin in 1960, the scientists who ventured through Huxley's 'Door in the Wall' were rarely using mescaline. By 1963, its research uses were tightly controlled and LSD was hitting the streets. From that bright May morning in 1953 the many threads of mescaline's story lead not forwards but back, into a past that Huxley simultaneously revealed and concealed.

In contrast to LSD, 'psychedelic' was only the latest of the many labels that had been attached to mescaline. The word had been coined to rescue it from the language of psychiatry, where clinical terms such as 'hallucinogen' and 'psychotomimetic' connected it to mental disease; but mescaline had many cultural lives before the psychiatrists claimed it. Over the previous decades it had been explored by artists, littérateurs and philosophers such as Jean-Paul Sartre, Walter Benjamin and Antonin Artaud, and its consciousness-expanding effects had been filtered through the gaze of modernist art, phenomenology and existentialism. It had arrived in interwar philosophy and the avant-garde via a series of psychological researches in 1920s Europe that placed it at the cutting edge of mental science, the strange visions and alterations of consciousness that it produced described by dozens of experimental subjects.

All this had been sparked by mescaline's chemical synthesis in an Austrian laboratory in 1919; but before then it had already been circulating across America and Europe for twenty years in the form of plant extracts, tinctures and alkaloid salts. It was introduced to western science during the late nineteenth century in the form of the peyote cactus, which originally reached the pharmacologists, neurologists and psychologists from the devotees of the peyote religion that had spread through devastated Indian tribes during their forced captivity in the reservations of Oklahoma. Peyote had reached the Plains tribes via the new Texas–Mexico railroad, and their ceremony drew on deep roots in Mexico, where peyote's recorded history stretches back to the earliest Spanish chronicles of the Nahua (Aztec) people.[15] Before that, an unwritten history attested by art and archaeology unrolls the story of mescaline-containing cacti all the way back to deep prehistory and the earliest temple cultures of the New World.

No mind-altering substance has been described more thoroughly and from such a variety of perspectives than mescaline. For decades there was no other drug known to western science that produced comparable effects on the mind or body, in particular its signature visions of unearthly colour and brilliance. Yet it remains impossible to give a simple answer to the simple-sounding question of what mescaline actually does. Hundreds of written descriptions attest to its unique spectrum of physical and psychic stimuli: dizziness, fullness in the head, nausea, time distortion, a rainbow sheen of visual trails, hyperventilation, an uncanny sense of double consciousness, physical prostration, auditory hallucinations, ineffable cosmic insights, a lazy euphoria, a pounding heart, scintillating patterns exploding across closed eyelids and the immanent presence of the sacred. But each experience is different. Not only do these stimuli occur in unpredictable combinations, but their meaning is different for every subject. There are many who have described mescaline as essentially a poison, an emetic or a deliriant that disorders the mind and sense of self like a high fever or a psychotic episode. There are many others who have used it as a medicine: sometimes as a specific such as a stimulant or cardiac tonic, sometimes as a panacea for mind and body that rebalances the metabolism and cuts sickness off at its root. Some have deployed it as a precision tool that offers a privileged glimpse into the hidden workings of the mind and brain, or as a catalyst to creativity and a portal to new dimensions of aesthetic awareness. For others it has been a sacrament, a direct connection to the energies of nature, the world of spirits or the mind of God.

Mescaline's signature visions, the phenomenon for which it is best known, exemplify the difference between describing its effects and explaining them. Already by the late 1920s psychologists had assembled hundreds of pages of first-hand reports of mescaline visions' dazzling colours and intricate geometrical forms that resolved at higher doses into otherworldly figures and landscapes. But where do they come from, and what do they mean? Some have seen them as a key to the subconscious or a revealer of hidden personality; others have concluded that they have no discernible relevance to the individual subject. Some have experienced them as transmissions from another world, others as deeply encoded or buried memories. For others still they are a trivial epiphenomenon, artefacts of a brain tricked into producing signal from noise. Western modernity has scrutinised them through every conceivable lens – neurological, literary, occult, psychodynamic, aesthetic, spiritual – but they remain as mysterious in their essence as the mind itself.

Indigenous cultures, by contrast, have paid mescaline's visions much less attention. Its traditional users commonly regard them as peripheral to the experience: distractions for the unwary or wandering mind, an indication that the subject is failing to grasp the deeper meaning of the experience.[16] The literature on mescaline-containing cacti is rich in stories and ethnographic detail but includes very few subjective descriptions, most of which have been given at the prompting of western interviewers. Non-western subjects are typically reluctant to share what is considered a private and often highly emotional experience. They have a strong presumption against reducing the experience to the psychoactive effects of the cactus, let alone to the mescaline the cactus contains. It is a teacher to be listened to, not an object to investigate. Its meaning is embedded in generations of culture, and at the same time specific to each individual.

In this respect western encounters with mescaline are quite different. When its subjects describe its effects, they are also seeking to discover, construct or invent a framework of meaning to explain them. This is a literature rich in detailed subjective descriptions by scientists, artists and other investigators, in most cases their first experience of this kind. Their reports are extravagantly diverse, as might be expected from a collection of individuals undergoing a profound and often life-changing experience for a wealth of different reasons. At the same time they have the commonalities that might be expected from a demographic that (whether strait-laced scientists or countercultural rebels) skews heavily white, male and intellectual. Together, they constitute a crowd-sourced journey through the modern mind and the many forms in which chemically altered consciousness was conceived before the label 'psychedelic' emerged to contain it.

The distinction between western and indigenous understandings of mescaline maps closely, though not exactly, onto the distinction between pure mescaline, the product of the twentieth-century laboratory, and its natural sources: two families of cactus, the peyote of Mexico and the San Pedro of the Andes. The various species have slightly different psychoactive profiles; all contain a mix of other alkaloids alongside mescaline, and in this their effects differ to some extent from those of the pure drug.[17] But these chemical distinctions are marginal in comparison to the range of individual responses and to the context in which the experience takes place. Being injected with mescaline in a clinic is quite different from eating peyote in a Native American tipi ceremony, or indeed from drinking a solution of its crystals in the Hollywood Hills on a bright May morning and contemplating a vase of flowers.

The stories of peyote and mescaline, the cactus and the crystal, have unfolded in parallel: sometimes entwining, sometimes diverging, each taking many unexpected turns. At times they inform one another, although, as with much else, the modern world has learned less from the indigenous experience than it might have done. The crystal's narrative has a more spectacular rise and fall, but the story begins – and ends – with the cactus.

CHAPTER ONE

CACTUS MYSTERIES

2000 BCE–PRESENT
ANDEAN SOUTH AMERICA

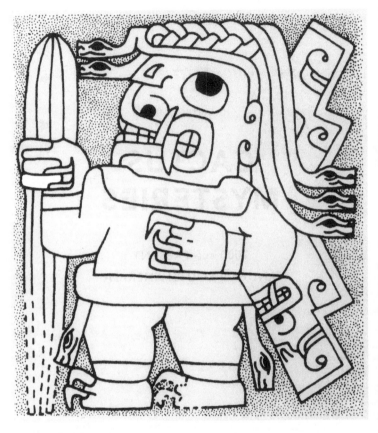

Figure holding a San Pedro cactus, Chavín, c. *1200* BCE.

In the opening paragraph of *The Doors of Perception* Aldous Huxley traced the story of mescaline back to the peyote cactus, 'a friend of immemorially long standing' to 'primitive religion and the Indians of Mexico and the American Southwest'.[1] But some scholars already suspected by that point that mescaline also had another ancient source, one attested in art, sculpture and architecture dating back hundreds of years further than the Spanish chronicles that offer the first cultural records of peyote. In 1947 the Peruvian pharmacologists Carlos Gutiérrez-Noriega and Guillermo Cruz-Sánchez published the first of a series of papers that tentatively identified the presence of mescaline salts in the family of tall columnar cacti known across the Andes in Spanish as San Pedro and in Quechua and Aymara as *achuma* or *huachuma*. In 1950 they documented its secret use on the Peruvian coast in traditional healing ceremonies that were still prohibited under laws against sorcery, and in 1959 the presence of mescaline was confirmed in *Trichocereus pachanoi*, the classic San Pedro.[2]

This identification dovetailed with recent discoveries made by the Peruvian archaeologist Julio Tello, who had been excavating since the 1930s at the mysterious temple site of Chavín de Huántar in the snow-capped range of the Cordillera Blanca in the high Andes. The temple structures at Chavín – a huge complex of sunken plazas and step pyramids, with evidence only of minor habitation and no trace of military fortifications – are surrounded by massive walls of faced stone blocks studded with elaborately carved heads, some up to half a ton in weight, held in defiance of gravity by concealed tenons. The heads are part human and part monstrous feline, with exaggerated jaws and fangs. Many are contorted and grimacing, and some have streams of mucus flowing from their nostrils. The oldest of the sunken plazas, dated to at least 1200 BCE, has a frieze running around its circular inner wall at knee height featuring a similar figure, snake-haired, sprouting fangs and claws and clutching an unmistakable San Pedro cactus.

Chavín had previously been assumed to be a far outpost of some Mesoamerican civilisation, perhaps Olmec or Maya, but a landslide in

1925 that altered the course of the Mosna river above which it perches enabled Tello to recover potsherds that pushed back the date of its habitation and revealed a three-stage construction spanning close to a thousand years. In the twisting network of subterranean chamber-galleries under the old temple he focused his attention on a carved stone stela (which he named the *Lanzón* for its lance-shape), its surface carved with a fanged humanoid figure that he identified with the deity Viracocha, later worshipped in a different form by the Inca. By the time of his death in 1947, just as the presence of mescaline in San Pedro was being revealed, Julio Tello had won acceptance for his theory that Chavín was far more ancient than previously assumed and represented a previously unsuspected pristine culture of monumental architecture in the Andes.

The evidence for this culture, now named Chavín or Early Horizon, has grown considerably in the interim, particularly since 1994 when Ruth Shady Solís of Peru's National Archaeological Museum began work on a complex of sites in the arid coastal valley of the Norte Chico around a hundred miles north of Lima. This barren desert, where rain never falls except in El Niño years, is dotted with huge mounds which were assumed to be natural formations but turned out to be complexes of plazas and pyramids, some older than any in Egypt. Like Chavín they appear to be ceremonial: they stand unfortified, situated away from the irrigated streams of snowmelt in the valley's heart, and appear to have been inhabited only by a small number of priestly functionaries. Caral, the first to be excavated, is now dated to 2700 BCE, and some of its neighbouring structures may be even older.

These coastal complexes are connected to Chavín not only by their monumental architecture but by imagery – depictions of tropical birds and monkeys, native to the highlands, decorate bone flutes found there – and by networks of trade. On the barren coast, in the permanent sea-mist that clings where the desert heat meets the cold Humboldt current, waste middens dating back millennia are exceptionally well preserved. They reveal a material culture founded on fishing the rich Pacific coast with cotton nets and gourd floats, technology that allowed a sizeable population to thrive in the harsh landscape. They also include objects that must have been sourced from the distant mountains and beyond including, alongside the pyramid complex of Las Aldas, the preserved skins of cacti, presumed to be San Pedro, rolled neatly like cigars.[3]

The switchback road up into the Andes gives a sense of the organisation and energy that the trade route would have demanded. The baked silt and pebble crust of the coastal plain stretches for miles inland without shade or water before the foothills begin to rise. The slopes are gradually colonised by scrub and bushes until, at an elevation of around 1,000 metres, the clouds forced upward by the desert heat coalesce and clothe the slopes in green. The arable land between the scree slopes becomes a patchwork of small farms growing subtropical fruit – guava, lime and lucuma – and stands of coffee and coca bushes beneath the shade of avocado trees.

At around 2,000 metres the air thins, the lush foliage dies away and the domain of the San Pedro begins. The cactus clings to the high, barren cliffs, sometimes as a single stem but often in clusters that fan upwards like organ pipes or collapse under their own weight and trail like cucumbers down the gravel slopes. For three months of the year they are wreathed in hanging cloud and drizzle; for the other nine they are blasted by the high tropical sun. Their skin colour ranges from a parched olive green to a rich emerald, often dusted with a delicate verdigris bloom that rubs off at the slightest touch and takes months to re-form. In the spring they flower magnificently, a dazzling explosion of life from a dull and apparently lifeless stem, usually a single bloom that unfurls from near the top. The flower is a luxurious frill of creamy white and yellow petals that opens at night with a lemony scent and is pollinated by hummingbirds and bats.

This is the ancestral domain of the cactus. The family evolved in the desert regions of South America some 30 to 40 million years ago, long before the southern continent became joined to the north. Cacti are part of a unique flora and fauna – sloths, tapirs, anteaters, llamas, vampire bats – that developed idiosyncratically in this self-contained world. Under the fierce sun they selected for ever smaller leaves and for thicker, leathery skin. To avoid losing moisture they opened the stomata that collect carbon dioxide for photosynthesis by night (rather than by day, as do other plants). During the day they synthesise their sugars, and San Pedro is usually harvested in the late afternoon when at its sweetest. The first cacti developed areoles, a unique feature from which their spines – modified leaves – emerge. Their stems became receptacles that could swell to hold huge volumes of water within their dusty and wrinkled exteriors, in the form of thick and often bitter mucus.

Why the San Pedro and peyote cacti should contain mescaline is a mystery – or, more precisely, a cluster of interlocking mysteries. Mescaline seems to occur in nature only within the cacti, and within the cacti only significantly in two families that are about as distantly related as it is possible for cacti to be.[4] Recent studies have identified it in a growing number of species, but mostly within the *Trichocereus* and *Echinopsis* genera, closely related to the San Pedro and usually present only in trace amounts.[5]

In outline the biochemistry is well understood. Mescaline is one product among many of the conversion by methylation or hydroxylation of the amino acids tyrosine and phenylalanine, which are widespread across the plant and animal kingdoms – present in the human body, and in many of our foods, such as meat, eggs and milk. It is an alkaloid, a type of compound commonly produced in plants from the building blocks of amino acids. The term 'alkaloid' derives from 'vegetable alkali', coined by the German chemist Friedrich Sertürner, who isolated the first of them – morphine, from the opium poppy – in the early nineteenth century. He had expected that the pure chemical would be acidic, but it turned out to be an alkaline salt. Over 7,000 alkaloids are known, and San Pedro and peyote both contain around fifty others beside mescaline.

The more difficult question, and presumably the key to unlocking the mysteries, is what purpose these alkaloids serve as far as the plant is concerned. Most alkaloids contain nitrogen, often in the structure of a benzene ring, and it was assumed for a long time that they were metabolic by-products whose purpose was to flush excess nitrates out of plants, the equivalent of animal waste chemicals such as urea. The picture now appears considerably more complex. Alkaloid levels in plants rise and fall during their diurnal cycles, suggesting they have a metabolic function. They are often shuttled from the sites where they are produced to other parts, such as leaves or roots, and between different types of cells. Some plants contain them but others, often closely related species, do not. Their overall distribution across the plant kingdom is without obvious pattern. Some studies suggest that they are unusually prevalent among the cacti, but there is a wide discrepancy between estimates.[6]

Mescaline, one of many plant alkaloids that are psychoactive in humans (like opium in poppies, caffeine in tea and coffee, and psilocybin in magic mushrooms), belongs to a chemical family known as the phenethylamines, which are readily synthesised from the amino acid phenylalanine (this is reflected in mescaline's full chemical name, 3,4,5-trimethoxyphenylethylamine). In this respect mescaline is different from the other compounds regarded as classic psychedelics – LSD, psilocybin and DMT – which are not phenethylamines but tryptamines, another family of alkaloids more similar in structure to the amino acid tryptophan. All share the same basic mechanism of action in the brain – binding to and activating the serotonin or 5-HT receptors – but, whereas the tryptamines' most pronounced alterations are cerebral, mescaline generates a wider spectrum of sensory and physical effects.[7] The phenethylamine family includes stimulants such as amphetamine and the human neurotransmitter dopamine, and mescaline shares some of their physiological properties: elevating mood, increasing the heart rate and banishing sleep. Its pronounced psyche-delic qualities are absent or muted in other naturally occurring pheneth-lyamines, but have in recent years been created in synthetic mescaline relatives such as 2C-B, DOM and 2C-T-7.

There is much more to be learned about mescaline's biosynthesis in cacti and its neurochemical activity in the brain, but none of it will solve the riddle of why a handful of cactus species should contain a potent psychedelic drug found nowhere else in nature. Mescaline is one of the few chemicals produced by plants in a dose concentrated enough to alter profoundly the way we think, feel and perceive the world around us. For the cactus, though, these properties may have no particular significance. Alkaloids, it seems, have no single and simple function in plants; they have probably evolved many times and for many different reasons. Recent research suggests that, in addition to their poorly understood metabolic roles, they may have coevolved with insects and animals: acting as poisons or deliriants for some and attrac-tors for others, and thereby shaping the plants' habitat in their favour.[8] Within their microscopic ecologies of fungi and bacteria, any plants that develop a distinctive chemical profile are likely to have some advantage over their neighbours. Mescaline may be a step in a coevolu-tionary dance with other inhabitants of the desert, one that began long before the arrival of our species.

＊   ＊   ＊

Human relations with the mescaline-containing cacti are ancient, complex, intimate and reciprocal. The much disputed taxonomy of the San Pedro family reflects the ease with which all cacti tend to hybridise, but it has probably also been shaped by localised human selection over millennia for short spines or high mescaline content. The deep valleys that rake across the Andes are ecological islands that breed their own distinctive varieties, with every imaginable combination of spine length, height, girth and skin colour. *Trichocereus pachanoi*, the classic

San Pedro, typically has short spines growing in tight, regularly spaced clusters; the closely related *Trichocereus peruvianus*, which contains mescaline at similar or slightly lower concentrations, has spines that can be several inches long and needle sharp. Some cactologists treat *T. peruvianus* and *T. pachanoi* as long- and short-spined versions of the same species, while others regard them as only two species among a much more extensive family. Since the 1930s cactologists have used *T. pachanoi* as a rooting and grafting stock on account of its small spines, rapid growth and tolerance to a broad range of conditions, and there are now countless cultivar varieties worldwide.

Indigenous classification recognises many more varieties than western botany, defining them by their context and habitat as much as by a specimen's individual characteristics. It also recognises different markers: for example, the number of ribs or columnar sections, ranging from four to eight, which meet at the tip and form a star shape when the cactus is cut into slices. Seven-ribbed specimens are highly favoured for magic and medicine but the four-pointed cactus, a rare variant analogous to a four-leaf clover, is regarded as the most potent. This is the form that appears to be carved in relief at Chavín.[9]

At 3,200 metres, Chavín stands at the upper limits of the San Pedro belt, beyond which the valleys rise above the treeline into the mist-shrouded grassland known as the *puna*. The cactus is a distinctive presence in the landscape: tall clusters are dotted outside the ancient site's walls and cultivated around the local houses as fences and windbreaks. San Pedro's precise role in Chavín's ancient culture is, however, not so readily identifiable. The distinctive flora of South America includes many psychoactive species whose use dates back into deep prehistory. Sites from the Chavín period are decorated with representations of *Brugmansia*, the angel's trumpet flower, whose leaves and seeds are a source of the powerful toxic deliriant scopolamine and its related alkaloids. Dried quids of coca leaves, found on the northern coasts of Peru together with the burnt lime with which to chew them, have been dated as far back as 6000 BCE. Tobacco's centre of origin may well have been the Peruvian Andes, and its earliest cultivation is estimated at 5000–3000 BCE. By the time of the Early Horizon culture, maize and manioc were being fermented into *chicha*, a beer-strength alcoholic brew to which other psychoactive plants could be added.

Uniquely, the flora of South America also includes a variety of plants containing high concentrations of DMT (dimethyltryptamine). Though widespread in nature, including in trace amounts in the human brain, DMT is rarely present at levels potent enough for human use without chemical extraction. It is inactive when eaten or drunk, since enzymes in the human stomach break it down rapidly, but when snuffed at sufficient dosage it produces a burning sensation, an intense bout of nausea and brief, dazzling hallucinations. In the Amazon a concentrated dose can be sweated out over hot coals from the resinous bark of the *virola*, a jungle tree of the nutmeg family, or squeezed from the soaked roots of the spiny *jurema* (*Mimosa hostilis*). The DMT-rich leaves of *chacruna* (*Psychotria viridis*), a shrub related to the coffee plant, have long been boiled together with the *yagé* vine *Banisteriopsis caapi*, whose beta-carboline alkaloids make DMT psychoactive when consumed orally, into the emetic and hallucinogenic ayahuasca brew. In the Andes not far from Chavín, DMT is present, along with other related tryptamines, in the papery, disc-shaped seeds of *Anadenanthera colubrina*, a leguminous tree known in Quechua as *vilca*.[10] Its close relative *Anadenanthera peregrina*, native to the Amazon, was brought to the Caribbean in around 500 BCE by the Taíno people; the first Spanish adventurers encountered it there under the name of *cohoba*.

The San Pedro cactus is the only psychoactive plant depicted in naturalistic style at Chavín,[11] but the presence of *vilca* is clearly attested by snuffing trays and tubes, artefacts that were widespread across the Andes in pre-Columbian times and are still in use by a few isolated groups today.[12] *Vilca* seeds, ground to a fine powder, were traditionally laid out on bone or wooden trays and snuffed forcefully with tubes, often made from the hollow bones of birds and sometimes combined into a Y-shape to propel the powder up both nostrils. Across Chavín-era sites from northern Peru down to northwest Argentina, these snuff trays and tubes have been found at many sites from 1200 BCE onwards. Trays made from whalebone have been unearthed hundreds of miles from the coast, alongside tubes fashioned from the bones of foxes and pumas as well as birds. It may be that *vilca* and San Pedro were also added to ceremonial *chicha* brews at this time, a practice witnessed in 1571 by Juan Polo de Ondegardo, a Spanish administrator in Cuzco.[13]

The consensus among its recent archaeologists is that Chavín was a temple built for large-scale ceremonies, and that hallucinogenic plant preparations were an important component of the rituals that took place there.[14] The architecture of the complex seems to have been designed to frame and create a spectacle in which the senses were manipulated by sound, light and spatial disorientation as well as consciousness-altering plant preparations. Rushing mountain streams were rerouted to create an artificial watercourse that echoed through the tunnels; conch trumpet shells have been found, and fragments of anthracite mirror that may have bounced light through the galleries along with sound. The expansion of the site over centuries, and the replication of Chavín's motifs in later sites hundreds of miles distant, suggest that the experience drew participants from great distances, uniting the cultures of the coast with those of the jungle on the Andes' eastern slopes into which the Mosna river descends. For Julio Tello this made Chavín the founding nexus of Peruvian culture. He described it as the trunk of a mighty tree out of whose three great limbs – the coast, the mountains and the jungle – the nation had been born.[15]

Chavín places mescaline at the origins of South America's first monumental culture, but in the company of too many other visionary plants to trace its signature clearly. The imagery that swarms across the temple's stone reliefs is, to modern eyes, intensely psychedelic: a chaos of claws, jaws, wings and huge dilated eyes that resolves into geometrical, tessellated abstracts and stacked vertical repetitions. But this style suggests not so much the characteristic visions of mescaline as the fractal, bejewelled mindscapes that feature so prominently in contemporary DMT- and ayahuasca-inspired art. Chavín's pantheon of fanged and bug-eyed deities are carved across *vilca* snuff trays and tubes from other, later cultural sites in Bolivia, Argentina and Chile. The consumption of DMT-containing snuffs is vividly suggested by the tenon heads on the walls that pour gouts of mucus from their noses as they grimace in ecstatic agony and shapeshift into feline predators, an ordeal still practised with similar snuffs by Amazonian shamans today.

The role played by mind-altering substances in the rites of long-vanished cultures can only be a matter for speculation, but the architecture of Chavín may offer some clues to how San Pedro was used. The pyramids, countersunk plazas and subterranean galleries constitute a vertical complex that appears designed for a sequence of ritual elements: a mass gathering, an ascent to the summit and a private ordeal or mystery, perhaps involving DMT snuffs, enacted in the labyrinths beneath. The imposing gate in the outer wall suggests a formal procession route into the temple's ceremonial core. The gatherings in the plazas might have taken the form of singing and dancing enhanced by a San Pedro brew, perhaps as an admixture to a ceremonial *chicha*. Mescaline, like its modern stepchild MDMA (ecstasy), encourages rhythmic and stereotypic movement: in Mexican traditions, peyote was commonly used to drive celebrants through all-night dancing ceremonies. As well as moderating the nausea and uncomfortable physical symptoms of the cactus, rhythmic group movement on mescaline helps to bond celebrants together in a euphoric trance state. San Pedro could have performed this role for those who made the pilgrimage to the high mountains, as an element in a ceremonial brew that subsumed the inhabitants of desert, mountain and jungle into an ecstatic group mind and a shared Andean culture.

🌺   🌺   🌺

To judge by the archaeological evidence, San Pedro remained a prominent feature of the pre-Hispanic cultures that succeeded Chavín. Ritual vessels with cactus motifs are found among the Wari and Tiwanaku cultures in the highlands of southern Peru and Bolivia, where it is used in traditional healing to this day.[16] The later Cupinisque, Lambayeque, Chimú and Moche cultures of Peru's northern coast also produced ceramics and pottery featuring the cactus's distinctive winding columns, working with the natural symmetry of its form. Stirrup-cups in which the San Pedro intertwines with the jaguar have been found in burial sites together with snuffing tubes and trays. In textiles on the coast further south, the cactus is commonly partnered with the jaguar or the hummingbird, a symbol today of the shaman's power to suck malignant darts out of the victims of sorcery.

After the Spanish conquest, archaeological evidence was supplemented by fragmentary written testimony. In 1653 the Spanish priest Bernabé Cobo, who spent most of his life in Peru as a Jesuit missionary, witnessed the use of San Pedro and wrote of it in similar terms to those used by the Inquisition in Mexico to describe peyote: 'this is the plant with which the Devil deceived the Indians of Peru in their paganism . . . transported by this drink, the Indians dreamed a thousand absurdities and believed them as if they were true'. (Cobo also recorded the use of *vilca* as an additive to *chicha* maize beer, and was one of the first Europeans to describe cinchona bark, the source of quinine. He suggested that San Pedro might share some of cinchona's medicinal properties: 'one can use its juice against fevers'.[17])

It was only in the 1960s, with the identification of mescaline in the cactus and a new anthropological interest in syncretic urban cultures, that Peruvian ethnographers, pharmacologists and social psychiatrists began to investigate the secretive traditions of *curanderismo* or folk healing that had previously been dismissed as superstition, or at best as corrupted forms of the 'pure' shamanisms found in pristine cultures. Today, San Pedro *curanderos* are a distinctive presence in Peru's northern coastal cities such as Casma and Trujillo. Large sections of the city markets are devoted to their trade – stalls crammed with wands, tablecloths and bottles of pungent floral scent, with thick stems of San

Pedro stacked behind the counter – and practitioners' painted signs, directing clients up narrow stairs to tenement rooms or back yards, jostle with those of astrologers, chiropractors and bus-ticket agents. In recent years a new genre of signs has emerged alongside them, lettered in English and illustrated with psychedelic designs of cactus stems and magical talismans, offering healing ceremonies in beach huts to western seekers. San Pedro shamans and healers are increasingly visible, too, in the jungle retreats of the booming ayahuasca tourist scene around Amazon towns such as Iquitos and Pucallpa.

San Pedro *curanderismo* as practised today incorporates many elements which are presumably of ancient provenance, but the ritual is shaped for modern sensibilities. It takes the form of a consultation between healer and patient in which a decoction of the cactus is drunk, sometimes by both participants but often only by the healer, as a catalyst to seek guidance from spirits or confront the powers of witchcraft. Prior to the ceremony, San Pedro stems are sliced into discs and boiled together with herbs for several hours in a metal pot. Unlike peyote, which contains a high enough concentration of mescaline to eat fresh or dried, San Pedro requires preparation to achieve a psychoactive dose.[18] The resulting liquid is bitter to the taste and viscous in texture, and the dose is typically no more than mildly psychedelic in its effects: a languid, dreamy state, accompanied by mild nausea, and an expansive turn of mind that casts a clairvoyant glow over the proceedings. The brew is often given a herbal admixture to provide 'heat': sharpness and focus, to stop the subject from becoming too 'cold' and withdrawn. Many *curanderos* stir in a leaf or two of *floripondio* (plants from the *Datura* or *Brugmansia* genus), which adds a substrate of feverish energy along with a horribly parched mouth.

The focus of the ceremony is a *mesa* or table on which are arranged objects of special significance and power to the *curandero*: family heirlooms, ancient artefacts, animal remains, wands, bottles, feathers, effigies of saints. The space is cleansed with prayers and invocations to *curandero* ancestors and Christian saints, and tobacco smoke blown in the four cardinal directions; a liquid tobacco snuff is often taken by both participants to clear the head and please the spirits. As the effects of the mescaline build, certain objects on the *mesa* 'catch the light', announcing their particular significance and calling for interpretation. *Curanderos* spray perfume – usually a strong artificial rose or gardenia – to sweeten the air and honour the spirits; the inner gleam from the San Pedro infusion heightens the sparkle of the objects and the heady transport of the smokes and scents. The magically charged moment allows the *curandero*, with the assistance of the talismans, to project their awareness beyond the human range, opening up a sixth sense that reveals the hidden causes of things. A rattle or music may be used to conduct the spirits or reach out to a relative living far away; the configuration of the objects on the *mesa* may reveal the location of a lost possession. In cases of serious illness or psychic assault, the *curandero* may grab a wand from the *mesa*, leap up and do battle directly with the invisible source of the evil. By the end of the ceremony, when the psychic space is closed with prayer, the patient has been 'opened up like a flower', and the cause of their troubles plucked from them.[19]

🌵   🌵   🌵

Several years ago I joined a San Pedro survey expedition, collecting specimens from the valleys of Peru's northern cordillera. We visited Chavín and Caral and the northern coastal town of Trujillo, where we bought cultivated stems of San Pedro, plump and glossy, from a herbalist in the market. Back in Lima on a rooftop terrace in the old Spanish district of Barranco, crowded with potted cactus specimens labelled by date, location and altitude, we sliced the stems and boiled them on the stove.

The internet teems with recipes for preparing San Pedro in more concentrated forms than the simple *curandero* method of chopping and boiling. Most of them are complicated, with several stages – freezing, skinning, boiling, reducing, fermenting – and their relative merits are vigorously disputed. We had no time for anything but the simplest: boiling chunks of cactus with the addition of cane sugar and lime to aid absorption and offset the bitterness. After a couple of hours the decoction was dark yellow, intensely bitter (a promising indicator of mescaline and its fellow alkaloids) and thick with ropes of mucus suspended in the liquid like raw egg white. Dosage was simply a question of how much we could hold down, in my case somewhere around half a litre.

We lay down on mats as the sun disappeared behind the roofs and over the ocean, and within minutes felt a sense of internal acceleration, gravity pressing us into the tile floor. Mescaline is notoriously slow to take effect, and it can often be two hours before the full measure of a dose is felt. Previously this type of simple brew had left me with little more than nausea, some physical heaviness and mild mental stimulation. This time, for whatever reason, I was immersed within twenty minutes in the paradoxical physical sensations of a strong mescaline dose. Languorous muscle relaxation combined with tremors, restlessness and nausea; fizzing euphoria with the ominous sensation of a fast-rising fever; a thrumming vibration in the chest with a cold heaviness in the limbs. As pleasure and discomfort mingled and intensified, it was easy to understand how some subjects feel themselves transported to the realms of the divine while others retire miserably to their sickbeds for the duration (a long wait). It was easy, too, to see why so many techniques had evolved to manage and work through these physical symptoms, whether by adding a stimulant to the brew or music and shuffling dance to the ritual.

As darkness fell, honeycombs of green and violet threaded across my vision. The cactus still sat queasily in my stomach but my blood pressure and circulation were recovering and the numbness and lassitude receding. In contrast to alcohol, as the peyotists of the Native American Church observe, with the cactus you get the hangover first. Standing up and stretching released warm rushes of energy, unlocking cramped muscles and pinched nerves. I thought of the thousands of cacti we had seen stretching and sprawling across the slopes of the mountain valleys as they luxuriated in the sun, each one a mescaline factory.

I walked over to the wall of the roof terrace, chest-high and surmounted with pots of cactus cuttings. It was Saturday night, and Barranco was coming to life. Below us was the dome of the ruined Spanish church of La Ermita, its beams visible through the collapsed plaster, and below it the ravine – *el barranco* – that leads through the cliff to a promontory over the ocean, a famous sunset spot from where crowds were slowly drifting back to the bars of the old plaza. In the centre of the view was the Puente de los Suspiros, spanning the ravine and connected to upper and lower walkways by stairs with black wrought-iron railings and balustrades. The panorama was mesmerising, and as I watched it took on the granular, hypnotic quality of a mescaline vision. The crowd seemed composed entirely of young couples, gazing off the bridge or strolling arm in arm; the bridges and railings became an Escher puzzle in which all were simultaneously ascending and descending. The streetlights against the tropical night made the scene into a rich chiaroscuro, balanced on the cusp between figurative and abstract. Like so many mescaline experimenters before me I reached for aesthetic references, and the sight obligingly moulded itself to fit them: Balinese shadow theatre, the silhouette animations of Lotte Reiniger, the technicolour abstracts by Oskar Fischinger that open Walt Disney's *Fantasia*.[20] Distant bubbles of laughter, chatter and accordion music resolved themselves into an orchestral soundtrack, then into tinnitus and back again.

Until this vision absorbed me, I had been entirely immersed in the strange alterations in my sensorium. Now I was nowhere in the scene, no more conscious of myself than when caught up in a movie. The scene in front of me might have been endless, or it might have been a short repeating loop; I had, in another familiar refrain of mescaline's subjects, stepped outside of time. At some point in the small hours the crowds filing across the bridge must have thinned, but my next distinct memory is of the sky brightening, the early morning jet trails slicing pink webs across it, as the spell of the San Pedro slowly faded.

CHAPTER TWO

THE DEVIL'S ROOT

1519–PRESENT

MEXICO

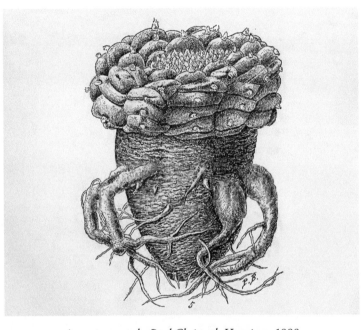

A peyote cacuts by Paul Christoph Hennings, 1888.

The western world's first encounter with mescaline came in the form of the peyote cactus, part of the astonishing complex of magical and medicinal plants to which the Spanish conquistadors were introduced on their arrival in Mexico. They had brought with them samples of spices such as cinnamon which they were surprised to discover that the local 'Indians' didn't recognise. Instead, they were presented with the richest psychoactive flora on earth. The *tabaco* already brought back to Europe by Columbus's crew was on sale in the markets as cigars, chewing preparations and snuff, together with an array of beautifully worked pipes, pouches and snuff tubes. Here, however, it was traded and consumed in conjunction with other plants that had even more powerful mind-altering effects. These included several species of hallucinogenic mushrooms; the seeds of the morning glory plant, containing alkaloids closely related to LSD; shrubs of the *Datura* and *Brugmansia* genera, cousins to the bewitching nightshade herbs of Europe; the toxic and deliriant red mescal bean; dream-giving varieties of mint and sage; and, most highly venerated of all, woven baskets filled with nubs of a small, wrinkled spineless cactus known in the Nahuatl tongue as *peyotl*.

The peyote is about as different from the San Pedro as a cactus can be. The latter's tall columns dominate the slopes of its Andean heartlands, while the peyote is all but invisible in its natural habitat, the mountains and high desert scrub of northern Mexico, extending across the Rio Grande into pockets of modern-day Texas. Its creased, leathery, spineless heads barely protrude above the sand and gravel, usually covered in dust, looking more like stones or deer droppings than plants. It becomes easily visible only during its brief flowering season, when each head produces a fountain of lustrous satiny pink and white petals.

Peyote's lifeless appearance is one of its many defences against predators, along with its thick, waxy skin, the bitter taste of its alkaloids and its well-hidden tap root. The heads, or buttons, are only the visible tip of a thick carrot-shaped body in which sparse desert moisture is held in a bitter, chemical-rich mucus. Compared to the irrepressible San Pedro its pace of growth is glacially slow. A button can remain visibly unchanged for years, often shrinking during the dry seasons, while slowly bulking out below ground. But when the head is damaged – trodden upon by a deer or cut with a knife – the enzyme channels that suppress budding are disrupted and new heads (or 'pups') rapidly form; long-established specimens can thus elaborate themselves into hydra-headed, coral-like colonies.

Like the San Pedro, there are several closely related species of peyote and their taxonomy has been no less contentious. *Lophophora williamsii*, the true peyote, was allocated to various different genera over many decades before the current classification was standardised. For a long time it was not differentiated from *Lophophora diffusa*, a similar-looking species that grows slightly further south, closer to Mexico City. *L. diffusa* contains some phenethylamine alkaloids but only trace amounts of mescaline itself; the early pharmacological investigators of peyote were confused for years by dried samples in which the two species were not distinguished. There is still no consensus about the number of species in the family, and in 2009 an entirely new one was discovered, *Lophophora alberto-vojtechii*, a miniature with buttons rarely reaching an inch in diameter and an alkaloid content yet to be officially established (though probably, like *L. diffusa*, richer in related compounds than in mescaline itself).[1]

Peyote has been collected and consumed for as long as San Pedro, perhaps longer. Dried buttons found alongside ancient rock art in the Shumla caves on the Texas side of the Rio Grande have been radio-carbon dated to around 4000 BCE, and shown still to contain mescaline at a concentration of around 2 per cent.[2] The first written evidence of its use by Spanish observers is found in *The General History of the Things of New Spain*, the twelve-volume compendium which the Franciscan friar Bernardino de Sahagún began to assemble after his arrival in Mexico in 1529, and which reached Florence around 1570 (it is commonly known today as the *Florentine Codex*). In it Sahagún mentions the peyote's drab physical appearance only briefly before moving on to its more remarkable properties: 'those who eat or drink it see visions either frightful or laughable . . . it stimulates them and gives them sufficient spirit to fight and have neither fear, thirst nor hunger, and they say it guards them from all danger'.[3] The effects appeared to him similar to those produced by the mushrooms to which the Indians were also devoted.

The perspective of the Nahua people (or Aztecs, as the Spanish called them) can be teased out a little further in the fragmentary written record of their songs and poems from the pre-conquest era. These include a handful of 'flower-songs', incantations received by their composers from the divine House of the Sun, that describe a paradisiacal garden in which 'The Cocoa flower gently opens his aroma / The gentle Peyote falls like rain'.[4] This paradise of the Nahua was conceived both as the source of their psychoactive flora and the place to which those who consumed those luxuries were transported. It was a bright world of radiant colour, the home of flowers, glittering gemstones, opalescent seashells, perfumes and incenses, and particularly the vibrant, iridescent feathers of birds such as the quetzal, the macaw and the hummingbird. It was the domain of the sun, in which nature was distilled into its quintessence. The Spanish missionaries seized on its similarities with the Christian heaven and drew on its imagery for their religious instruction: the songbook translated by Sahagún and published in 1583, entitled *Psalmodia christiana*, embedded songs of the Nahua flower-world among biblical texts and passages from the lives of the saints.[5] But the bright world of the Nahua was not a transcendental realm or a future state. It was reality, the here and now, stepped up to a higher energetic level in which colour became dazzling light and time dissolved into an eternal present. Those transported to it were intoxicated, enraptured, bathed in fragrance and lifted up sunwards on shimmering wings.

Early Spanish accounts of peyote focused on the Nahua belief in its miraculous properties, which they interpreted in a variety of ways. The naturalist Francisco Hernández de Toledo, personal physician to the king of Spain, considered Mexico's psychoactive plants in detail in his botanical survey of 1577, giving a supernaturally tinged account: 'this root scarcely issues forth but conceals itself in the ground, as if it did not wish to harm those who discover it and eat it'. The Nahua attributed 'wonderful properties' to it, including the power to 'foresee and predict things; such things, for example, as whether the weather will continue favourable; or to discern who has stolen from them some utensils or anything else'.[6] Others interpreted the local beliefs in more sceptical and natural terms, notably the physician Juan de Cárdenas. In his 1591 treatise *Problems and Miraculous Secrets of the Indians*, Cárdenas asserted that the effects of the peyote were not supernatural or demonic but due to the pharmacology of the cactus, which disturbed 'the interior sense of the cerebrum' and generated visions of 'monsters, bulls, tigers, lions and ghosts, that is, painful and horrible things'.[7]

The Indians' relationship with their visionary plants presented the Spanish with profound problems of interpretation. The parallels with the Christian Eucharist were unmissable. They fasted before taking them, stood with their heads bowed as their priests dispensed them, and mumbled prayers as they chewed them. They perfumed their ceremonies with the fragrant tree resin *copal* just as the Spanish did with frankincense; they even referred to their psychedelic mushroom as *teonanacatl*, the 'flesh of the gods'. Since their Christian mission was the justification of the conquest, it was crucial for the Spanish clergy to interpret these practices correctly. Some missionaries argued that God been using these plants to prepare the heathen to receive the Gospel. Others countered that the Devil was mocking them with a parodic inversion of the true Sacrament. The supposed miraculous powers of the peyote were dismissed by some as a primitive delusion, but taken by others as evidence that the Devil stalked the New World as cunningly as the old.

Sahagún's monumental survey expresses the mix of wonder, fear and practicality that the first western observers brought to peyote. His project was essentially descriptive, modelled on the classics, particularly Pliny's *Natural History*, spanning botany, zoology, geology, agriculture and medicine, and aiming at an objective presentation of the Mexican world for the Spanish reader. He interviewed hundreds of native subjects, often former members of the nobility, and trained scribes to record huge quantities of data in Nahuatl; the eventual codex was presented in parallel Nahuatl and Spanish text. He strove to present Indian beliefs and practices in their own terms, free from doctrinal interpretation, but he did so in the interests of domesticating Indian culture under Spanish rule and providing missionaries with the tools they needed to combat its beliefs. He drew some of his information from tribunals of the Inquisition and cited the example of Saint Augustine, who described pagan beliefs in Book VI of his *City of God* specifically in order to furnish the godly with weapons for spiritual conquest.

Missionaries accounted for much of Sahagún's early readership, and they paid close attention to his descriptions of how Indian idolatry was practised and the rituals, objects and plants that accompanied it. Confession manuals were structured around his work, guiding penitents to a full accounting of the deities they worshipped and the festivals they held in their honour. Sahagún's intention was not to damn his Indian subjects but to exculpate them. By describing their beliefs dispassionately, and separating evidence from judgement, he presented them as innocents who had been duped by the forces of evil. The act of confession, by instilling a sense of personal identity and responsibility, allowed them to rescue their consciences and their souls from the practices that had previously enslaved them. The evil of their beliefs was projected onto the practices and the plants intrinsic to them. One early seventeenth-century catechism, the *Camino del Cielo* (Road to Heaven), included in its questions: 'Hast thou eaten the flesh of man? Hast thou eaten the peyotl? Do you suck the blood of others? Do you adorn with flowers places where idols are kept?'[8]

Under peyote's influence the Devil was summoned, and it was he who worked its magic and whispered knowledge of the future. The communion with the cactus had to be extirpated because, as one priest put it, 'the devil neither sleeps nor has forgotten the cult that these Indian natives offered him in the past, and that he is awaiting a suitable conjuncture to return to his lost lordship'.[9]

Alongside missionaries, however, Sahagún's readership included many who were fascinated by the New World's intoxicants. Their classical inheritance fed an appetite for marvels, myths and monsters, and for possession of new dominions of knowledge. In particular, some of these miraculous plants had great potential for trade and profit. Nahua knowledge of plant pharmacy was in many respects more advanced than that of the Spanish, who from Cortéz onwards had chosen to adopt local remedies in preference to their own. Even the strangest of their medicines might be worth its weight in gold. By the time Sahagún's work was published in Europe, the physician Nicolás Monardes was growing tobacco in his gardens in Seville and it had begun to command a high price as a panacea against infections and fevers. By 1590 the Spanish were cultivating chocolate, first encountered among the luxuries of Moctezuma's court, using Nahua techniques and exporting it to Europe as a precious substance said to enrich the blood. In both cases the cultural barriers to adopting a savage practice were overcome by developing new preparations more acceptable to the European palate and claiming medical benefits unique to the constitution of Christians.

Tobacco and chocolate were, in the paradoxical term, 'sober intoxicants' that found a niche in the trading spheres and social spaces of the European world. But more powerful psychoactives such as peyote were harder to assimilate. They were regarded as agents of *borrachera*, 'drunkenness', a descent into animal nature to which Indians were regarded as particularly prone.[10] Alcoholic intoxication among Indians was governed by very different rules from the Spanish. It was highly visible but, less obviously, also more compartmentalised. Spanish customs permitted solitary, regular and moderate drinking, all of which were foreign to Indian culture. Peyote ceremonies often incorporated alcohol and climaxed in drinking to the point of unconsciousness. In consequence the Spanish saw Indian sacred rituals as no more than drunken orgies in which the worst aspects of their savagery – idolatry, human sacrifice, cannibalism – were given free rein. They observed psychedelics through the lens of alcohol, while the Indians treated alcohol like a psychedelic.

*　　*　　*

The Spanish encounters with the intoxicants of the New World, framed as they were in religious language, are often treated as a superstitious prelude to the modern prohibition of peyote and other drugs that began in earnest in the nineteenth-century United States. Yet a continuous line can be drawn from these first contacts to the contemporary 'War on Drugs', which still retains the vestiges of its origin in religious and racial taboo. The use of peyote became a marker that separated the civilised from the savage, and with the advent of racial science a symptom of hereditary degeneration and inferiority. In response, the cactus became ever more tightly bound into Indian identity and sacred practices. By the time anti-peyote campaigns emerged in the United States in the late nineteenth century, government policy was largely conducted in the modern language of public health and social progress, but it was still shaped by missionaries for whom the suppression of peyote had long been a crucial aspect of the war for souls. The language that resulted was a hybrid that blurred the medical, the religious and the moral: peyote was a plague, a heathen cult and a menace to civilisation.[11] Texts from this era's anti-drug crusades were incorporated into the international treaties of the twentieth century and still underpin them today. The 1961 United Nations Single Convention on Drugs, the foundation of the global drug control system, is unique among UN documents in its use of the word 'evil' to describe the dangers that drugs pose, a term not deployed in its official definitions of child abuse, terrorism or genocide.[12]

Peyote was not easily suppressed. Abandoning their vision-giving plants proved one of the most stubborn doctrinal obstacles to the

Indians' conversion. As the sixteenth-century Jesuit missionary José de Acosta observed, 'the people venerate these plants so much that they do all in their power so that their use does not come to the attention of the ecclesiastical authorities'.[13] Just as the mescaline-containing cactus traditionally known in the Andes as *huachuma* was renamed San Pedro, peyote worship persisted under the aegis of Jesus and Mary, the saints and the angels, which gave it cover as well as imbuing it with Christian magic. In some localities a liquid decoction of the cactus was surreptitiously used to baptise infants. The danger that it posed to Indian backsliders extended to the Spanish and mestizo populations, who took to using it in witchcraft, love magic and pacts with the Devil.[14] In 1620 the Mexican Inquisition issued an edict to prohibit it, on the grounds that 'the use of the herb or root called peyote' was 'an act of superstition condemned as opposed to the purity and integrity of our Holy Catholic Faith'. Its intoxicating properties were designated as supernatural: in them could be 'plainly perceived the suggestion and intervention of the Devil, the real author of this vice'.[15]

Between 1620 and 1779 the Inquisition heard seventy-four cases against what they referred to as *raíz diabólica*, the 'devilish root'. In some cases the context of its use was described in detail, and a picture emerges of two distinct forms of peyote ritual. More common was that described by Sahagún and the early chroniclers of the Nahua: a consultation or healing between a *curandero* or shaman and their patient, in which the clairvoyant power of the peyote trance was used to reveal the location of a missing object, the cause of an illness, the source of a bewitching, prognostication of weather or the outcome of battles. But, particularly in the north, in the cactus's ancestral homeland among the semi-nomadic Chichimeca peoples, missionaries also witnessed group ceremonies in which an entire village or community would sing and dance all night under its influence. In 1649 a Coahuiltecan community in the desert around the Rio Grande were said to have assembled en masse – at least a hundred men and women – singing so harmoniously that 'it seems a single voice'. They drank peyote 'ground up and dissolved in water', along with wine, and scratched their bodies 'with some beaks of a fish called *aguja*' until blood flowed, which they smeared all over themselves. Dawn revealed them lying exhausted 'on the ground like dead persons', where they remained until they were 'over their drunkenness'.[16]

The fullest description of a ceremony of this kind was received by the Inquisition in 1760 from a Franciscan mission in the remote ranges of the Sierra de Tamaulipas along the Atlantic coast, an unruly border zone where Spanish writ had never run more than intermittently. A tribe in the area were in the habit of spending two or three days gathering peyote in advance of a seasonal festival to which neighbouring communities were invited. The 'feast' was held at night, around a 'great bonfire'; the 'poetic enthusiasm of the guests' was ignited by 'the first fumes of peyote' that was served by the young girls and old men on a table improvised from a tree trunk. A deer or coyote skin drum struck up, and the party danced in a circle around the fire, 'alternately raising one foot and then the other' and breaking out in 'discordant howls'. These feasts always ended 'with the complete drunkenness of the guests, who, exhausted moreover by the dance, fell asleep around the almost burnt-out fire'.[17] To the hostile eyes of priests and missionaries these 'feasts' were no more than drunken orgies. More sympathetic witnesses would reveal them as ritual practices of astonishing complexity, woven deep into the fabric of the participants' lives.

✼　　✼　　✼

In the northern borders of Mexico, where its use dated back millennia, peyote traditions clung on. The Spanish had never fully established themselves beyond the main roads and mining towns, and their scattered and poorly supported missions left much of the Sierra Madre's remote canyon country undisturbed. After the Pueblo Revolt of 1680, the horse was adopted by Indian tribes from the north and the mountains came within range of Apache warbands who ambushed travellers, raided forts and made isolated settlements unsustainable.

In 1890 the Norwegian traveller and ethnographer Carl Lumholtz mounted an expedition through an eerie landscape of abandoned mines, crumbling churches and empty pine forests to the ravines and ridges of the northern Sierra Madre where a white man had never yet set foot. He was looking for the surviving descendants of the Indians who had built the mysterious ruined pueblos and temples in the deserts of New Mexico; he found a people called the Tarahumara who had retreated into the most inaccessible canyons to evade the Spanish and who held ceremonies under the influence of small cacti they called *hikuli*. 'The eating of them causes great ecstasy,' Lumholtz recorded. 'They are therefore treated as demi-gods, who have to be treated with great reverence, and to whom sacrifices have to be offered.'[18]

Hikuli, or peyote, permeated Tarahumara life. They were chewed as a medicine against snakebite and fever, and when carried in a man's belt they gave him energy for running and watched over him to ensure he was not poisoned or ambushed. The more Christianised members of the tribe made the sign of the cross when they encountered one, and Lumholtz was told to lift his hat in their presence. People sang to them in the desert as they passed them, and collected them reverently for their feasts. At these the cacti were welcomed with music, the sacrifice of a sheep or goat, dancing and maize beer: 'peyote wants to drink beer, and if the people would not give it, it would go back to its own country'.[19] A fire was lit, and a shaman took his seat to the west of it; assistants carried censers filled with *copal* incense. The shaman sang, describing how peyote 'walks with his rattle and his staff of authority; he comes to cure and to guard the people and to grant a "beautiful" intoxication'.[20] A brewed peyote liquor circulated and the dance continued till daybreak, when the shaman turned to the rising sun and made passes towards it with his notched stick. 'By this act, three times performed, he waves peyote home.'[21]

Lumholtz was inspired to try peyote for himself, though 'only a small cupful'. It gave him an immediate rush, 'similar to coffee but much more powerful' followed by 'a depression and a chill such as I have never experienced before', which even a night huddled next to the fire failed to dispel.[22] He took some away with him, adding it to the baggage on his mule train, which included canvas tents, folding camp furniture, scientific instruments and boxes of dynamite for unblocking mountain passes. A shaman named Rubio, 'the great *hikuli* expert' of the tribe, fed his samples with *copal* smoke to keep them safe from 'sorcerers, robbers or Apaches' on their travels.[23] Lumholtz headed south, where after several hundred miles – and many adventures – he arrived among the windswept cliffs and canyons of another people famous for their peyote rites, the Huichol.

Wandering the Huichol country, Lumholtz met small groups of peyote hunters, easily recognised by the happy smiles on their faces and the peculiar gleam in their eyes. 'They are always merry, and they sing much.'[24] He tried the cactus again during a strenuous hike to some sacred caves in the distant cliffs, and was surprised to discover that in these circumstances it was no longer a depressant but 'refreshing, quenching thirst and allaying hunger . . . I felt stimulated, as if I had had some strong drink'.[25] A great peyote feast was being prepared, and Lumholtz waited impatiently as trees were hung with 'large bundles of deer meat threaded on strings, as well as large coils of fresh *hikuli*'.[26] The ceremony was to take place at a temple, or *tuki*, one of a network that extended across Huichol country, positioned in cardinal directions to face the sun at solstices and equinoxes and keep the ritual universe in balance. But it turned out that renovations had to be completed at another *tuki* in a neighbouring village before the feast could begin, and after weeks of delay the ceremony was eventually held in a fierce dust storm that turned the proceedings into blind chaos. Lumholtz lost his guide, on top of which a group of Mexican traders arrived with strong liquor and 'of course all present got drunk, and it was impossible to do anything with them'.[27]

🌿   🌿   🌿

A full picture of the Huichol's peyote rites was only obtained in 1966, when two anthropologists joined for the first time the annual pilgrimage that members of the tribe make to their aboriginal lands to collect it – or, in their terms, to hunt it – for their temple ceremonies. Barbara Myerhoff, together with her UCLA colleague Peter Furst, had studied for some time with an apprentice *mara'akame* or shaman named Ramón Maria Silva, with whom they negotiated the unprecedented problems raised by bringing a non-participant on their journey. During this process Myerhoff discovered that despite its 'rude technology and simple social organisation . . . in aesthetics, mythology, oral tradition, symbolism, and cosmology, Huichol culture is highly developed, rich, and especially beautiful'.[28] The world of the Huichol was one where sacredness was not something 'set apart' from daily routine but a 'natural condition' that imbued every aspect of it. Unlike other semi-settled Mexican tribal groups which moved between their own culture and that of the wider world, all Huichol participated fully in this symbolic existence, at the core of which was the elemental trinity of deer, maize and peyote. As Ramón expressed it to her: 'These things are one. They are a unity. They are our life. They are ourselves.'[29]

Myerhoff's narrative of the ritual journey, *The Peyote Hunt* (1974), is vividly complemented by the documentary film *To Find Our Life*, shot by Peter Furst on a second pilgrimage in 1968. Ramón and his Huichol band of pilgrims process through the bleak, parched desert margins in wide-brimmed straw hats glinting with embroidered tassels, red and white tunics and ponchos flapping in the biting wind; their belts and pouches are decorated with votive images of saints and woven yarn emblems; they are hung with garlands and carry guitars, fiddles and single-stringed bows. The journey from their village to the peyote hunting grounds at Wirikuta, in the high mesa above the former colonial mining town of Real de Catorce, is around twenty days' walk, though it is mostly now travelled in trucks and buses. As the pilgrims progress toward their sacred destination, every landmark is a sign imbued with memories and symbolic meanings. Ramón establishes an improvised language of nonsensical reversals, by which the familiar is rendered strange: he becomes the pope, their destination is Los Angeles, their van is a donkey. He later explains that 'everything should be upside down and backward', as they cross over into the world of the peyote.[30]

When they arrive in Wirikuta, they speak not of collecting cacti but hunting deer. The first peyote is spotted among thorny brush and agaves, its head almost invisible in the dust of the gravel plain. It is described as the deer's footprint. Before disturbing it, the pilgrims surround it and transfix it with four feathered arrows at each of its cardinal points. When they begin harvesting, they cut the cactus tops delicately while speaking to them, addressing them as 'our elder brothers' and informing them 'we shall eat your body'.[31] Myerhoff theorises that the deer–maize–peyote complex speaks of a transition, still in progress, from a hunter–gatherer culture to one of sedentary farming. The deer is the food of the former, the maize of the latter, with peyote the mercurial agent that transcends time and permits a deeper vision in which past and present are brought together.

After the hunt, darkness falls and the pilgrims gather round a camp-fire in the open desert. Ramón feeds them peyote which they receive as a sacrament, hands folded and heads bowed. Fiddle and guitar music strikes up as they stare at the fire, 'waiting to see the beautiful flower in the centre'.[32] Their visions unfold in silence. For the pilgrims, Ramón told Myerhoff, the visions are primarily 'for beauty': they see 'little animals, beautiful colours, and occasionally some of the creatures told of in the myths'.[33] For the *mara'akame* they have more profound meanings, but these are not to be spoken of. For shaman and pilgrim alike, they are private gifts; to share and compare them would diminish their power to nourish 'that part of a man's life which is private, beautiful and unique'.[34]

In Myerhoff's assessment, 'peyote occupies no utilitarian place on any level of Huichol life. Even the visions obtained by it are not used for religious illumination, or didactic purposes.' The peyote hunt is a return to paradise, through which the pilgrims become their own ancestors and their own gods. They have stepped outside time, into a world before creation and individual consciousness, where the past and the future are the same. In the mundane world of modern Mexico they 'are aware that they are destitute while outsiders prosper',[35] but their annual return to Wirikuta creates for them an alternate reality. In the peyote hunt they inhabit an eternal present in which all things are in harmony.

🌿   🌿   🌿

The work of Myerhoff and Furst was instrumental in bringing the Huichol, and particularly their use of peyote, to a global audience. They have become an archetype of traditional psychedelic shamanism and, though peyote is only one element in their highly elaborated cosmology and ritual, it now dominates western perceptions of them. Some scholars regard them as surviving exemplars of an archaic peyote culture that spanned northern and central Mexico centuries before the Spanish conquest: Peter Furst, along with Weston La Barre, the twentieth century's leading authority on peyote religion in the USA, argued that the Huichol peyote rituals are 'probably the closest extant to the pre-Columbian Mexican rite' and 'may well be virtually unchanged since Cortéz'.[36] Others have proposed a direct connection via the Huichol's ancient community temples, known as *tuki*, which they regard as the last surviving remnant of 'a vast network of regional trade and ceremony' that from at least 200 CE spanned much of pre-Hispanic Mexico, setting seasonal cycles for deer hunting and maize growing and governing the trade in sacred items such as peyote, conch shells and feathers.[37]

Barbara Myerhoff, however, was less convinced. In the early Spanish accounts the Chichimeca peoples of Mexico's northern deserts were culturally distinct from the urbanised Nahua further south, and in her view Huichol traditions 'appear unrelated to Aztec [Nahua] peyotism . . .

nor do the other Mexican Indian groups have comparable symbolic associations between deer, maize and peyote. Further, they have no ritual
which corresponds to the Huichol peyote hunt.'[38] The theories are not
entirely exclusive: the world of the Huichol may be a uniquely rich source
of pan-Indian motifs without referring to any other culture beyond itself.
The hazards of interpreting it as a relic from prehistory are illustrated by
the Tarahumara, whose use of peyote has evolved strikingly even since
Lumholtz's day. John Kennedy, an anthropologist who lived among them
in the 1970s, described the central role in their culture of *tesgüino*, their
maize beer, which is deeply entwined with sociality, cooperative labour
and reciprocal obligations. *Hikuli* (peyote), which used to be part of this
complex, is now used only by shamans and is predominantly associated
with sorcery. It has the malign reputation of 'a spiritual substance having
an independent soul' that spies on its subjects and foments feuds and
grievances.[39]

The other facet of Huichol culture that has risen to global prominence along with peyote is its art. It seems obvious from first glance
that the two are intimately connected. The yarn paintings that are
synonymous with Huichol art today – dazzling coloured fibres pressed
onto boards spread with beeswax – are, to the western eye, quintessen-
tially psychedelic. Animals, birds and plants, often outlined in vibrant
red and gold, dance across fields of stars, jewels, feathers and geometrical shapes, often in radial symmetry around a central solar burst of
retina-scorching yellows, pinks and purples. Among the most common
motifs is the peyote: clusters of blue-green heads attached to tapered
roots that arrange themselves into kaleidoscopic mandalas, edged in
fluorescent threads that throb and pulse like op-art illusions. These are
among the world's most popular indigenous artworks, from small
pieces sold by the hundreds to tourists in Puerto Vallarta and Acapulco
to wall-sized galaxies of imagery that command many thousands of
dollars in the galleries of the southwestern USA, Spain or Japan.
Huichol artists are flown across the world to create murals, from San
Diego airport to the Paris Métro. Art has become the mainstay of the

Huichol's economy, their passport to protection by the Mexican state and their lifeline to cultural survival and the preservation of their ancestral land.

It should not, however, be taken for granted that these images are straightforward visual transcriptions of their creators' peyote experiences, the flowers that they see in the fire. Like the peyote rites of the Tarahumara, their style has altered markedly within the span of a lifetime. The work collected in the 1930s by Robert Zingg, the anthropologist who first introduced Huichol art to the west, was quite different. Most of his pieces, recently exhibited at the Museum of Indian Arts and Culture in Santa Fe, New Mexico, were votive objects – crosses, gourd bowls and painted sticks adorned with feathers – to be left on rock shelves at sacred spots in the desert. Today's synthetically dyed threads were unknown: most were decorated with precise but simple patterns in a subdued range of earth-toned reds, greens and browns. Very few were yarn paintings, a medium that may have evolved as a portable version of the more valuable stone disks. The handful of examples that Zingg collected were used as altar mats rather than hung on walls. The psychedelic brilliance that resonates so clearly with mescaline's visions has emerged only in recent decades, in symbiosis with the western commercial market.

After his stay among the Huichol in 1934–35, Robert Zingg concluded that Huichol art was an altogether different activity from that practised in the west. 'Every adult is an artist,' he wrote, just as 'every man is a shaman of sorts.' In modern societies, 'civilised art is the most specialised and individualised aspect of the whole gamut'; the quest of the artist is to 'torture his spirit into some new quirk or style'. The Huichol were not artists of this kind: they were far closer to 'another theoretical pole in art, the primitive'. Civilised art is 'not only specialised and individualised, but also secularised . . . Primitive art, as currently exhibited by the Huichols, reveals art brought under the principle of the sacred.'[40] The core of Huichol experience is the deer–maize–peyote complex: like 'transubstantiation in the Mass . . .

this sort of mystic participation is the strongest sort of social device for moulding the individual into the likemindedness of the group pattern'. In medieval Europe it produced the Crusades; 'among the Huichol it induces pilgrimages'.[41]

At the time of Zingg's visit the idea of Huichol art created for sale, like the presence of foreign observers on the peyote hunt, was outside the bounds of possibility. Today there are workshops where yarn paintings are produced for the international art market and noted individual artists whose work commands the highest prices. Yet sacred art still exists. Votive works are constantly produced for ceremonies, on a scale that would be unsustainable were it not for the proceeds of commercial art that support it. As Barbara Myerhoff wrote, 'The Huichol notion of the sacred is elusive and in many ways difficult for a westerner to grasp . . . it is a dynamic condition of balance in which opposites exist without neutralising each other.'[42] Huichol art, both new and old, epitomises this state of creative contradiction: in ceaseless flux, yet always contained within an overarching geometry and harmony. Western descriptions of the mescaline experience often revolve around the same tension, and it seems fitting that peyote should preside over a visual aesthetic that expresses it so eloquently.

CHAPTER THREE

MAKING MEDICINE

1880–93

OKLAHOMA, TEXAS, DETROIT, BERLIN

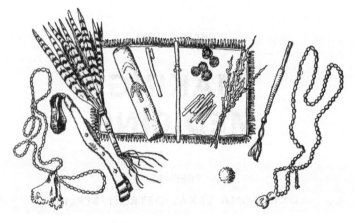

Peyote ceremony, ritual objects.
Left to right: mescal bean necklace, necktie, pheasant feather fan, smokestick,
eagle bone whistle, drumstick, peyote buttons, corn husk cigarettes, sage,
powdered cedar, drumstick, mescal bean necklace.

W hile Carl Lumholtz was negotiating the precipitous trails over the Sierra Madre towards Tarahumara country, another white man's encounter with peyote set in motion the events that within a few years led to its systematic investigation by western science and the isolation of mescaline.

February 1891 found James Mooney, of the Smithsonian Institution's Bureau of Ethnology, in residence at the Bureau of Indian Affairs' agency at Anadarko, southwest Oklahoma, from where several tribes including the Wichita, the Caddo and the Kiowa were managed. Mooney was, as always, racing against time to record and preserve centuries of Indian language, culture and tradition that were vanishing before his eyes as white pioneers colonised what had previously been designated as Indian country. He had learned to speak Kiowa, a five-toned language isolate barely known outside its own people, as well as the sign language developed among the Plains tribes as they mingled for the first time in their forced captivity. The Kiowa way of life, he reported back to Washington, was 'all unstudied except as I have given it attention . . . their heraldry, name system, military organisation, myths and songs, religion and ceremonials, are all interesting and worthy of close study'.[1] He had recently discovered that the Kiowa kept pictographic calendars that recorded the series of cataclysmic events that had overtaken them over the previous generation.

At the same time he was being pressured by the Smithsonian to assemble material for a display of Indian culture at the World's Fair scheduled for Chicago in 1893, a project with which he was becoming 'thoroughly sick & disgusted'.[2] He had also recently stumbled on the Ghost Dance and become one of the few white men permitted to witness its mesmerising mass ceremonies in which dancers would assemble in a huge circle, decked in costumes never seen before, and sing the newly channelled 'Messiah songs'. One by one they were taken by the spirit and broke out of the rings, staggering and collapsing unconscious, and 'as each one recovered from his trance he was brought into the centre of the ring to relate his experience'.[3] The ceremonies persisted night and day, with 'some in a maniac frenzy, some in spasms & others stretched out on the ground stiff and unconscious. They lie where they fall, like dead men, sometimes for an hour or longer while the dance goes on.'[4]

Mooney sought out clandestine ghost dances around Anadarko and collected the new songs. He spent as little time as possible at the agency, staying mostly in the Kiowa camps 30 miles to the south where the Wichita Mountains rose out of the rolling prairie like piles of red rubble, enclosing a hidden landscape of stunted post-oak forests, fast-running creeks and valleys of long grass in which the last remaining buffalo had taken refuge. He was moving too spontaneously for his living expenses to be reimbursed, and by the summer of 1891 would be reduced to sleeping on the ground in a dirty tipi and living on crackers and coffee. Briefly back in Anadarko on administrative business, he was approached by a young Kiowa who 'came to tell me in a guarded manner that his people intended to eat mescal that night at a camp about ten miles up the Ouachita and would probably be willing to have me present'.[5]

As dark fell Mooney was met by two men, a Comanche and a Mexican who had been brought up by the Kiowa as a child captive. On their walk upriver he was told he must remove his hat when he entered the tipi, and not look at anyone while they were eating the *seni*, as peyote was called in Kiowa.[6] Eventually they arrived at a copse beside the river where a tipi had been erected. As the door flap was drawn open he saw a group of about thirty men, a mix of Kiowa, Comanche and Apache, seated in a circle around a central fire enclosed within a horseshoe of banked earth on which had been placed a large peyote button. At 10 o'clock a master of ceremonies, known as the roadman, rolled a smoke of tobacco in a dried corn shuck and offered an opening prayer before passing twelve dried buttons to each participant. They ate them, plucking the downy tuft from the centre before chewing carefully and swallowing. If Mooney respected protocol by not watching, he would have plenty of opportunities to do so over the months and years to come. On this occasion he declined the cactus, 'as I did not feel sure that I could keep my brain clear for observation otherwise'.[7] It was a mistake he never made again.

At this point a small water-filled drum and rattle were unveiled and passed around the group. Each participant in turn sang in their own language, 'with full voices, at the same time beating the drum and shaking the rattle with all the strength of their arms'. The songs continued till midnight, when the roadman blew an eagle-bone whistle and water was passed around. Participants were allowed to leave the tipi to stretch their legs: 'few, however, do this as it is considered a sign of weakness'. The singing and drumming resumed, now interspersed from time to time with 'earnest prayers' from 'some fervent devotee' moved to address the Creator, casting his eyes up through the tipi chimney to the stars while 'stretching his hands out towards the fire and the sacred mescal'.[8]

At one point in the dark hours that followed, 'the door flap was suddenly lifted and a man stepped in, carrying in his arms an infant, a 'child sick almost to death'. Mooney watched with profound emotion 'the pathetic earnestness of the father as he watched the priests praying over his child, which seemed in stupor and made no sound', after which 'he left as silently as he entered'. The songs and prayers continued through to first light, when a group of women from the camp entered with water, bread, dried meat, sweetened maize and coffee. The ceremony ended with the roadman requesting of Mooney that he 'should go back and tell the whites that the Indians had a religion of their own which they loved'.[9]

Mooney spent much of his subsequent career honouring this request, which went to the heart of his lifelong commitment to preserving the essence of Indian culture in a white world committed to its eradication. Growing up in Indiana not long after the defeated tribes had made their final journey through the Midwest to the reservations, Mooney had always been fascinated by Indians, with whom he felt a strong kinship through his own Irish heritage. His family had left

Ireland during the famine, and his father found work as a ditch digger in Richmond, Indiana. As a teenager he rejected Catholicism as a faith but cherished it as an identity, writing long and scholarly essays on Irish folk medicine, funeral customs and calendar days. In one of his early lectures on the subject, to the American Philosophical Society in 1887, he described Ireland pointedly as a nation 'crushed into the ground by an alien tyrant'.[10]

At the age of twelve Mooney began to compile an inventory of all the tribes, and rapidly absorbed the available ethnographic literature on them. At eighteen he took a job in the print room of the local newspaper but his sights were set on the newly founded Bureau of Ethnology in Washington, a division of the Smithsonian Institution established on the urging of John Wesley Powell, the distinguished geographer and explorer of the American West, that a proper understanding of Indian cultures was a vital component of any humane solution to the 'Indian problem'. Mooney wrote to the Bureau, enclosing some of his researches and boldly asking for a job. In 1885, at the third attempt, he was offered an unpaid post in Washington.

He proved his worth on his first field trip to visit the remnants of the Eastern Cherokee people in the forests of the Great Smoky Mountains on the border of North Carolina and Tennessee, where he was shown books of sacred rituals written in an indigenous script entirely unknown to western scholars. The calendars of the Kiowa were another revelation, equally unknown, as was the peyote religion. By early 1891, however, the consequences of the Ghost Dance had overtaken all of Mooney's other priorities. The tensions it had built up had exploded in the massacre at Wounded Knee on the Pine Ridge reservation in South Dakota on 29 December 1890, and Mooney's insight into the phenomenon was urgently sought by the administrators of the reservations through which it had spread like brushfire during the previous two years.

🌲   🌲   🌲

The 'great underlying principle of the Ghost Dance doctrine', James Mooney would later write in his definitive study of the phenomenon, 'is the time will come when the whole Indian race, living and dead, will be united upon a regenerated earth, to live a life of aboriginal happiness, forever free from death, disease and misery. On this foundation each tribe has built a structure from its own mythology.'[11] The movement was inspired by a vision received by a Paiute man named Wovoka during the solar eclipse on New Year's Day 1889. As the sun died, Wovoka was raised up to heaven and told by God that a new world had been set aside for the Indian tribes in which the white man would have no part. Jesus Christ had already returned to earth in the form of an American Indian, and Wovoka was shown a ritual dance that would bring cleansing rains and call the new dispensation into being.

White settlers, missionaries and government officials were terrified by the dances convened to realise Wovoka's vision. Government agents warned that the dancers might be working themselves up to violent insurrection; some Lakota warriors wore 'ghost shirts' that were said to render them bulletproof. On 15 December the Lakota spiritual leader Sitting Bull was arrested in an attempt to break up what US troops were calling 'the Messiah craze'. Two weeks later a detachment of the 7th Cavalry Regiment attempted to disarm a group of 350 Lakota and escorted them to Wounded Knee Creek, where in response to a still-disputed provocation – the commencement of the Ghost Dance, a refusal to hand over a rifle, an order that went unheard – the troops surrounding them began firing indiscriminately at close range, killing over 250 men, women and children.

Shortly after his first peyote meeting Mooney left Oklahoma for Washington and thence for South Dakota to visit the scene of the atrocity. He interviewed a teacher at the Pine Ridge school, who recalled 'the most fearful, heart-piercing wails I have ever heard' as hundreds were subsumed in 'crying, moaning groaning and shrieking out their grief'. He was deeply moved to see the mass grave, now enclosed with sacred painted stakes. He was not surprised to find that witnesses were reluctant to speak about the events, or about the Ghost Dance itself. After a long search he tracked down the prophet Wovoka in Nevada. Wovoka related his vision of the restored world but disclaimed any responsibility for the confrontation: he had advocated non-violence towards whites and had no knowledge of the ghost shirts. Mooney felt 'he seemed to be honest in his belief' but 'I knew that he was holding something in reserve, as no Indian would unbosom himself on religious matters to a white man with whom he had not had a long and intimate acquaintance.'[12] He returned south to the wide prairie country of Darlington, Oklahoma, seat of the Cheyenne and Arapaho agency, where news that he had met Wovoka was greeted with great excitement by the tribes. He brought back magpie feathers, sacred to the Northern Plains people, and letters in which the prophet stated that there was no violent intent in his words.

To most white observers the contagious mass possession of the Ghost Dance was a mark of the primitive mind, yet another compelling argument for assimilating Indians into the culture of the white majority. Mooney, in his official report, shocked many by tracing at length its parallels in civilised history. 'What tribe or people has not had its golden age?' he asked. 'The doctrines of the Hindu avatar, the Hebrew Messiah, the Christian millennium and the Hesûnanin of the Indian Ghost Dance are essentially the same, and have their origin in a hope and longing common to all humanity'.[13] The New Testament was 'full of inspirational dreams and trances' that served the same function as Wovoka's prophecies, generating hope for an oppressed people.[14] Similar scenes of mass trance possession ran through European history from Joan of Arc and the medieval Flagellants to the Fifth Monarchy Men of the English Civil War and the early Quakers; John Wesley could scarcely make himself heard above 'the groans and cries of suffering and raving enthusiasts'.[15] Nineteenth-century white America had been filled with revivalists, Methodists and Baptists whose mass spirit-possessions 'far surpassed the wildest excesses of the Ghost Dance'.[16]

Such opinions made him enemies in the Bureau of Indian Affairs and among the missionaries on its reservations, some of whom would carry their grudge against Mooney till the end of his life. But he was no supporter of the Ghost Dance: it was predicated on a miracle that was bound to be disappointed, and embracing it could only lead deeper into cultural despair. Against this background the peyote religion assumed for him a crucial importance. As he had witnessed at his first meeting, it was pan-Indian, drawing on the shared traditions of formerly hostile peoples obliged to live cheek by jowl, and deepening the intertribal networks the Ghost Dance had forged. Rather than awaiting a transformation of the world, it gave its worshippers a means to transform themselves from within. It created a sacred world beyond the sphere of white civilisation, but one that could coexist with it. Within the outward form of the Christian service, a solemn and dignified occasion devoted to prayer and songs of praise, it created conditions in which the old medicine could be summoned. Those who now worshipped the Christian God could sit and pray alongside those who still addressed the Great Spirit. Rooted in ritual practices older by millennia than the United States, it opened a path to the survival of Indian identity.

Mooney was well aware that the goal of preserving Indian culture ran against the grain of a US federal policy predicated on the assumption that within a generation there would be no more Indians, only Americans. He presented peyote in his Smithsonian reports as a source of religious and moral inspiration, not the enemy of the missionaries but their ally. He also stressed its utility as a medicine that deserved a place in the western pharmacopoeia. As he put it in an 1896 article for the *Therapeutic Gazette*, the medical journal published in Detroit in association with the pharmacists Parke, Davis, 'the Indians regard the mescal as a panacea in medicine, a source of inspiration, and the key which opens to them all the glories of another world'.[17] The last phrase was characteristic of the ambiguity his advocacy demanded: those preoccupied with the salvation of the Indian soul would read it in Christian terms, but for Mooney it meant the old tribal ways.

He was, however, genuinely convinced by peyote's medical powers, especially against infectious and consumptive diseases.[18] He often cited the case of Paul Setkopti, his Kiowa interpreter, whom he had seen restored to health by the cactus when seemingly on his death bed, after four years' coughing up blood. It was commonly used to treat a wide range of conditions, including pneumonia, liver disease, diabetes, sores and other skin conditions, eye inflammations and mental distress. But Mooney's insistence on peyote's medical virtues also had a tactical component. While the old charges of heathen superstition and sorcery were still levelled by missionaries, government agencies and medical officers confidently deployed the language of public health against it: peyote was toxic and addictive, enfeebling the nerves and leading to degenerate collapse. Mooney countered these arguments with evidence from his personal experience that 'mescal is a powerful stimulant and enables one to endure great physical strains without injurious reaction'. When he abstained from it at his first meeting, 'the result was that from cold, numbness and exhaustion I was hardly able to stand up on my feet when it was over'. Since then he had always taken three or four buttons, and on occasion as many as seven, his limit both on grounds of nausea and 'keeping my mind constantly tense and alert for observation'.[19]

His fellow participants, he admitted, tended to take rather more. He had once witnessed a Kiowa man eating ninety, but most Indians 'admit that such a quantity is excessive and extraordinary' and 'the habit never develops into a mania, but is always under control'.[20] Aware that peyote was all too easily conflated with stereotypes of Indian drunkenness, Mooney stressed that a meeting was not a dissolute orgy, as some missionaries and Indian Christian groups claimed but, as he later described it in the Bureau of Ethnology's official handbook, 'a ceremony of prayer and quiet contemplation'.[21] Peyotists were, indeed, the moral core of their communities and fiercely opposed to the scourge of alcoholism. The cactus was essentially a catalyst that enhanced the ritual power of songs, drumming and firelight, though 'it is evident that marked psychologic effects are produced by the plant itself without any of these aids'.[22]

※   ※   ※

James Mooney was the first white man to attend a peyote ceremony, but not the first to take peyote. The stimulant effects that he noted had already brought it to the attention of botanists, physicians and the pharmacy business.

The trade in the cactus beyond the limits of its natural range is ancient, perhaps as ancient as its indigenous use. The tradition of annual pilgrimage and harvesting established in prehistory among the Huichol and their neighbours had long made peyote into a commodity that was preserved, stored, transported and traded. Fresh buttons are heavy, and bruise and spoil easily, but once dried – simply by hanging them up on strings in the desert sun – they are light, easy to transport and retain their potency for years, even decades. By the mid-nineteenth century a trading network was well established on both sides of the Rio Grande, particularly in the parched plains and hillsides around Laredo, Texas, that are still referred to as the 'peyote gardens'.

These gardens drew visitors from many tribal groups and became a centre for cultural exchange. Peyote rarely changed hands for money: it provided the impetus for a barter economy in which a constellation of goods, artefacts, ideas and practices circulated. By the 1870s the trade was partially monetised by local Hispanic traders known as *peyoteros*, who typically sold to Indian visitors from more distant tribes without local connections, and was focused around Los Ojuelos, an old ranch 40 miles west of Laredo which was both a wagon-train rest stop and a prime harvesting spot. After the Texas–Mexico railroad was opened in 1881 trains stopping at the station in Aguilares, 10 miles west of Ojuelos, were regularly filled with barrels of dried peyote for transport to Laredo and on as far as Oklahoma.[23]

In April 1887 a Texan doctor and crusading medical journalist named John Raleigh Briggs published an article in the *Medical Register* on 'Muscale [*sic*] buttons . . . a Mexican fruit with possible medicinal virtues'.[24] He had heard that Indians were in the habit of eating six or ten of these buttons, settled in their tipi 'as does an opium smoker', after which they lapsed into unconsciousness and remained thus 'for two or three days'. On awakening they related 'many remarkable adventures in the "spirit world", and the return to the prairies of innumerable herds of buffalo and wild horses'. Briggs had procured some buttons from a Mexican *peyotero* who 'makes it a business to furnish the wild tribes of Indians with it'[25] and had smuggled them across the border. He ate a third of one, which he assumed would be a tiny dose, but the effects were 'violent and rapid'. His heart raced and breathing became difficult; he briefly lost consciousness and, convinced he was about to die, rushed to the office of a doctor friend who revived him with ammonia and whisky. It was, he concluded, 'well worth the trouble to investigate . . . I know of nothing like it except opium and cocaine.'[26]

Briggs's article was reprinted in the *Druggists' Bulletin* the following month and drew an immediate response from George S. Davis, the flamboyant and energetic general manager of the Detroit pharmacists Parke, Davis, who sent a memo asking his staff to contact Briggs and ask 'when a supply of this fruit can be obtained and any other facts regarding it he may be acquainted with'.[27] The reference to cocaine was particularly tantalising. Pharmacies were now well stocked with sedative drugs such as bromides, chloral hydrate and morphine, but cocaine was, apart from caffeine and alcohol, the only stimulant on the market and by far the most effective. It was Parke, Davis's current blockbuster: by 1886 they were the leading US supplier, marketing it enthusiastically in powders, solutions and lozenges as 'the most important therapeutic discovery of the age'.[28] Concerns about its addictive properties were, however, starting to tarnish its image and Davis was seeking out alternatives.

Ever since its foundation in 1866 Davis had built the company through drug discovery and entrepreneurship. By 1874 its catalogue listed 254 types of fluid extract, 300 different pills and dozens of solid extracts and elixirs.[29] In 1876 it had its biggest commercial success to date with the laxative cascara, derived from a bark long used by the native people of the Pacific Northwest. Now Davis and his colleagues were dispatching researchers to Mexico, Fiji and South America in search of further miraculous 'vegetable drugs'. They developed their discoveries for market by supplying prominent physicians with regular 'Working Bulletins', pamphlets on new plants and drugs, accompanied by samples and requests for feedback.

Davis passed Briggs's article on to his leading authority on medicinal plants, Henry Hurd Rusby, a physician and pharmacist who in 1889 would be appointed professor of botany and materia medica at Columbia University. In 1884 Parke, Davis had commissioned Rusby to travel to Bolivia to obtain a large supply of coca leaves, from which the company had developed their most profitable product range and Rusby made his name as a botanical adventurer with a two-year overland trek through deserts, jungles and mountains. When pressed by Rusby for more information, Briggs prevaricated. There was, as far as he was aware, 'absolutely no literature in English on this plant'.[30] The buttons grew only in Mexico; his supplier was unimpressed by the name of Parke, Davis and was demanding $75 up front for further samples. Eventually Briggs discovered a supplier in Vernon, Texas, who was able to order the buttons and he sent a cigar-box full of them on to Detroit.

✿   ✿   ✿

Around the same time, peyote was also brought to Parke, Davis's attention by a Laredo dealer in ornamental cacti, Anna Nickels, whose nurseries boasted several thousand cactus specimens ready for shipment to the emerging domestic market. Nickels was one of the first commercial

63

mail-order cactus suppliers, and the only woman among them. She offered 'almost any cactus found in Mexico' to a clientele that became international after her display won a 'Highest Award' at the Chicago World's Fair. She travelled extensively across Mexico, hiring mules and soliciting specimens from local villagers. In her handsomely produced catalogues she described to her customers 'the weary weeks, months and years spent in crossing vast arid wastes, climbing almost inaccessible mountains, and exploring dense forest jungles'.[31] One of her Mexican travelling companions, she discovered in 1887, had sold 30,000 dried mescal buttons to a local trader. She wrote to Parke, Davis, who she thought would be interested to learn that the buttons were being 'used by the Indians as a drink', apparently with medical properties.[32] She had begun supplying fresh specimens at 5¢ each to local Mexican customers who, they told her, used it to treat headaches: 'they pound . . . and soak them in water, then strain and drink the water. They use the pulp left to bind any sort of sores.'[33]

Parke, Davis found it difficult to square these wildly differing accounts. According to John Raleigh Briggs's reports of Indian use, mescal was a powerful opium-like sedative that induced a two-day coma; according to his alarming self-experiment, it was a violent poison that accelerated the heart rate to a terrifying degree. Anna Nickels' evidence, by contrast, suggested a mild tonic and poultice. Its botanical taxonomy was equally unclear. According to some testimonies it was a dried mushroom (a confusion that would persist into the twentieth century).[34] The terms 'mescal' and 'peyote' were used interchangeably by some and differentiated by others. 'Mescal' or 'muscale' was a particularly unhelpful term since it was applied to three quite different plants: the peyote cactus; the strong spirit distilled from the roasted heart of the agave; and the 'mescal bean' (*Sophora secundiflora*), a bright red toxic seed used by various peoples of Mexico and the American Southwest as a medicine and a stimulus for vision quests.[35] As a result, 'mescal' blurred the alcoholic, the toxic and the psychedelic, and was used loosely by some, especially law enforcement officers, as a portmanteau term for all local plant intoxicants. It was believed by James Mooney among others that the term derived from the Mescalero Apache, but there was no consensus on whether their name related to the cactus, the agave, the red bean or something else entirely.

Despite Briggs's insistence that there was no information in English on peyote, it had over previous decades been observed, collected, depicted and its effects recorded under other names. Two botanists, Charles Lemaire and Prince Joseph de Salm-Dyck, had described it in the 1840s and classified it as *Echinocactus williamsii*; it had been handsomely illustrated for *Curtis' Botanical Magazine* in 1847 and subsequently grown as an ornamental by European collectors. Its psychoactive properties were unknown to these experts, but it was recognised in Texas under the name of 'whisky-root': there were Civil War anecdotes of imprisoned Texas Rangers, deprived of whiskey, boiling it up into an intoxicating brew. Its effects were first described in print in the *New Orleans Picayune* in 1857, where a correspondent wrote that 'the Indians eat it for its exhilerating [*sic*] effect on the system, producing precisely the same as alcoholic drinks', though 'giving a rather wilder scope to the imaginations and actions'.[36] The letter was reprinted over the following weeks in local newspapers from South Carolina to Ottowa, and the explorer Sir Richard Burton included a reference to 'whisky-root' in his 1860 travelogue of the Wild West.[37]

Parke, Davis forwarded some of the buttons from Briggs's cigar box to Harvard University where Professor Sereno Watson, curator of Harvard's Gray Herbarium, identified it conclusively as a cactus and tentatively as a member of the genus *Anhalonium*, of which five species were known in Mexico, though he suspected this might be a new one. They also sent some of Briggs's sample to the world's leading specialist in intoxicating drugs, Dr Louis Lewin at the university of Berlin. Lewin was a charismatic figure who held packed lecture theatres spellbound with his magisterial command of chemistry, mythology, botany, history and medicine. He had published studies of dozens of drugs, from opium to arrow poisons, cyanide to cannabis, antiseptics to poison gases and the narcotics mentioned in Homer. Yet beyond his lecture-ship he held no academic position and conducted his research not in the university laboratories but at his Berlin home, to which pharma-cists and toxicologists made pilgrimage from across the world. An outsider who remained an active member of Berlin's Jewish Society throughout his life, Lewin had little interest in establishment honours and an active distaste for commercial exploitation of his discoveries.

The peyote samples arrived just as Lewin was about to visit the United States to study the opium scene in San Francisco's Chinatown, and en route he stopped off in Detroit to visit Parke, Davis's grand new offices. He marvelled at the new age of pharmacy that was opening up in America. At the ever-expanding manufacturing plant on the river-side, plant materials were extracted and pills were rolled; all prepara-tions were subjected to chemical assay, making them the first drugs in medical history with a standardised dose. Products were methodically tested on animals, and batch numbers on labels allowed every pill or droplet to be traced to its source. 'I had not expected such a magnitude and such a skilled exactitude of workmanship,' Lewin wrote back to Berlin; 'the manufacture of pharmaceutical preparations is worthy of the American genius'.[38]

Lewin was given further peyote samples and on his return to Germany extracted a mixture of alkaloids and resins from them. Somewhere within these fractions must lurk a stimulant or vision-producing drug, but they also contained powerful toxins: frogs and pigeons given large doses passed from vomiting and twitching to muscular spasms and eventually death. His initial findings, published in the April 1888 issue of the *Therapeutic Gazette*, identified an active principle he named 'anhalonine'.

Lewin also passed some dried buttons over to a botanist at the Botanical Society of Berlin, Paul Christoph Hennings, who announced that, despite its close kinship with the familiar *Anhalonium williamsii* (as *Echinocactus williamsii* had been renamed in 1886), this appeared to be a new species. He named it *Anhalonium lewinii* in Lewin's honour, 'as you are the actual discoverer of the plant as well as of its toxic nature'.[39] It was a famous discovery, the first known example of an intoxicating cactus. Rusby and the Parke, Davis pharmacists, however, were not entirely convinced: Hennings was a mushroom specialist, and had made his identification on the basis of a single dried button which Lewin had rehydrated by boiling into a pulpy mass. Lewin was aware that more work was required to isolate the drug or drugs involved but nevertheless claimed priority, announcing that 'I expressly reserve to myself further investigations in this area.'[40] In the meantime Parke, Davis went to market with a fluid extract, 'tincture of anhalonium', which they offered in their 1893 catalogue. It had, they claimed, 'a marked physiological action similar to strychnine' and was recommended as a depressant, respiratory stimulant and cardiac tonic.[41]

＊　　＊　　＊

By this time James Mooney had extended his peyote researches in Oklahoma beyond the Kiowa. He built a strong relationship of trust with the Arapaho, who recognised his sympathy at the collapse of the Ghost Dance religion and invited him to witness their Sun Dance. His exploits were becoming known to the wider public: in August 1893 he was first referred to in the press as 'the Indian Man', a sobriquet that would accompany him for the rest of his life.[42] In October he wrote to the Bureau of Ethnology from Darlington, asking for an extension of his trip to visit the agency of the Caddo people at Anadarko and the army post of Fort Sill, 20 miles further to the south in the foothills of the Wichita Mountains, from where tribes including the Comanche were now administered.

According to Mooney's sources, the Kiowa had first learned of the peyote religion from the Comanche, whom he believed to be among the earliest adopters of the tipi ceremony he had now attended several times. The lines of transmission by which it had travelled were obscure and tangled. As in the first ceremony he witnessed, it seemed from the beginning to have been a pan-tribal affair. Prior to the Indian Wars, the Comanche sphere of control across the Southern Plains had been vast, extending at times well into Mexico and the cactus's natural habitat. But as with the horse, of which the Comanche became undisputed masters, it seemed they had originally received the peyote rite via intermediaries, probably one of the Apache bands who had raided deep into the homeland of the Huichol and the Tarahumara before being forcibly settled in Oklahoma alongside the Comanche. Mooney believed that the Mescalero Apache were the conduit, and that their name reflected their use of peyote; they were said to have used it in healing rites with a shaman, in the Mexican fashion, in the days before the tipi ceremony.[43] (Subsequent scholarship and oral histories have found stronger evidence of early peyote use among the Lipan Apache, who in the early nineteenth century were resident in the peyote gardens around Laredo and whose influence has been detected in the musical style of the peyote songs.)[44]

The many Comanche, Apache and Kiowa tales of the discovery of peyote all place it in the distant south. In the version that Mooney recorded from the Kiowa, two young men failed to return from a raid in Mexico and their distraught sister set out to find them. Sleeping in the desert, she was directed by a spirit to the small cactus button beside her head, which she dug up and took back to her people. She passed on to them the spirit's instructions to set up a tipi, eat the cactus, pray and sing, and all received a miraculous vision of the young men wandering in the Sierra Madre, close to starvation. A search party set out and rescued them, and 'since then the peyote is eaten by the Indians with song and prayer that they may see visions and know inspiration'.[45]

In November 1893 Mooney arrived at Fort Sill, originally a frontier garrison and now the administrative centre of the Kiowa–Comanche reservation. It was intended as a cradle of civilisation for the people regarded by white society as the wildest and most savage of all the Plains tribes, the last to be brought to heel. But the rules of white civilisation on which their captors insisted made little sense to the Comanche. They had at first been issued with rations of cornmeal, which they had never eaten and instead fed to their horses. When the government built them houses they camped outside and left them standing empty. In an attempt to awaken their civilised urges the reservation was broken up and each individual allotted 160 acres of land to cultivate – or, the local white settlers hoped, to sell. For a nomadic people who had never planted a seed or conceived of land being owned, there was little appeal in a life-time of hard labour for vegetables that they barely considered food. They quickly became dependent on beef rations, which they wanted delivered as live cattle to be butchered and eaten raw. But this was a small part of their allowance to begin with and, after all the graft and pilfering along the chain of government employees and contractors who provided it, they were left languishing in near starvation.

These were similar conditions to those under which the Ghost Dance had spread across many reservations, but among the Comanches a leader emerged who rejected the prophecies of Wovoka and embraced the peyote religion. Quanah Parker had grown up on the Southern Plains as the son of a Comanche chief, Peta Nocona, and a white mother, Cynthia Ann, who had been captured as a child from her settler family. When he was fifteen she had been found and forcibly returned to civi-lisation, where she spent the last ten years of her life begging without success to be returned to her tribe. Though despised for his white blood – Quanah, the name given him by his elders, meant 'bad odour' – he submitted to mockery without complaint and proved himself in battle, becoming a member of the feared Quahada warband.[46] He was barely more than a child when the Plains tribes were finally forced onto the reservations by the Treaty of Medicine Lodge in 1867, but he was among those who refused to submit and became an outlaw. When the campaign to eradicate them escalated into the Red River War, they hid out in the sandstone bluffs and canyons of Palo Duro in far northwest Texas. In 1875, after the ruthless cavalry commander Colonel Ranald Mackenzie shot a thousand of their horses, Quanah's band finally submitted to forced captivity.

Quanah proved remarkably adept at navigating his new world. He took the lead in negotiations with the agency at Fort Sill, insisting that white cattlemen's trails through the reservation be closed and organising his people to resist attempts to buy out their 160-acre plots. 'All red men are at one in this,' he told the council, 'and wish to hold their country in common.'[47] He negotiated personally with the Texas ranchers who wanted to use the rich Comanche grasslands for pasture and watering, and insisted on being paid directly by them rather than via the agency. By 1884 this arrangement was bringing considerable income into the reservation, and to Quanah personally. He began to use his white surname, dress in western suits with his long hair braided back and made the first of four visits by train to Washington. He met President Roosevelt, who later accepted a return invitation to visit Quanah at his house. He accepted the title of chief of the Comanches, a role that had never existed in their days of freedom.

Quanah's authority rested on the delicate balancing act of remaining a trusted broker to the federal government while also defending his people against exploitation and the existential threats to their culture. In 1890, unlike many other tribal leaders, he firmly rejected the Ghost Dance. Such messianic prophecies had cost him dearly once already: the destruction of his warband had been set in motion by their failed raid on a US Army battalion at Adobe Walls in 1874, into which they had been enticed by a medicine man named Eschiti, who had prophesied that Quanah and his fellow warriors would be immune to the white man's bullets. Quanah had no interest in following Wovoka down the same road. 'Having just got fixed to live comfortably,' he remarked, 'I would be worse than an idiot to incite my people to do something that would make beggars and vagabonds of them.'[48]

By this time he was a prominent advocate for the peyote religion, which had become established in the reservation after the Texas–Mexico railroad opened. It was said that Quanah first encountered peyote in 1884 when he was cured by it of a serious stomach illness; he may also have learned its rites from one of his wives, who was a Lipan Apache.

Some histories credit him as the originator of the Plains peyote ceremony, and he was certainly one of its most effective proselytisers: during the 1890s he presided over meetings among many tribes including the Cheyenne, the Arapaho, the Pawnee, the Osage and the Ponca. But it was no one's invention; it was at once a creation of all and none. Setting the ceremony within a tipi was in part a response to the new strictures of forced captivity that included prohibitions on openly singing and dancing, though the form of the tipi circle took its charter from older traditions such as the Kiowa sacred stones ceremony. Many of its elements were of great antiquity. The water drum and gourd rattle, the sacred space purified with sage and cedar incense, the beaded feather fan and the eagle-bone whistle were the patrimony of every Plains Indian.

Quanah, like Mooney, saw peyote as an alternative to the self-destructive path set by the Ghost Dance. The federal government, however, treated it from the beginning as another movement to be crushed. An 1886 report on 'Gambling and Other Crimes' in the Fort Sill reservation described it as a vice that 'produces the same effect as opium'.[49] In 1888 the trade in peyote was banned on the reservation but it remained on sale at nearby trading posts, and the clandestine nature of the tipi ceremony made it impossible to police. 'They keep it hid out like the whites do whisky in Kansas,' the exasperated new agent Charles Adams wrote in 1891.[50] Quanah stood his ground, insisting to the agency and to the missionary council that it was both a sacred tradition and a valuable medicine. Picking his battles carefully as always, he relaxed his opposition to Christian schooling but insisted firmly on his right to peyote, as he did with his polygamy. He counted on the government to recognise that persecuting him on either count would be more trouble than it was worth.

The Methodist minister John Jasper Methvin, who arrived on the reservation in 1887 and founded a church and an Indian school, remained for decades peyote's implacable enemy, unshakeable in his conviction that its use was 'more of a drug habit and a dissipation than a worship'.[51] There were plenty of Comanches who shared his view. At least half had converted to Christianity, and many of them regarded peyote as a relic of the heathen world they had chosen to leave behind. There were others who adhered stubbornly to the old ways, suspicious of Quanah's dealings with the government and of the new ceremony's pretensions to tradition. But for its adherents, mostly men of the younger generation, it was a microcosm of the old ways within the shattering trauma of captivity. The tipi was a sacred space within which men raised as warriors could speak from the heart, confessing their fears, their failures and their sufferings to the Creator and drawing solace and support from their fellows.

Like Mooney, Quanah recognised that the peyote religion needed to accommodate itself within the Protestant culture that surrounded it. He presented the tipi ceremony not as a rival of the mission school and the prayer meeting but a complement to them. Unlike in tribal Mexico, there was no caste of shamans who cultivated their spiritual power: the roadman who led the ceremony was merely a facilitator, humble in his role and careful to pass the sacred wand, rattle and drum around the circle for every participant to touch. Peyote made every man his own conscience and his own priest. Quanah resisted Christian conversion to the end but he spoke its language fluently, and he presented peyote as a distinctively Indian expression of the same higher truth: 'the white man goes into his church house and talks *about* Jesus, but the Indian goes into his tipi and talks *to* Jesus'.[52] Christ's crucifixion was the white man's sin, and Indians had no need to atone for it. Peyote, the form in which God had always been with them, was their communion.

Quanah came to embody the archetype of the Comanche roadman. When he conducted a ceremony he placed on the raised earth altar around the fire his personal 'grandfather' peyote, a huge and perfect dried specimen that he kept beside his bed in a polished wood box with a glass lid, originally made for a fob watch. To his right would sit the drum chief, who provided the instruments to accompany the singer, and to his left the cedar chief, who offered the incense to the fire. Opposite them across the circle was the fire-man, who fed the central fire and opened and closed the tent flap when required. He would roll and light a smoke, then open the meeting with thanks and prayers as the tobacco was passed round. The peyote circulated after it, as it would do several times during the night. The meeting proceeded much like the one that James Mooney had first witnessed among the Kiowa, with songs and prayers alternating until dawn, when the fire-man would fetch a woman with a bucket of water who smoked and prayed over it before passing it round. At this point the roadman might preach a lesson, directly or indirectly to members of the circle. Quanah was particularly known for his advice and admonishments at this point, which could be stern and lengthy.[53]

The Comanche rite is the classic form of the ceremony, known as the 'half-moon' for the horseshoe shape of the dirt mound that circumscribes the altar. From the beginning there were variants: individual roadmen positioned the ceremonial objects differently and interpreted the symbolism in their own way. Among the Kiowa the altar was crescent shaped and a line drawn in the dirt through its centre to represent the 'peyote road' its disciples should follow. A significant variant was introduced by the Caddo medicine man John Wilson, who had been caught up in the Ghost Dance and in its wake took to eating peyote alone. He was vouchsafed a series of visions in which Christ and the peyote walked together in the sky, and was shown a form of the ceremony with new songs, costumes and ceremonial roles, and more overtly Christian elements. Its differently shaped altar, based on Wilson's arrangement of the spiritual energies of moon, sun and fire, led to its name of the 'full moon' or 'big moon' ritual, distinct from the half-moon that became identified with Quanah.

※　　※　　※

James Mooney's arrival at Fort Sill in November 1893 brought the white man with the deepest knowledge of Indian culture together with the Indian who had learned how to negotiate the white world as none before him. Twenty-five years later Mooney testified to the US House of Representatives that Quanah, who died in 1911, had been 'altogether the ablest man in the history of the western tribes of Oklahoma',[54] and certainly 'as shrewd and able as any white man'.[55] Quanah, for his part, referred to Mooney as 'the only white man who knows our religion'.[56] They had come to it from different worlds but both recognised the peyote religion's unique potential to square the circle of tradition and assimilation. They had settled independently on the same strategy for presenting it to white audiences: as a medicine and a sacrament rather than an intoxicant, and a companion rather than a rival to the Christian faith in which privately neither of them believed.

For their peyote meeting, Quanah nominated as roadman one of the oldest members of his tribe, Puiwat, whom he told Mooney was the first Comanche peyotist. Puiwat was married to an Apache and was said to have learned the rite from the Mescalero some fifty years previously. Quanah said he wanted to convince his guest that peyote 'does not age men prematurely or make them weak-minded or crazy'.[57] Mooney recalled later that Puiwat 'was blind and very feeble' but 'when his turn came to sing the midnight song he took the rattle and sang as vigorously as any of the others'.[58] Mooney accepted the peyote as it circulated and entered the state in which, as he later wrote:

> One seems to be lifted out of the body and floating about in the air like a freed spirit. The fire takes on glorious shapes, the sacred mescal upon the crescent mound becomes alive and moves and talks and you talk to it and it answers. You look around on your companions and they seem far away and unreal, and yet you know they are close by your side. At times the songs and the drum-beat fill the tipi like a burst of thunder ... then the sound comes up from the ground and out of the air and is all around you like spirit whisperings.[59]

After the daylight song that concluded the ceremony, the group of eleven men and two women, huddled in blankets in the freezing dawn, posed for Mooney's camera beside Quanah's large two-storey clapboard house, in front of the Wichita peak now known as Quanah Mountain.[60] Quanah kneels, second from the left in the front row, with Puiwat to his right, his face obscured by his eagle feather; two of Quanah's wives, Chony and Tonarcy, stand behind them. After taking the photograph Mooney conversed with Puiwat, who 'gave me a long interview through an interpreter without showing any unusual signs of fatigue'.[61] Quanah walked straight from his ten hours in the tipi into a meeting with two Texas cattlemen to discuss an important pasture lease, clearly 'perfectly confident in his ability to transact the business'.[62] As Mooney would later observe in defence of peyote, Quanah 'is entirely too smart a man to attend to business when his brain is not in working order'.[63]

After concluding his business, Quanah presented Mooney with the wand that Puiwat had used during the ceremony. Mooney also negotiated the purchase of a large burlap sack of dried peyote buttons, 50 pounds in weight, which he brought back with him to Washington. Its contents had already passed through many hands on their journey from the peyote gardens of Laredo and would pass through many more, launching the first scientific trials of peyote on human subjects and being consumed by America's leading authorities in pharmacy, neurology, psychology and philosophy. It was an exchange that cemented a bond of trust between peyote's two great advocates, but it was also a transmission between worlds: from millennia of sacred tradition to the clinical gaze of western modernity.

CHAPTER FOUR

BRILLIANT VISIONS

1895–98

WASHINGTON, DC, PHILADELPHIA,
LEIPZIG, LONDON

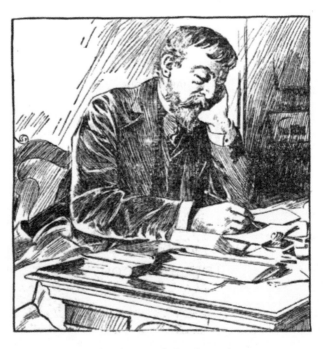

Silas Weir Mitchell in his study.

The first scientific trial of a major psychedelic took place in 1895 in Washington, DC, at the medical school of Columbian (now George Washington) University. Its initial subject was a twenty-seven-year-old male, identified only as 'Chemist'. Between 9 and 11 p.m., in student residential rooms under medical supervision, he chewed three of the dried peyote buttons supplied to James Mooney by Quanah Parker. He noted a slight nausea; he stretched out on the bed and, as it faded, he closed his eyes and found he could see 'all sorts of designs in brilliant and ever-changing colours'. Encouraged, he chewed a fourth button and part of a fifth. 'Then followed a train of delightful visions such as no human ever enjoyed under normal conditions.'[1]

'My mind was perfectly clear and active,' the subject recalled; he spent part of the time sitting at his desk and making notes. At other points he luxuriated, eyes closed, as 'an ever-changing panorama of infinite beauty and grandeur, of infinite variety of colour and form, hurried before me'. He found that by the act of concentration he could exert some control over the visions: the most satisfying sequence was coaxed to life by recalling Imre Kiralfy's electrically illuminated stage extravaganza *America* which he had witnessed two years previously at the Chicago World's Fair, and which brought the dazzling filaments that coursed across his closed eyelids to a peak of intensity. Such moments 'so far passed the more ordinary realms of delight as to bring me to that high ecstatic state in which our exclamations of enjoyment become involuntary'. He probed the limits of pleasure by turning his imagination to the dark side and conjuring 'myriads of horrible crawling monsters' and gruesomely distorted human shapes, but these 'merely added another item to the list of the inexpressible delights of my remarkable night's experience'.[2] He lost track of time and external space until around 4 a.m., when the effects began to wear off. They were succeeded by a slight depression and an insomnia that persisted until the following evening.

On his return to Washington Mooney had turned a quantity of his peyote buttons over to Daniel Webster Prentiss, the professor of materia medica and therapeutics at the university's medical department, for human testing. He gave rather more, about half, to Dr Harvey Wiley, head of the Department of Agriculture's chemistry division. Wiley was known as the 'Crusading Chemist' for his campaigns against food adulterants, which would eventually lead to the Pure Food and Drug Act of 1906 and the reconstitution of his division as the Food and Drug Administration. His laboratories provided chemical analyses for the entire department, and at this time were predominantly focused on establishing a self-sufficient American sugar industry. Wiley believed that a high sugar diet was a mark of civilisation and its consumption should be maximised, particularly for children: his maxim was that 'childhood without candy would be heaven without harps'.[3] He passed the dried cactus buttons on to a junior chemist in the division named Erwin Ewell.

Ewell approached cacti with an intense fascination that he believed to be in tune with the spirit of the age. 'Among civilised and uncivilised peoples, old and young, scientific and unscientific', who was not, he asked, 'inspired with awe' by their 'weird forms' or 'moved by the mysterious beauty of an opening blossom of the "night-blooming cereus"'? Thanks to the recent efforts of collectors and suppliers such as Anna Nickels and Albert Blanc, whose nursery in Philadelphia was at this point the largest mail-order supplier in the world, there was now 'scarcely a housewife in the land that pretends to maintain a conservatory or a window-garden without numbering one or more cacti in her collection'.[4]

The chemistry of the cactus family was for Ewell their most mysterious and fascinating aspect. Most botanical chemists, vaguely aware that their juices were sometimes drunk by thirsty desert travellers, assumed them to be devoid of active constituents, but Ewell had collected examples of the medicinal use of cacti in various cultures, particularly as cardiac stimulants. Now the most prominent experts around the globe – Louis Lewin in Berlin, Sereno Watson at Harvard and his own network of Washington researchers centred around the Bureau of American Ethnology – were all turning their attention in the same direction: the 'one or more species of cacti that are used by the American Indians for ceremonial and medicinal purposes'.[5]

Meanwhile Daniel Webster Prentiss and his assistant Francis Morgan proceeded to a second human trial, this time on a twenty-four-year-old male subject identified as 'Reporter'. After Chemist's complaints that chewing the peyote buttons had made him nauseous, they were ground to a coarse powder for easier digestion and wrapped in wafer paper for swallowing. The subject's physical examination before the dose revealed a rather high pulse, which Prentiss and Morgan attributed to the glass of whisky he had just taken with supper. Between 11.30 p.m. and 2.30 a.m. he consumed the equivalent of seven buttons. By 1.30 a.m. his pupils were dilated and by 2.30 he was feeling 'decidedly lazy and perfectly contented'. He closed his eyes and was enveloped by visions which he described to the doctors as they unfolded: 'a host of little tubes of shining light' down which red and green balls were rolling, then shaping them-selves into letters, then revolving rapidly, the spaces between them filling with shifting seas of green. The patterns evolved 'through rich arabesques, Syrian carpet patterns, and plain geometric figures, and with each form came a new flash of colour'.[6]

From this point, however, his experience took a disagreeable turn. He had an intermittent, highly discomfiting feeling of 'double personality – to be outside of himself looking at himself'. He became acutely aware of his 'mental inferiority' towards the doctors surrounding him, and evinced 'a feeling of great distrust and resentment'. His supervisors recorded that he 'firmly believed that we were secretly laughing at his condition. He believed that we intended to kill him, and for this reason he refused to take the eighth button.' In the intervals between these 'paroxysms' his hostile feelings disappeared entirely and he apologised for his outbursts. In a later interview he maintained that the drug had made him 'perfectly "insane"', and he 'would have attempted violence had it not seemed to him too much trouble in his lazy and depressed condition'.

This was a confounding result. It was a basic assumption of phar-macy that drugs produced broadly predictable and replicable reactions.

Even with psychoactive drugs, the effects of which could be influenced by the subject's personality and mental state, there were clear tendencies: a stimulant such as cocaine never sedated its subjects any more than a sedative such as chloral hydrate ever stimulated them. Yet as the peyote trials continued, the contradictions mounted. Every dose seemed to produce a different response. 'Reporter' agreed to a second trial, and this time 'no disagreeable symptoms appeared'.[7] The third subject suffered 'a most marked depression of the muscular system' and 'became unable to walk without assistance'.[8] The fourth barely noticed any visions at all. The fifth found his visions wonderfully enhanced by music and drummed time on a table for hours, reminding the doctors that 'a constant beating upon drums is a regular part of the taking of mescal buttons by the Indians'. The universal symptoms amounted to little more than trivial side effects: dilation of the pupils, loss of the sense of time and an inability to sleep.

Prentiss and Morgan's report, published in September 1895 in the *Therapeutic Gazette*, was tentative in its conclusions. The experiences they witnessed contradicted not only each other but also the only prior report, that of John Raleigh Briggs, whose racing heart and breathing difficulties were not observed in any of the subjects. The closest comparison Prentiss and Morgan could adduce was cannabis, which also 'produces visions, with dilated pupils, and with slight effect upon the circulation', but that was a hypnotic sedative that tended to sleepiness rather than insomnia. The cactus seemed to share some of cocaine's stimulant effects but little else. The most plausible hypothesis was that the active principle in the cactus bore no relation to anything currently known to science. Its unusual effects might, if they could somehow be harnessed and standardised, support a range of therapeutic applications. 'It may prove of value,' Prentiss and Morgan suggested in a follow-up paper, 'as a cerebral stimulant in depressed conditions of the mind, such as melancholia, hypochondriasis, and in some cases of neurasthenia.' It might also be of value as a tonic for 'general "nervousness", nervous headache, nervous irritable cough', or as a substitute for opium in the treatment of 'active delirium and mania', given the advantage that its use was 'not followed by the unpleasant effects which often attend the use of that drug'.[9]

It was a lengthy list, but lacking in detail and tepid in its enthusiasm: much more research would be needed before any medical application could be recommended. In the meantime the underlying problem of peyote's unpredictability was highlighted by an unscheduled experiment. Erwin Ewell, as he became absorbed in his attempts to extract resins and alkaloids from his cactus specimens, was unable to resist sampling them. In November 1895 he took two buttons in his rooms on Upper Fourteenth Street. What happened next is recorded in two sharply differing accounts, both dating from twenty years later. Harvey Wiley recalled that Ewell had mentioned he was thinking of making a self-experiment with peyote and Wiley had advised him against it. The next he knew was at 2 a.m. on the night in question when Ewell's roommate, alarmed at his condition, brought him to Wiley's house. Ewell was 'constantly talking and saying, "Oh, how beautiful; oh, how splendid; oh, how magnificent . . . I see the angels in the streets of gold"'.[10] Wiley concluded that the cactus was a deliriant poison.

James Mooney recalled the event clearly but rather differently. Ewell's dose was a small one – Mooney himself had taken much larger – but rather than 'having his mind at ease, and his body at ease also, as most people do when they take medicines', he had panicked, convinced himself he was dying, written his will and gone wandering out into the street in the middle of the night. In Mooney's version Ewell had met a policeman who, making sense of the situation as best he could, had escorted him to Wiley's house. Mooney had spoken to Ewell the next day, by which time he had recovered and 'although he was rather excited, he knew what he was doing and could talk in a very interesting fashion of what had happened to him'.[11]

To Mooney, if not to the doctors and chemists, one point was obvious: the experiences that they and their subjects were having were quite different from those of any traditional peyotist. The 'horrible visions and gloomy depression' reported under medical supervision were 'entirely foreign to my own experience or that of any Indian with whom I have talked'. As he explained, 'the Indian is familiar with the idea from earliest childhood'; peyote was not an adventure into *terra incognita* but a journey to the deepest source of their culture and its power. Such journeys were undertaken in a regular manner, in keeping with tradition, with plenty of time allowed afterwards to recover and integrate the experience. This was why the ceremony was typically convened 'on Saturday night in order that he [might] rest and keep quiet on Sunday'. The trial subjects, by contrast, undertook their experiments with little idea of what to expect and no attempt to prepare their minds; often they seemed 'to have hastily swallowed a sandwich and plunged at once into exciting action'.[12] The investigators assumed that trials on randomly selected subjects would allow them to reduce the drug's action to a uniform set of symptoms. But the cactus confounded this expectation: the outcomes it produced seemed as random as the subjects themselves.

※　　※　　※

In Germany, the parallel attempt to isolate peyote's active chemical compound had by this point flared into controversy. Despite reserving the field for himself, Louis Lewin had made little progress since 1888 and in 1891 a Leipzig chemist named Arthur Heffter began his own investigations. He bought samples of peyote from two different dealers at a horticultural fair, and subsequently requested and received from Carl Lumholtz a small sample of the *hikuli* he had brought back from his visit to the Huichol people. Heffter concluded from these samples that there were at least two species of peyote, similar in physical appearance but with very different chemical profiles. One he identified as *Anhalonium williamsii*,[13] from which he extracted an alkaloid he called 'pellotine'; experimenting with it on himself, he noted only a slight sedative effect. *Anhalonium lewinii*, by contrast, yielded at least two alkaloids with properties as yet undetermined.

Heffter was a gentle and retiring character whose work had thus far excited little attention outside his specialist fields. He had begun his career as an agricultural chemist, taken some medical training and worked on the biochemistry of lactic acid and the metabolism of iodine. He was sensitive to Lewin's exalted reputation and did his best to present his findings in a conciliatory manner. In March 1895, however, the renowned cactologist Karl Schumann stirred controversy with a lecture on poisonous cacti that cast doubt on Heffter's claim that *A. williamsii* and *A. lewinii* were two separate species. In the *Pharmaceutische Zeitung*'s synopsis of the lecture Heffter's views were summarised inaccurately and he responded with a correction, in which he acknowledged Lewin's priority in the field but pointed out that he had been the first to isolate a pure alkaloid from the cactus.

Lewin was furious at the breach of what he regarded as his prerogative. He wrote a letter to the *Pharmaceutische Zeitung* complaining that 'I have neither time, nor do I feel inclined, to make Mr Heffter understand the results of my research.'[14] Lewin's personality and profile made the contest unequal. As one student who attended both men's lectures recalled, Lewin's were packed: he was a 'tremedously stimulating, flamboyant orator . . . who always carried his audience away with his enthusiasm'. Heffter, by contrast, was 'not very verbal, awkward, frankly, in the presentation of his material', and his lectures were dull and poorly attended.[15] But Lewin was losing interest in peyote: the tincture with which Parke, Davis went to market in 1893 had attracted little interest, and Prentiss and Morgan's inconclusive trials suggested no obvious medical applications. Heffter, however, was puzzled and intrigued by the tangled botany and lengthening list of resins and alkaloids, and continued to dig deeper.

✿   ✿   ✿

There was one medical scientist in whose opinion Daniel Webster Prentiss was particularly interested, and he had set aside some of Quanah

Parker's buttons especially to send to him. Silas Weir Mitchell was nearing the end of a long career specialising in the disputed territory between mind and body that was known as 'nervous illness', during which he had become almost as dominant in American neurology as Freud's mentor Jean-Martin Charcot, 'the Napoleon of the neuroses', was in France. The son of a distinguished physician, Mitchell had taken an early interest in the subject because it was so poorly understood. During the Civil War he specialised in the nerve damage and paralyses caused by shells and artillery, and in 1872 was the first to describe phantom limb syndrome among amputees. After the war he had become one of America's first and most distinguished specialists in neurasthenia, the condition of shattered nerves, fatigue, depression and hysterical symptoms that was so prevalent it became known as 'the American disease'.[16] By 1896 he was Philadelphia aristocracy, married to a wealthy and well-connected wife, easing into retirement and travelling extensively with a retinue of servants. He had recently embarked on a second career as a novelist and his most recent work, *Hugh Wynne*, set against the backdrop of the American Revolution, was currently at the top of the bestseller lists and on its way to selling half a million copies.

Prentiss guessed correctly that despite his advancing age – he was now sixty-seven – Mitchell would find peyote a tantalising prospect. He had a longstanding expertise in toxicology and had studied rattlesnake venom and South American arrow poisons; more recently he had taken a keen interest in new psychoactive drugs such as chloral hydrate, ether, bromides and opiates. He was a bold self-experimenter who had over the course of his career frozen his own ulnar nerve, requested samples of hashish from his colleagues and submitted to a straitjacket, an experience that prompted in him 'a half-frantic desire to fight for freedom'[17] and made him a committed advocate for asylum reform. He was a firm believer that 'there are yet triumphs to be won in medicine by therapeutic boldness, and by the use at times of enormous doses'.[18] He had read Prentiss and Morgan's reports on peyote with interest and his powers of imagination and description, allied to his vast medical knowledge, made him uniquely qualified to produce a subjective account of its effects. On 24 May 1896, 'at 12 noon of a busy morning',[19] he took a decoction containing the equivalent of one and a half buttons. An hour later he repeated the dose.

Between 2 and 4 p.m., while holding consultations with a succession of patients, Mitchell began gradually to feel a 'pleasing sense of languor' stealing upon him, together with some discomfort in the stomach. He drove home and took another, larger dose. By 4.30 p.m., making notes, he 'became aware that a transparent, violet haze was about my pen point'.[20] He felt 'a decisive impression that I was more competent in my mind than in my everyday moods', and dashed off a letter of advice on a questionable diagnosis. By 5 p.m. such tasks seemed too effortful and he retired upstairs to lie in a darkened room.

'The display which for an enchanted two hours followed,' he wrote, 'was such as I find it hopeless to describe in language.' His 'first vivid show of mescal colour' was a shower of stars, succeeded by floating films of pink and purple, then by electric zigzags such as those described by migraine sufferers. Then came objects such as 'a tall, richly finished gothic tower of very elaborate and definite design' dripping with gemlike drops of colour. Time and space unrolled before his eyes in a vast immensity, 'miles of rippled purples, half transparent, and of ineffable beauty'. Without thinking he opened his eyes and to his consternation the vision vanished. He attempted to conjure up human figures, but without success; later he was rewarded with a scene of 'two little dwarves, made, it seemed, of leather . . . blowing through long glass pipes of green tint, which seemed to me to be alive, so intensely, vitally green were they'. His energy waned, and he drifted between sleep and waking. Settling into his visions once more, he saw a scene he recognised from waking life: the beach at Newport, with waves rolling in, 'liquid splendours huge and threatening'. He 'wished the beautiful terror of these huge mounds of colour would continue', but 'a knock at my door caused me to open my eyes, and I lost whatever of wonder might have come after'. After dinner the visions faded, leaving only the odd shimmer of colour.

The following day their magnificence was still vivid in his mind; he also had a headache and 'a smart attack of gastric distress'. 'These shows,' he noted, 'are expensive.' His mind began to turn on the questions raised by them, and the mechanisms in the brain and nervous system that might account for them. Uncanny as they were, they had parallels in the stranger dimensions of neurology: 'even my most brilliant visions' were not different in kind from the searing optical symptoms described in migraine or epilepsy. There was some overlap, too, with the visions of hypnagogia and the 'phantasms' of hysteria, with their uncanny detail and independence from conscious control. He saw 'no obvious therapeutic uses for mescal in massive doses' – the physical ordeal made it unsuitable for neurasthenic patients – but was struck by the rich possibilities for psychological research. 'Here is unlocked a storehouse of glorified memorial treasures,' he concluded.[21] The visions, at their root, seemed to be enhanced and transposed creatures of memory, though he recognised nothing from his direct personal experience except the sudden appearance of Newport beach. He wondered whether the visions 'of the navvy would be like those of the artist, and above all, what those born blind could relate'. He noted that 'no one has told us what visions come to the Red Man'. However, he concluded his account with a caution: 'I predict a perilous reign of the mescal habit when this agent becomes attainable. The temptation to call again the enchanting magic of the experience will, I am sure, be too much for some men to resist after they have once set foot in this land of fairy colours, where there seems to be so much to charm and so little to excite horror or disgust'.[22]

♣   ♣   ♣

Mitchell himself had no difficulty resisting the temptation of another dose. The experience 'was worth one such indigestion and headache, but was not worth a second'.[23] He was eager, though, to pass it on to an old acquaintance, one of the few figures in America whose authority on matters of the mind compared to his own. William James was now professor of philosophy at Harvard, having made his reputation with his two-volume *Principles of Psychology*, published in 1890. The two men had been friends for many years, though not close ones. Their mutual esteem had been punctured during the 1880s by a subject that threw their differences into sharp relief: spiritualism. They had attended a séance together, which James had witnessed with an open mind – perhaps a will to believe – but Mitchell had pronounced 'inconceivable twaddle'.[24] James had taken offence, and Mitchell had attempted to make amends by offering to pay for another séance, commenting that 'we did find the Spirits costly'[25] and thereby offending James further.

Where Mitchell looked primarily for the physiological correlates of altered consciousness, James set his sights beyond them. He had, for example, been the first psychologist to take up Mitchell's observations of phantom limb syndrome, but his 1887 paper on the subject, 'The Consciousness of Lost Limbs', focused not on their neurological basis but their similarities to clairvoyance and telepathy. His pluralist philosophy aimed to encompass domains beyond the material and accept classes of mental phenomena that resisted conventional scientific investigation. Psychoactive drugs had always interested him because they offered the prospect of chemical, measurable and repeatable journeys into dimensions of the mind typically dismissed as subjective and unverifiable. More personally, they held out for him the possibility of a long-sought illumination. His father, a Swedenborgian theologian, had instilled in him a conviction that mystical experience was profound and meaningful, but his own mental character had from an early age tended towards the logical and he had only known such revelations at second hand. Drugs were for him pregnant with the possibility of transcending the prosaic habits of mind that barred his entry to an important facet of human psychology.

Mitchell's gift of peyote was part peace offering, part challenge. His covering letter spoke, in James's summary, of 'the most gorgeous stimulation of the visual centres, magnificently colored hallucinations, pure fairyland pictures such as earth cannot afford'.[26] Here was a ticket to another world whose reliability Mitchell could vouch for, and which he believed would offer more substantial phenomena than the spirits. It was an intriguing test for the approach that James had formulated in the first volume of his *Principles of Psychology*: a study of the mind that built on the natural sciences but aimed beyond measurable data at a more faithful representation of its mercurial and often contradictory operations. In his chapter 'The Stream of Thought' he had argued that mental events cannot be treated as objective facts, discrete and logically connected, nor do they proceed in a linear fashion: consciousness is rather 'a teeming multiplicity of objects and relations', a crowd of overlapping rational and subconscious selves in constant flux and dialogue.[27] If peyote had thus far defeated the doctors and pharmacologists with its paradoxical and unpredictable effects, perhaps James's more capacious theories might make sense of it.

One of the few effects reliably exhibited by all Prentiss and Morgan's subjects, for example, was the subject of a later chapter in James's book, 'The Perception of Time'. Every one of them had been astonished to discover that their epically unfolding panoramas and visions had occupied only a few minutes at most. James theorised that false perceptions of this kind might be more than mental impairments: they offered clues both to the action of the drug and to the workings of the mind in normal states. They showed that subjective time, as opposed to 'clock time', was elastic, tending to reflect the number of mental events that were taking place: 'awareness of *change* is thus the condition on which our perception of time's flow depends'.[28] This explained why time seems to slow at moments of crisis, and it suggested that under the influence of peyote the mind was being subjected to a flux of perceptions many times more rapid than in its normal state.

However he interpreted Mitchell's offer, James was more than ready to accept it, and he repaired promptly to his family's cottage in the hills of New Hampshire. At 6.30 the following morning he took a peyote button and was rewarded with immediate nausea, followed by vomiting and diarrhoea that continued all day and finally abated at four the next morning. He described the ordeal to his brother, the novelist Henry James, as a '*Katzenjammer*' – a screaming hangover – and concluded ruefully, 'I will take the visions on trust!'[29] It was an oddly violent reaction to a tiny dose from which many subjects would have noticed nothing at all. Among the experiences thus far recorded, it most closely resembled that of John Raleigh Briggs: did the two men share a peculiar constitutional quirk, exacerbated perhaps by over-eagerness or suppressed anxiety? It was a reminder, if another were needed, of peyote's unpredictability and of the toxic reactions that it could manifest.

If the physiology or psychology that produced his *Katzenjammer* remained beyond the reach of his own theories, James nevertheless kept faith with the potential of mind-altering drugs and the mystical epiphany he had experienced with a less physically demanding substance: nitrous oxide. His experience engendered the famous insight in his 1902 masterwork, *On the Varieties of Religious Experience*, that 'our normal waking consciousness, rational consciousness as we call it, is but one special type of consciousness, whilst all about it, parted from it by the filmiest of screens, there lie potential forms of consciousness entirely different . . . no account of the universe in its totality can be final which leaves these other forms of consciousness quite disregarded'.[30] It was an insight he might equally have reached with peyote, had his constitution permitted him, and one on which later experimenters with mescaline would draw deeply.

🌢   🌢   🌢

Silar Weir Mitchell's report on peyote was published in the *British Medical Journal* in December 1896, bringing it to the attention of an international readership. It was read with great interest by Havelock Ellis, who was intrigued enough to look for a source for the cactus. He discovered that Parke, Davis, who had opened a London office in 1890, supplied dried buttons via Potter & Clarke, the London pharmacists best known for

'Potter's Asthma Cure', a greenish powder to be burned and inhaled that contained the dried leaves of the highly toxic datura plant.

Ellis was a qualified doctor but he made his living as a litterateur and art critic. He was an example of the modern renaissance man he had called for in his 1890 book *The New Spirit*, the manifesto for a movement in which the arts, sciences, politics and religion would all be reinvented and rejoined. He was an aesthete, an individualist and a feminist, a member of the Progressive Association and an intimate of London's tightly knit *fin-de-siècle* artistic coterie. He was in the process of writing, in correspondence with the art historian and advocate of 'male love' John Addington Symonds, the taboo-shattering multi-volume study of sex that would become his enduring achievement. He was staying, as he often did, in the rooms rented by his friend Arthur Symons, the literary critic and Decadent poet, in Fountain Court, a red-brick mansion block in the Middle Temple district beside the Thames Embankment. At that moment Symons was in Paris with their mutual friend W.B. Yeats. 'On Good Friday,' Ellis began in a tone similar to Mitchell's, 'I found myself entirely alone in the quiet rooms in the Temple which I occupy when in London, and judged the occasion a fitting one for a personal experiment.'[31]

Ellis's first report of his experience appeared in the *Lancet* in June 1897 and concentrated on the aspects that would be of most interest to medical readers. Peyote was not a physically dangerous substance, he reported: 'the only two really unpleasant symptoms of the experiment' were 'motor incoordination and cardiac and respiratory depression'. Its positive symptoms, by contrast, were remarkable: 'a saturnalia of the specific senses, and chiefly an orgy of vision'.[32] It was a tantalising advertisement for the much fuller account that he published six months later in a progressive literary quarterly, the *Contemporary Review*.

His title – 'Mescal: A New Artificial Paradise' – announced its line of descent from Charles Baudelaire's essay on hashish, *Les Paradises Artificels*, perhaps the century's most admired literary account of a drug experience after *Confessions of an English Opium-Eater*, written by Baudelaire's hero Thomas De Quincey. Ellis began with a summary of peyote's known history, citing Lumholtz's visit to the Tarahumara and James Mooney's encounters with the Kiowa, the experiments undertaken by Prentiss and Morgan and Mitchell's 'very interesting record of the brilliant visions by which he was visited under the influence of the plant'.[33] He proceeded to describe how he made a liquid decoction of three buttons and drank it slowly over two hours, after which he felt faint, his pulse weakened and he lay down to read. Like Mitchell, he first noticed peyote's effects as they impinged on the note-taking process: 'a pale violet shadow floated over the page around the point at which my eyes were fixed'. As evening closed in he was gradually enveloped, as Mitchell had been, by 'a vast field of golden jewels, studded with red and green stones, ever changing'. From this point on 'the visions continued with undiminished brilliance for many hours'.[34]

Having fulfilled his obligations to medicine with his previous report in the *Lancet*, Ellis felt free to discuss the experience in primarily aesthetic terms. The previous year he had written a paper on 'The Colour Sense in Literature', comparing the imagery invoked by authors such as Shakespeare, Chaucer, Coleridge, Poe and Rosetti. Now he brought a similar critical sensibility to bear on the peyote cactus. Every part of the spectrum competed in his visions, but 'there was always a certain parsimony and aesthetic value in the colours presented'. He was 'further impressed, not only by the brilliance, delicacy and variety of the colours, but even more by their lovely and various textures – fibrous, woven, polished, glowing, dull, veined, semi-transparent'. He compared the patterns that gradually took form and life to the 'Maori style of architecture' and 'the delicate architectural effects as of lace carved in wood, which we associated with the mouchrabieh work of Cairo'. They were 'living arabesques', with 'a certain incomplete tendency to symmetry, as though the underlying mechanism was associated with a large number of polished facets'. When he became exhausted by the visions in darkness Ellis turned on the gas light, and the shadows that leapt to life reminded him of the 'visual hyperaesthesia' of Claude Monet's paintings. It was a feast for the eyes, and an education for them. Writing months later, he maintained that 'ever since this experience I have been more aesthetically sensitive than I was before to the more delicate phenomena of light and shade and colour'.[35]

🌵   🌵   🌵

Ellis's description was the flowering of a tendency that established itself almost immediately in western encounters with peyote: to describe its effects primarily in terms of the visual sense. Over centuries of indigenous use, this dimension of the experience had been acknowledged as beautiful but rarely described in detail. Among its early western investigators, by contrast, only James Mooney resisted – or lacked – the urge to focus on peyote's optical effects and to narrate them in the first person. Unlike the others, Mooney's experiences took place in a communal ceremony rather than a darkened room: the primary focus was ritual, song and prayer, and to dissect one's private sensations was to miss the point. The distinction connects, perhaps, to the 'great divide' between orality and literacy theorised by Walter Ong, according to which the advent of print in the Renaissance fostered a distinctively 'ocularcentric' western culture: as text took precedence over the spoken word, the objective was privileged over the subjective, the individual over the communal, the fixed over the fluid and the visual over the aural.[36] This tendency entrenched itself further in the twentieth century after the synthesis of mescaline, and once the term 'psychedelic' was coined, it quickly became first and foremost the signifier of a visual style.

The ocularcentric turn may be characteristic of western modernity in general, but it was also a specific response to the *fin-de-siècle* moment at which peyote made its first appearance. The critic and philosopher Walter Benjamin, who would himself take mescaline in a clinical trial in 1934, wrote that the nineteenth century 'subjected the human sensorium to a complex kind of training'.[37] Visual illusions – from kaleidoscopes to magic lanterns to photography – made the transit from dazzling novelties to staples of mass culture. Magicians, mediums and psychic investigators all probed the limits of the real, blurring the line between optical trickery, the subconscious mind and the spirit world. The very first subject of peyote's scientific trials found an analogue for his visions in novel and spectacular displays of electricity. At the moment when Ellis made his experiment the world was being exposed for the first time to X-ray images and the cinematograph. 'Visual hyperaesthesia' was a property not only of peyote but of the culture in which he was consuming it, and to which Monet and the Impressionists were responding. Like the bright world of the Nahua, the electric age of the *fin de siècle* distilled matter to its quintessence of colour and light.

As with electricity, there was danger in this brilliance. By the late 1890s, mind-altering drugs that enhanced and intensified modern life were stronger, cheaper and more available than ever before. A substance such as cocaine made the world glow with preternatural brightness but those who used it incautiously could also be consumed by it. Ellis concluded his essay in the *Contemporary Review* with the assessment that 'the enjoyment of the colour visions produced' by the cactus meant that 'there is every likelihood that it will become popular': a new artificial paradise for a new age. He anticipated fears about its abuse but regarded them as misguided. Unlike the everyday poisons that delivered immediate pleasure, the peyote experience was a physical ordeal that demanded 'organic soundness and good health', and its rewards were conditional on occasional use. Ellis assured his readers it was 'not probable that its use will easily develop into a habit'.[38]

This assurance was greeted with scepticism in the *Review of Reviews* of January 1898, which predicted that 'in a year or two we shall probably find that mescal mania is an even more insidious and deadly malady than those caused by morphia, opium or whisky'.[39] The following month, under the headline 'Paradise or Inferno?', the *British Medical Journal* warned gravely in an editorial that 'such eulogy of any drug is a danger to the public', especially one 'the use of which has been suppressed by law in America' (a reference to the prohibitions on Indian reservations). Ellis might be a qualified doctor but he had crossed a line. Unlike Mooney or Mitchell, he was not simply a scientist taking peyote for ethnographic or medical research: he was a tastemaker who must be held accountable for 'putting temptation before that sector of the public which is always in search of a new sensation'.[40]

Ellis's immediate circle was more dedicated in the pursuit of new sensations than most and his encouragement brought into being mescaline's first informal artistic scene. Curious as to what a visual artist would make of mescal, he persuaded one of his acquaintances to try it. The first dose was too weak and the second far too strong, inducing, in his friend's words, 'a series of attacks or paroxysms, which I can only describe by saying that I felt as though I was dying'. Visions alternated with strange and disturbing physical sensations, and sometimes combined with them: when Ellis passed him a piece of biscuit to relieve his nausea, it 'suddenly streamed out into blue flame', an electric conflagration that spread across the right-hand side of his body. 'As I placed the biscuit in my mouth it burst again into the same colored fire and illuminated the interior of my mouth, casting a blue reflection on the roof. The light in the Blue Grotto at Capri, I am able to affirm, is not nearly as blue as seemed for a short space of time the interior of my mouth'.[41]

Ellis made a further experiment on himself to test the effects of music, and found that when a friend played the piano 'the music stimulated the visions and added greatly to my enjoyment of them'.[42] He also 'made experiments on two poets, whose names are both well known' and can be identified with reasonable certainty as W.B. Yeats and Arthur Symons. While Ellis was reading Weir Mitchell's account of peyote in December 1896, the pair were taking hashish together in Paris, an experiment that Symons memorialised in poetry[43] and Yeats referred to later and more obliquely in his memoir *The Trembling of the Veil* (1922). Symons had first visited Paris with Ellis in 1889, and the two had subsequently worked together as editors of the Mermaid series of Elizabethan plays. Throughout 1896 Symons had edited the short-lived but influential *Savoy* magazine, with Aubrey Beardsley as illustrator and both Ellis and Yeats among the contributors.

The peyote experiment caught both poets at a moment of transition and reinvention. Symons had been working for some years on essays and a book about the Decadent Movement, but under Yeats's influence he was distancing himself from the term and its jaded pursuit of 'learned corruption' and the 'deliberately abnormal'.[44] In Paris the two had embraced the term 'Symbolism' to capture the numinous aspects of experience which escape language and the occult techniques that Yeats used to pursue them. The artist was to become something closer to a defrocked priest and art a 'sacred ritual', as Symons announced in the introduction to *The Symbolist Movement in Literature*, his master-work which appeared in 1899 with a dedication to Yeats. The world of symbols connected directly to the art and literature of antiquity, and had been brought to a creative peak by French writers of the previous generation; but 'what distinguishes the Symbolism of our day from the Symbolism of the past is that it has now become conscious of itself'.[45] It was an appropriate moment to explore a new artificial paradise and its power to awaken the poet to mysteries beyond language.

The first subject, presumably Yeats – a poet 'interested in mystical matters, an excellent subject for visions' – was impaired by a weak constitution. 'He found the effects of mescal on his breathing some-what unpleasant; he much prefers hasheesh.' But Symons, on a modest dose of a little under three buttons, was transported. 'I have never seen such a succession of absolutely pictorial visions with such precision,' he reported. Dragons balancing white balls on puffs of their exhaled breath swept past him from right to left; playing the piano with closed eyes, he 'got waves and lines of pure colour'.[46] Like Ellis, however, he found the experience a saturnalia of vision rather than a descent into the deeper realms of the symbolic and the sacred. It would be another few years before London's artistic–occult milieu would produce its defrocked peyote priest.

Late that evening, Symons walked from Fountain Court down to the nearby Thames Embankment. As he gazed across at the South Bank, he found himself 'absolutely fascinated by an advertisement of

"Bovril", which came and went in letters of light on the other side of the river'.[47] The brilliance of electricity was the ruling metaphor for peyote's scintillating visions, but it was a literal stimulus too: it seemed that nothing delighted the eye of the mescal eater so much as the new electrical sublime. They arrived together as avatars of a new world of visual spectacle, equal parts scientific discovery and sensory delight.

🌵　🌵　🌵

While Ellis and his friends refined their descriptions of peyote's visions, another experimenter was probing their source. In Leipzig, Arthur Heffter was progressing systematically with his extractions, following the assumption that the active principle was not (as Prentiss and Morgan had theorised) one of the resins that could be extracted from it, but one of the alkaloids. He had thus far identified five, and arranged them into 'a sort of periodic table'.[48] At one end was what he was calling lophophorine, which he took to be a strychnine-like stimulant; at the other was a compound he had christened mescaline, which he suspected was a morphine-like depressant, responsible for the languorous sedative sensations. In between these poles were pellotine, anhalonidine and anhalonine. He decided that the quickest and simplest route to determining their effects was by self-experiment.

He began on 5 June 1897, the same day that Ellis's report was published in the *Lancet*, by taking an alcoholic extract of 16.6 grams of dried cactus, equivalent to around five buttons. He felt his pulse drop, together with 'nausea, occipital headache, intense dizziness and clumsiness in moving'. He lay down in a darkened room and was rewarded with visions 'which consisted partly of mosaics, and partly of winding coloured ribbons moving with the rapidity of lightning'. Gradually they resolved themselves into scenery – 'a richly decorated banquet hall, where the friezes, walls and chandeliers were ornamented with jewels, opals and pearls' – which had a tendency to flip upside down, adding to his dizziness and nausea.[49] His sense of time was scrambled;

he estimated a few minutes as half an hour. All in all, his experience correlated closely with previous reports. He began to suspect that the visions, the signature effect of the cactus, might be produced by mescaline, the most abundant of its alkaloids.

On 21 July he carried out a second self-experiment. He extracted all the alkaloids from the cactus with ammonia and chloroform, leaving a slurry of resins behind. He wrapped these in wafer paper and swallowed a portion equivalent to the amount in his previous dose of peyote. He felt some initial weakness and nausea but within two hours it had gone, and no abnormal sensations remained. The resins, he concluded, might be responsible for some of the physical symptoms but the visions were produced by one or more of the alkaloids.

Two days later he tried a third experiment, drinking the combined alkaloids dissolved in water and sitting down to read. Soon enough, telltale green and violet patches spread across the paper, evolving into the now-familiar kaleidoscopic display and accompanied by 'dilation of the pupils, dizziness, very distressing nausea'. He had demonstrated to his satisfaction that 'the alkaloids produce the same physiological effect as the drug, and the peculiar actions of peyote on the visual apparatus must, therefore, be produced by one of its alkaloids'.[50]

Cautiously, Heffter began to experiment with small doses of mescaline hydrochloride, starting with 20mg and working by increments up to 100mg. At this higher dose he experienced mild physical symptoms – heaviness, slight headache and nausea – and the faint traces of visions when he closed his eyes. On 23 November he took 150mg. The violet and green spots came first, then 'images of carpet patterns, ribbed vaulting etc.'. Soon he was immersed in the visionary 'landscapes, halls and architectural forms' of peyote. 'The results,' he concluded, 'show that mescaline is exclusively responsible for the major symptoms of peyote (mescal) poisoning. This applies especially to the unique visions.'[51]

The singular focus of western experimenters on peyote's visions had unlocked its chemical secret. Mescaline crossed another great divide into modernity: from plant spirit to chemical compound. Against all expectations, Heffter had beaten Lewin to the discovery on which he had staked his claim. Lewin had entered the field first, with an unsurpassed knowledge of psychopharmacology, a dazzling cross-disciplinary range that allowed him to draw insights from cultures ancient and modern, and the muscle of the American pharmaceutical industry behind him. What made the difference was Heffter's experimental method. Lewin, alone among peyote's early investigators, was not prepared to take it himself. This was with him a long-standing point of principle. While making his pioneering studies of morphine addiction in the 1870s he had been deterred for life by encountering 'men who first took a narcotic remedy from pure curiosity, and later, overcome by its influence, became habitual drugtakers'.[52] He had proceeded by making experiments on frogs and pigeons that allowed him to measure the physiological and toxic effects of different extracts, but laboratory animals could not reveal to him their alterations in consciousness. Heffter made the breakthrough in the laboratory of his own mind.

Lewin never publicly acknowledged Heffter's achievement. The magisterial survey of psychoactive drugs he produced at the end of his career, *Phantastica* (1924), relates that 'my first investigations of the plant proved that it contained alkaloid substances, especially a crystallized alkaloid called by me anhalonine'.[53] Heffter goes unmentioned. Lewin continued to refer to peyote as *Anhalonium lewinii*, the tribute of which he had been so proud, even though it had by then been shown to be identical with *Anhalonium williamsii*; by 1900 the scientific community had standardised its Linnaean name to *Lophophora williamsii* (the new genus name, created in 1894, meaning 'crest-bearing' and referring to the species' hairy tufts). Lewin concluded his summary with a caution that he considered it probable that 'the habitual administration of this substance . . . like morphinism, produces a modification of the personality by a degradation of the cerebral functions'.[54]

Heffter's own conclusions were characteristically modest. 'Physiologists and experimental psychologists,' he observed, 'should find work in this field rewarding.'[55]

CHAPTER FIVE

HIGHER POWERS

1899–1918
LONDON, MISSOURI, NEW YORK,
TAOS, OKLAHOMA

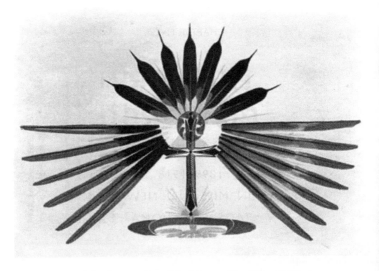

The Peyote Ritual *by Monroe Tsa Toke, 1957.*

Thus far peyote, and now mescaline, had proved to be of surpassing interest to western science but no obvious practical use. The panacea of the Indians was listed in the Parke, Davis catalogue and recommended by a handful of pharmacists as a stimulant tonic, but it had yet to find a defining medical application. Prentiss and Morgan had made broad suggestions that it might have value in nervous and mental conditions, but even robustly healthy-minded subjects were exhausted by its duration, unpleasant physical symptoms and relentless barrage of mental stimuli. Arthur Heffter concluded his 1898 paper by asking whether any of the peyote aklaloids might have therapeutic value and suggesting 'the answer is probably no'. He was equally doubtful about Havelock Ellis's prediction that it might become a popular recreation, on the grounds that 'the side-effects are so pronounced that they considerably spoil the appreciation of the beautiful visual images'.[1]

The following year saw the first thorough physiological trial of mescaline by Walter Dixon, one of Britain's first pharmacological specialists at a time when there was still no university chair in the subject (he would later become professor of materia medica at King's College London, and end his career as the first reader in pharmacology at Cambridge University). Dixon was simultaneously studying the effects of cannabis, which he concluded was a 'useful and refreshing stimulant and food accessory'.[2] He had paid close attention to the reports by Mitchell, Ellis and Heffter and enlisted Edmund White, pharmacist at St Thomas' Hospital, to follow Heffter's extraction method. White presented him with mescaline, anhalonidine, anhalonine and lophophorine 'in a beautifully crystalline condition'.[3]

Dixon proceeded through a systematic series of experiments on dogs, cats, rabbits and 'as far as practicable on the human subject', himself.[4] In animals the peyote alkaloids stimulated salivation, occasionally produced vomiting, lowered blood pressure and heartbeat, and quickened respiration at high doses. 'Occasionally, after an intoxicating dose', he discerned in cats 'most of the physical elements of "terror" ... the ears are drawn back, the hair over the body, especially the tail, becomes erected, there is twitching of the superficial muscles, the respiration being shallow and hurried, and the heart weak and irregular'.[5] In humans he found, in accordance with William James's theories, that 'as in cannabis indica, time is over-estimated, possibly as a result of the rapid flow of ideas and the inability to fix the attention'. On two occasions, after a high dose, he remarked on the 'indescribable feeling of dual existence' that had been mentioned by Prentiss and Morgan's second subject: after sitting with eyes closed, absorbed in the coloured visions, he opened them to find 'a different self, as on waking from a dream'.[6] The inner world and the outer were each so enthralling that one forgot the other existed; opening and closing the eyes was like jumping between two parallel streams of time.

As well as overlaps with cannabis, Dixon noted passing similarities with strychnine, nicotine, digitalis and cocaine, but in each case the contrasts were equally marked and he concluded that ' "mescal" acts differently from any known substance'. He sensed some therapeutic promise, especially at low doses, which elicited a gentle exhilaration and sense of well-being. It might have potential as a general tonic, or turn out to be 'of special use in melancholia'.[7] But even the most exacting physiological investigation with the purest chemical extracts advanced the medical practicalities no further than Prentiss and Morgan had. Mescaline undoubtedly had potential as a mild stimulant and mood elevator, but these qualities appeared inseparable from a spectrum of undesirable effects that stretched from queasiness to anxiety and physical collapse.

As the new century turned, however, peyote attracted the interest of another class of western investigators. For many the modern world had become, in the terms conceived at that time by the sociologist Max Weber, an era of disenchantment: an iron cage constructed by the demands of capital, industry and bureaucracy in which humanity and its inner life had no place. Modernity was haunted by the loss of the sacred; religion, the music to which every previous human society had danced, had been silenced by the tyranny of reason and its restless extension of human power and control. By the same token it became an era of resistance to the forces of modernity and their abolition of mystery: the disenchanted embarked on utopian projects, experimenting with new forms of thought and ways of living to rekindle the power of the sacred.

Over the twentieth century the spiritual dimensions of peyote and mescaline would repeatedly re-enchant western culture, at various times and places eclipsing their roles in science, medicine and therapy. This process began in its opening decades, though only among a small number of scattered individuals. The social and political movements of the Progressive Era, as it became known, conceived drugs in general and alcohol in particular as sources or consequences of dehumanisation, and campaigned vigorously for their prohibition. Most westerners who were aware of peyote regarded it as a degenerate and dissolute Indian habit, no different from the strong spirits that were ravaging the shattered tribes, a disease from which they needed to be cured before they could attain the benefits of civilisation. Yet there were a few, most but not all with some connection to Indian culture, who attempted in different ways to harness the spiritual power implicit in peyote. At the same time the peyote religion of the Plains tribes, beset by persecution and prohibition, found a new form that forced the modern world to accommodate it.

🌿   🌿   🌿

In August 1910 the London *Daily Sketch* reported on a ceremony to invoke Saturn conducted in an apartment at 124 Victoria Street, the home of the notorious occultist Aleister Crowley. Tickets had been sold, and visitors arrived to find the rooms in semi-darkness with thick curtains drawn. The ceremony began with the 'Banishing Ritual of the Pentagram and the Consecration of the Temple with Fire', after which Crowley's disciple, the poet Victor Neuburg, passed around a 'cup of Libation', a golden bowl that Crowley later described as a cocktail of fruit juice, alcohol, 'alkaloids of opium' and 'the elixir brought by me to Europe': an extract of peyote or, in Crowley's preferred terminology, 'anhalonium'.[8] The draught was reported to have an unpleasant taste, like rotting apples, a description suggestive of the sour and bitter undertones of a cactus brew. The ceremony began; Neuburg danced, Crowley's 'Scarlet Woman' Leila Waddell played the violin, and Crowley recited his poetry interspersed with selections from Swinburne. The cup was passed around again, and guests took second and third libations – enough, it seems, for some to notice a psychoactive effect. The poet and novelist Ethel Archer recalled later that she and her husband felt 'pepped up and lively' after drinking, a feeling that persisted for a week.[9] The *Sketch* reporter, Raymond Radcliffe, was entranced: 'We were thrilled to our bones ... if there is any higher form of artistic expression than great verse and great music, I have yet to learn it.'[10]

Ethel Archer was a friend of Victor Neuburg who later joined Crowley's magical order the A∴A∴ and wrote poetry for its journal the *Equinox*, which was published by her husband, Eugene Weiland. Her novel *The Hierophant* (1932) contains a retrospective account of the evening that, though fictionalised, gives a vivid sense of the impression it made on her. The protagonist Iris and her husband receive a narcotic-scented invitation to a ceremony being held by Vladimir Svaroff – an amalgam of Crowley and George Gurdjieff – who with his 'latest drug, a sedative tonic from Mexico ... had hopes of penetrating the future and overcoming time and space'.[11] On arrival she is offered a 'dark brownish liquid' in a glass phial; 'the odour of the stuff was certainly not inviting, it suggested bad apples and laudanum'.[12] Iris and her husband pass into a dimly lit room furnished with cushions, 'heavy with the haze of smoke and filled with the murmur of many voices'.[13] She feels a powerful throbbing energy inside her; meanwhile her husband has a vision of time 'unwinding backwards' through the Bronze and Stone Ages, with 'dancing figures brandishing stone-knives, flints, clubs, antlers of animals'.[14] Another guest, a 'tall youth', confides, 'It's a pretty stiff dose for a kick-off. I've been several times – it's quite good fun.'[15] Svaroff begins to 'intone in some strange tongue', and Iris is suddenly 'seized with a deadly nausea'. She is discreetly dosed with a white powder 'and the next thing she remembered was lying back in a chair in the inner room and Svaroff pouring her out some tea'.[16]

Sifting fact from fiction in Aleister Crowley's use of peyote is a delicate business. His habitual self-aggrandisement and mystification is compounded by a reticence about the precise details of his magickal practices that he maintained in correspondence even with his closest associates.[17] He never referred to the peyote experiments of Havelock Ellis, Arthur Symons and W.B. Yeats, of which he must have been aware; he and Yeats were both members of the small and close-knit fraternity of the Golden Dawn, but disliked one another cordially and Crowley was hardly likely to acknowledge Yeats's precedence. The corroborating evidence from others is equally unreliable. Crowley was using his anhalonium as part of an arsenal of mind-altering drugs that by the 1920s included hashish, morphine, ether, chloroform, cocaine and heroin, most of which were at this time only vaguely understood even among his immediate circle. Those who experienced the hallucinogenic effects of his potions at first hand were often unclear whether they had been given peyote, or hashish, or opium, or some combination of Crowley's devising. He was certainly not the first European to take peyote, nor to make a liquid decoction of its buttons, though his claim that his anhalonium elixir was 'brought by me to Europe' may be accurate in the narrow sense that his extracts were prepared to his own recipe. It is, however, probably true to say that he was the first westerner to take peyote methodically over a period of years, and the first to adopt it as a ritual sacrament.

Crowley's interest in peyote had little to do with its native use in the Americas, though he may have heard of it, and possibly encountered it, during his visit to Mexico in 1900. He approached it rather as a latter-day alchemist. He was initiated into drugs around 1898 in the company of Allan Bennett, a fellow member of the Order of the Golden Dawn who was also an analytical chemist. They sought the Elixir of Life, as Crowley wrote, 'by fruitless attempts to poison ourselves with every drug in (and out of) the Pharmacopœia'.[18] The first reference to anhalonium in his diaries, dated 12 March 1907, describes a commerically supplied tincture, presumably that of Parke, Davis. He had earlier that day visited Messrs Lowe & Co., the pharmacy in Bond Street run by his friend Edward Whineray, who specialised in supplying obscure drugs to the bohemian set. Whineray had a keen interest in the occult: he wrote an article on hashish for Crowley's journal, the *Equinox*, and placed advertisements for his 'oils, perfumes, unguents, essences, incenses, and other chemical products' in several of its issues.[19] Crowley experimented carefully with the drops, working his way up from one to ten, the maximum dose specified on the label, from which he still felt little effect.

He persisted, a process probably reflected to some extent in his short story 'The Drug', published in the January 1909 issue of the *Idler*, in which the narrator calls on a friend who is synthesising a mysterious potion he calls 'the drug that giveth strange visions', which plunges him into a phantasmagoric episode of temporary insanity. In his personal copy of his own 1922 *Diary of a Drug Fiend*, Crowley wrote in the margins of the passage on peyote 'I made many experiments on people with this drug in 1910, and in subsequent years.'[20] This supports the contention that the anhalonium extract was an element in the sour-tasting cup of libation at the Saturn ceremony that year. In 1913 Crowley dosed Katherine Mansfield with either peyote or hashish, upon which, according to a friend, 'up, up rose the spirit into a pink and paradisiacal contentment, whence she viewed space with a rosy rapture'.[21] Mansfield herself found Crowley 'a very pretentious and dirty fellow'.[22]

In 1915 Crowley visited America, where one of his first stops was Detroit. 'Parke Davis were charming,' he recalled in his memoirs, 'and showed me over their wonderful chemical works.' Like Lewin a genera-tion before, he was astounded by the 'countless and ingenious devices'; in particular 'a great mass of pills in a highly polished and rapidly revolving receiver was infinitely fascinating to watch'. Crowley charmed the pharmacists in turn, telling them about his anhalonium researches and they 'made me some special preparations on the lines indicated by my experience which proved greatly superior' to their standard line, and with which they supplied him from this point onwards.[23] The new elixir made its public debut at a party in New York, where he offered it to the writer Theodore Dreiser, who asked casually before drinking whether there was a doctor in the neighbourhood; Crowley replied that there was 'a first-class undertaker on the corner of 33rd Street and Sixth Avenue'. 'I don't like that kind of joke, Crowley,' Dreiser replied, before sampling the elixir and proceeding to describe his visions *in extenso* to the assembled company.[24]

Crowley's magickal diaries of 1915–16 make regular mention of the Parke, Davis extract, usually abbreviated to *Anh. Lew.* or simply *A. L.* In 1919 the *Equinox* advertised that the following issue would include 'Liber CMXXXIV [934]. The Cactus. An elaborate study of the psychological effects produced by Anhalonium Lewinii (Mescal Buttons), compiled from the actual records of some hundreds of exper-iments; with an explanatory essay'.[25] But the promised secrets of anhalonium never appeared. By 1921, during his residence at Cefalù in Sicily, Crowley's magickal drug experiments were in full flood: he was using the Parke, Davis extract along with opium, ether, cocaine, laudanum, heroin and hashish in nightly trials during which he forced himself to 'fathom the Abysses of Horror, to confront the most ghastly possibilities of Hell'. The process, he explained, was similar to psycho-analysis: 'it releases the subject from fear of reality and the phantasms and neuroses thereby caused, by externalising and thus disarming the spectres that lie in ambush for the Soul of Man'.[26] By 1922 in Paris the regime was devolving into a twin dependence on cocaine and heroin; the latter would be his companion until the end.

✿　　✿　　✿

In 1915 the new prophet-president of the Reorganized Church of Jesus Christ of Latter-Day Saints, Frederick Madison Smith, spoke to his followers for the first time about the peyote ceremonies of the Plains Indian tribes. Over the next few years it became a regular theme in his calls to renew the Mormon faith. Smith described in glowing terms 'the peculiar and esctatic state' generated by the ceremonies with their 'beautiful visions', and 'the wonderful and beneficial therapeutic effects' that followed.[27] In 1919 he published an article in the *Saints Herald* entitled 'A Trip among the Indians of Oklahoma' in which he stated explicitly that, despite the church's strict prohibition on alcohol, he regarded peyote as a potent stimulus to the elusive state of genuine religious ecstasy, and that he himself had taken it in all-night rituals with Indian tribes including the Omaha and the Cheyenne.

Frederick Smith was the grandson of Joseph Smith, the church's founder, and had become the prophet-president of the newly-founded Reorganized Church after his father's death in 1914. He was a man of the new century, eager to breathe fresh inspiration into the Mormon community and integrate the church more fully into the modern world. He created an imposing new centre of worship in Independence, Missouri and devoted his church to progressive social issues, expanding local sanitariums and building residential complexes for the elderly. He decided to educate himself in psychology and studied for a doctorate under one of the founders of the discipline, G. Stanley Hall, a professor at Johns Hopkins University. He became interested in the field of 'mind expansion', the search for techniques to maximise mental resources, efficiency and stamina. The world, he believed, had entered an era of efficiency in industry, agriculture and social organisation, but it was a 'soulless efficiency' that treated humanity simply as machines and failed to engage the spirit.[28] Hall suggested that Smith should focus his doctoral thesis on the ecstatic practices of primitive people, which might offer useful perspectives on the range and limits of man's psychic potential. Since the church was already involved in missionary work among the Indian tribes of the Southwest, Smith decided to concentrate in particular on their use of peyote in religious ceremonies.

At an early stage in his studies Smith came under the spell of Stanley Hall's colleague William James, in particular his essay 'The Energies of Men', originally delivered as a lecture to the American Philosophical Association at Columbia University in 1906. In it, James considered the phenomenon of 'second wind', in which perseverance at a task past the usual limits of exhaustion seems to tap an unsuspected reserve of energy. James had long been considering what the physiological basis for this might be, and why it should be that 'men the world over possess amounts of resource which only very exceptional individuals push to their extremes of use'.[29] He proposed that 'we live subject to arrest by degrees of fatigue which we have come only from habit to obey'.[30] The key to unlocking this hidden potential was to slip the chains of habit with unusual stimuli, unusual degrees of excitement, unusual ideas and unusual efforts.

Smith's doctoral thesis, published in book form as *The Higher Powers of Man*, extended James's ideas into a survey of the ecstatic rites employed by primitive religions around the world and throughout history. Ecstasy was typically pathologised within psychology as a form of neurosis or mental weakness and yet, from the Dionysian cults of ancient Greece to the yogis of Hinduism, it had played a central role in most societies and generated 'the "more than highest" conditions of pleasure, inspiration and the boldest flights of thought'.[31] 'Many are the agents of ecstasy', Smith discovered, and chemical inebriation, along with hypnotism, trance, rhythm and dancing, was a common tool in traditions across the globe. He was careful to bracket alcohol as a special case: although it had the capacity to incite ecstasy, it 'is essentially an exaltation of feeling followed by a depression',[32] reclaiming with interest the energy it temporarily loans and leading to dependency and dissolution.

The peyote of the Indians was quite different in this respect. Smith cited most of the published sources to date – Mooney, Lumholtz,

Lewin, Ewell, Prentiss and Morgan, and Mitchell – but based his extensive account on the testimony of two Cheyenne in Oklahoma, Philip Cook and Chief Three Fingers, who introduced him to their ceremony. Smith was struck by 'the universal extent of this movement among the Indians and the tenacity with which they held to it in the face of the combined opposition of the various church representatives and the government agents'.[33] This seemed to him strong evidence for the social value of the ecstasy it generated. He learned that the Oklahoma Indians avoided the ban on trafficking the cactus across state lines by 'the very simple expedient of sending a man with several trunks to El Paso, and from there he goes to where it can be gathered'.[34] He was particularly struck by the centrality of a 'Creator or Great Spirit'[35] that, in contrast to most primitive religions, seemed so easily compatible with Jesus Christ, the perfect exemplar of the divinity to which man's second wind might ultimately lift him. Jesus's forty days in the wilderness, Smith believed, were the moment when He 'entered the ecstatic state' and 'from these ecstatic moments sprung the nascent consciousness of his great powers'.[36]

Smith's researches seem to have won broad acceptance from his Mormon congregation, among whom the mission to the Indian tribes was regarded as highly important. Any thought of introducing peyote into its liturgy was, however, derailed by a crisis of authority that enveloped the church in the 1920s. Smith's reforming programme was opposed by the more traditionally minded members of its General Conference, and he responded by pushing through a decree of Supreme Directional Control that made his presidential decisions binding on the church at large. The decree resulted in further schisms and breakaway Latter-Day Saints churches, and was effectively reversed in the 1930s.

Smith, however, continued to work with Indian peyotists and lobbied in Washington, DC, against federal attempts to outlaw their ceremonies.[37] He also promoted peyote in non-Indian circles. His wife Ruth had joined him in peyote meetings in 1918 and when his daughter Alice went to Harvard University the following year Smith introduced the cactus to her classmates. After dinner one evening he described its effects to her friend Virgil Thomson, a prodigiously talented musician and composer whom Smith helped with a loan for his college fees. Thomson asked to try peyote, and Smith agreed on condition that he wrote a report of his experience that he could add to his files. Thomson described a series of rapturous visions 'each as complete in color and texture as a stage set . . . each one, moreover, had a meaning, could have been published with a title'. In sum they 'constituted a view of life not only picturesque and vast but all mine and all true'.[38]

Thomson subsequently introduced various members of his Harvard scene to peyote, including the socialist and poet Sherry Mangan, who started buying dried buttons by mail order from New Mexico. Their informal researches devolved into what would later in the century be termed 'recreational use'. Mangan and Thomson were members of a heavy-drinking coterie that convened in the Harvard dormitory buildings and they introduced peyote to these sessions, grinding the dried buttons up in water. Students stricken by nausea stuck their heads out of windows to relieve it and on one occasion the toilet seat in Mangan's rooms was mysteriously burned.[39] The group experiments soon ran their course. Thomson took peyote several more times in private but although his 'adventures were always surprising and sumptuous . . . in none did the heavens so definitely open as they had for me that first time alone in my room'.[40]

   ✼ ✼ ✼

In New York in the spring of 1914, a year before Aleister Crowley's anhalonium party was held there, the heiress Mabel Dodge hosted a peyote meeting – part salon, part ceremony – in her exquisite home at 23 Fifth Avenue. It remains the best-remembered western encounter with peyote from this period, thanks to the full and candid description she included in her memoirs. The episode is by turns bizarre, whimsical and harrowing, and rendered unintentionally comic by her naïve and breathless prose, but this mystically inclined socialite's report provides much that is passed over by the male medico-scientific gaze. Rather than descriptions of her visions, Dodge gives us an intensely emotional account of a social gathering dissoving into chaos and the personal fallout that resulted. It seemed at the time to most observers, including Dodge herself, a foolish and regrettable incident, yet it turned out to have momentous consequences, setting off a chain of events that would transform not only her and her circle but federal Indian policy.

Born Mabel Ganson in 1879, the daughter of a wealthy banker from Buffalo, she had grown up among the upstate New York elite before marrying Edwin Dodge, a prominent architect, and spending eight years in Europe, where she became a patron of the arts and attended Gertrude Stein's salons. She separated from her husband and in 1912 returned to New York, where she took up residence in a brownstone on the east side of Greenwich Village that she decorated sumptuously in white, with a polar-bearskin rug in front of a marble fireplace overhung with a white porcelain chandelier, lit through clouded and coloured glass panels in the doors and windows. It became a bohemian salon *par excellence*, with Dodge in her own words 'a species of head-hunter', gathering up 'socialists, trade unionists, anarchists, suffragists, poets, lawyers, murderers, old friends, psychoanalysists, artists, clubwomen ...'[41] She identified strongly as a New Woman and a spiritual feminist, and devoured Havelock Ellis's writings on the psychology of sex. She began a passionate affair with John Reed, poet and radical journalist (and yet to witness the Russian revolution), who captured the tenor of their life in his poem 'The Day in Bohemia': 'Blazing our nights with arguments uproarious / What care we for a dull old world censorious / When each is sure he'll fashion something glorious?'[42]

It was into this world that Dodge's friend, the poet and anarchist Hutchins Hapgood, introduced his cousin Raymond Harrington, an ethnographer who had been following in James Mooney's footsteps by studying the peyote religion among the Kiowa in Oklahoma.

Harrington enthused about peyote, explaining (in Dodge's words) that 'it was not a drug at all, but a marvellous vehicle of the Indian life enabling one to be deeply and wholly and concisely what one inherently was'. It emerged that he had brought some buttons with him and offered to host a ceremony: 'We were all thrilled.'[43]

The participants were a more or less random selection from Dodge's coterie: her effervescent young cousin Genevieve, who had just returned from China 'full of a mystical elation'; the political activist Max Eastman and his wife; the early Cubist painter Andrew Dasburg; and a 'grand anarchist' named Terry, who had long ago 'passed up the capitalistic system and swore that he would never take a job or do a day's work under it, and he had carried out his vow'. Harrington set a serious tone, carefully constructing a facsimile of the Kiowa tipi space with eagle feathers, a green branch for an arrow, a peyote path made of a folded white sheet and a light bulb with Dodge's red Chinese shawl over it to take the place of the fire. On his instructions they fasted for supper and dressed their best. ('Like Church, I thought to myself.')[44]

Harrington chewed a button and began to sing; he sounded to Dodge like a howling dog. The rest of the company took their buttons, including Dodge ('But it was bitter! Oh, how it was bitter!'). When they were passed around again, she secreted hers behind her back. The impulse to giggle became irresistible. At the same time, her friends all seemed to be subtly transmuting, one into a Persian miniature, another into a Lutheran monk. The singing went on, 'monotonous and outlandish, and gradually my laughter wore itself out and I grew weary and longed to leave'.[45] She caught the eyes of several of the others and they quietly withdrew, leaving Harrington with Genevieve and Terry, who both appeared entranced by the ceremony.

Dodge retired to bed, where she felt fury building inside her at the way she had lost control of the evening: 'To think that it was going on there in my house and *I could not stop it* if I wanted to!' As she prayed for the ritual to end, she heard loud footsteps from the other end of the house: Dasburg, bursting back into the ceremony. She opened her bedroom door and found Genevieve outside it, pale and wide eyed, gasping 'Oh Mabel! It is *terrible!*' In the living room, Dasburg was trampling the altar and scattering the peyote, Harrington shouting 'Stop, man! That is terribly dangerous!' and Dasburg violently insisting 'I *had* to break it up!'[46] Terry sat motionless in the centre of the scene, contemplating the end of his cigarette.

They realised abruptly that Genevieve had vanished. Harrington gathered up the peyote buttons, in case the police were called. ('Police! Heavens, I *was* scared!') Genevieve was eventually found outside a window, gibbering and insisting she had to go and find her father. They called a discreet 'East Side Jewish doctor who is a friend of all of us', who examined the peyote with curiosity. He hadn't heard of it, but wondered if it was the same thing as 'mescal': if so, he pronounced, 'a highly strung girl like this might easily be injured by it'. Harrington broke into Terry's reverie, and the anarchist 'smiled the most illuminated smile I have ever seen. His eyes were blue like gentians. "Harry," he said, "I have seen the Universe, and Man! It is wonderful!" '[47] He left without a word, and Dodge never spoke to him again (though she did glimpse him one more time, at one of Eugene O'Neill's parties in Provincetown).

Genevieve was now mute, blank and sobbing on the chaise longue. They called for a nurse and an urgent discussion began about how the story could be kept out of the papers, and whether they should call the police. They decided instead to summon John Collier, a crusading lawyer who was widely admired in bohemian circles for his work in support of New York's immigrant communities. Collier's response was anything but reassuring: 'Undoubtedly you could all be indicted under the illicit drug act.' It dawned on Dodge that the evening might be represented as 'a "Dope Party". Horrors! I had heard of such gatherings and they were the antithesis of all I wished to stand for. The level of my life, at least in my own eyes, was infinitely raised above such sordid sensationalism.'[48]

✤   ✤   ✤

Mabel Dodge never saw her cousin Genevieve again, though she did receive incomprehensible letters from her 'composed of symbols and hieroglyphs' and was not surprised to learn that she had become *persona non grata* with that branch of the family.[49] The episode precipitated a rocky period in her own life, and her mental health became fragile. In August 1914 John Reed left for Europe as a war correspondent and she retreated into herself, searching for a 'mind cure' that could offer equilibrium in the face of civilisation, the 'great machine' that seemed intent on its own destruction.[50] She tried Freudian talking cures and New Thought, a popular movement that drew on the Hindu philosophy of Vedanta together with Zen and Sufi traditions of healing by integrating the individual with the 'Divine Mind'.[51]

In August 1917 she married the sculptor Maurice Sterne, who had left Gertrude Stein's circle in Paris to search for a 'Garden of Eden'. After a few months he departed New York to continue his search in the deserts and mountains of the American Southwest. Dodge visited a medium who predicted she would soon be surrounded by Indians, and she had a psychic vision of Sterne at the same moment that he arrived in Santa Fe. She joined him there for Christmas, trading the dour New York winter for the snow-capped desert mesa, a decision that transformed her life. Soulless, mechanised modernity melted away in a landscape that seemed to be made of light. When she visited the ancient adobe pueblo at Santo Domingo (now Kewa) and witnessed the centuries-old Christmas dance in its plaza, she was transported entirely. 'For the first time in my life,' she wrote, 'I heard the voice of the One coming from the Many.'[52]

In 1918 Sterne left to continue his travels and Dodge moved further up into the mountains to Taos, where the Pueblo Indian community had subsisted on the sagebrush plateau for at least a thousand years, its adobe dwellings stacked like living cells beneath the cloud-wreathed sacred mountain. The town beside it was centred on a seventeenth-century

Spanish plaza, expanded by pioneer trappers and traders such as Kit Carson and more recently colonised by artists drawn to the play of light across the mountains and the exquisite, timeless aesthetic of the pueblo's architecture and cultural life. Over the next forty years Dodge would collect around her a commune of artists and Indian activists – in her words, a 'fabulous honeycomb, irresistible and nourishing'[53] – that drew the likes of Georgia O'Keeffe, Ansel Adams, D.H. Lawrence, Carl Jung and Aldous Huxley. In partnership with the Pueblo community leader Tony Luhan, who after Dodge's divorce from Maurice Sterne became her next and final husband, she bought a traditional adobe farmhouse set under a huge cottonwood tree in 12 acres of sagebrush desert adjoining the pueblo's ancestral land. Adding a series of adobe extensions that fused Tony's traditional building techniques with her modern arts-and-crafts aesthetic, they elaborated it into the first example of the style that would become known as Pueblo Revival.

In time, many from Dodge's Greenwich Village set followed her, including some of those who had participated in the peyote episode. Andrew Dasburg relocated to Taos, discovering a productive fusion of his emerging Cubist style with that of the pueblo's architecture and remaining there until his death in 1979. By far the most consequential arrival, however, was that of the community lawyer John Collier, who by 1920 found himself under government surveillance in New York during the Red Scare that followed the Russian Revolution and accepted Dodge's invitation to join her. She found him a house in the artists' colony next to D.H. Lawrence, and he transferred his activist energies from the immigrant communities of New York to the native population of the Southwest. He would later be appointed commissioner of Indian Affairs for the federal government by Franklin Roosevelt, from which position he launched the 'Indian New Deal' that turned federal policy away from assimilation and towards the preservation of Indian culture and religion.

Collier, like Dodge, felt passionately that modern industrial society was destructive to the human spirit. He was at once a radical and a deeply conservative thinker who rejected the individualist goals of social Darwinism and laissez-faire economics in favour of social and spiritual collectives. Taos pueblo became for him a living example of the alternative to twentieth-century materialism, wealthy instead in beauty, comradeship and godliness. He believed this had been the natural state of man in prehistory and developed a vision of Indian culture as a font of ancient wisdom, humanity's last chance of redemption from a brutal modernity that was consuming itself in war. In 1921 he coined the term 'Red Atlantis' to capture the sense, developed over long evening discussions at Dodge's house with her bohemian and Theosophical neighbours, that the Pueblo culture at Taos was the surviving remnant of a lost high civilisation, 'the quest through art expression of an ecstasy communally realised'.[54]

This vision of Red Atlantis was, however, strictly drug-free. Unlike the counterculture of the 1960s, for which peyote was a major attractor towards native American cultures, Dodge and the Taos art colony maintained a horror of it. Prohibition was one of the few causes that united social progressives with the reactionary elements of religion and politics. Missionaries to the Indian reservations and pueblos equated peyote with the foreign 'dope' habits of ethnic minorities: Chinese, blacks and Mexicans. The prohibitions on Indian peyote use that had begun in 1886 on the Kiowa–Comanche reservation in Oklahoma and escalated to statute law in 1899 were advanced by prohibitionist politicians on the national stage who attempted to add peyote to the laws prohibiting intoxicating liquors on reservations.[55] When the Harrison Narcotics Act was passed in 1914, prohibiting the unlicensed sale of opium and cocaine, the Bureau of Indian Affairs classified peyote as a narcotic in an attempt to bring it under the same federal controls. Sensational press coverage established the term 'peyote cult', along with 'peyote séance' and 'peyote debauch'. In 1923 the *New York Times* ran the headline 'Peyote Used as Drug in Indians' Cult of Death' above an article arguing that its worship originated in the Aztec cult of human sacrifice.[56]

For the white admirers of Indian culture, the use of peyote was – like that of alcohol – a tragic response to the miseries of captivity and a degeneration of its once proud traditions. This was also the view of many Pueblo Indians in Taos, where peyote meetings were a recent arrival and a source of communal tension.[57] They had been introduced from Oklahoma by nomadic peoples such as the Comanche, into whose culture they fitted much more easily. Comanches had long been in the habit of forming impromptu groupings for camps and warbands, and it was relatively straightforward for one family or faction to adopt the peyote religion without creating friction in the wider tribe. Pueblo cultures such as Taos, by contrast, were sedentary, with a structure of recognised roles and hierarchies centred round the kiva, a sacred space for ceremonies in which the entire community was expected to participate.

As the anthropologist and folklorist Elsie Clews Parsons observed when studying Taos pueblo in the 1930s, religious innovations were 'fundamentally contrary' to the 'general temper of Pueblo ceremonialism'. In Taos, peyote acted as a wedge between traditionalists and innovators. It appealed to the progressive tendency as it 'emphasizes individual emotional experience against communal, ritualistic performance'; as a result it 'became associated with a group of Americanized individuals inclined to rebellion against the hierarchy'. Its leaders, often the better educated and travelled members of the community, were on occasion expelled from the kiva hierarchy, which made them 'bitter, hostile and more ardent in supporting the foreign cult'.[58]

The conflict played out in miniature in Dodge's blossoming relationship with Tony Luhan. The two of them became, in her eyes, a dyad in which his deep-rooted wisdom and her transcendental modernism fused to become a beacon for humanity. She did not immediately appreciate that Luhan was among the pueblo's leading peyote devotees. One day, while they were working on the house, Tony looked at the purple ribbon Dodge was wearing and purred, 'Ni-i-i-ce colour!' She recognised that 'he saw more in it than I did', and 'a queer magic that opened windows in my imagination soon filled the room and I drifted upon it'.[59] But it was not until some months later that the question became explicit, when Tony produced some peyote buttons and showed them to her. 'You know Him?' he asked.

'"Do you Indians out here eat peyote?" I asked tremulously.' Tony replied that they did, but 'This peyote . . . he not *ours*. The Plains Indians gave him to us. Maybe he belong to all Indians a long time ago but not now . . . this is Montezuma's medicine.'[60] Dodge was profoundly shaken. She recognised that this was 'a terribly important issue between us, perhaps actually the most important adjustment we had to make'.[61] She told Tony about 'that evening at 23 Fifth Avenue' and he seemed unsurprised that events had spun out of control: 'You got to do it right, or peyote get mad.' Dodge was still troubled: 'It seems to me you go away from yourself when you eat peyote; you lose yourself.' 'And seem to me I find myself more and more,' Tony replied.[62]

Some time later Dodge fell ill and Tony told her that there was a traditional medicine for her sickness: peyote. With trepidation, she accepted a dose. 'The medicine ran through me, penetratingly,' she wrote, and 'the whole universe fell into place . . . all the heavenly bodies were contented with the order of the plan, and system within system interlocked in grace . . . I was not separated and isolated any more.'[63] It was more than relief of her symptoms: it was medicine that went to the root of her sickness, in spirit as much as in body, and rebalanced her whole being.

Yet she was still unwilling to accept peyote into her life as a spiritual practice, or to permit it in Tony's. 'Anything that tampers with consciousness always frightens me – consciousness is all we have . . . I am afraid the peyote will make it unreal, make you seem unreal if you are using it. If I come together with you, won't you give up the peyote?' she asked, 'terribly in earnest'.[64] Tony conceded, and it became the bride price of their dyad. But their house still bears its traces. The adobe chimney surround sculpted by Tony in one of the grand downstairs rooms is known to this day as the 'peyote fireplace', and a peyote bird, a symbol associated with the Plains Indian ceremony, can be discerned among the frescoes in his bedroom.

✳   ✳   ✳

At the point when Dodge moved to Taos, peyote was facing its most serious legal challenge to date: the prospect of a federal ban. Over several days in February and March 1918 the US House of Representatives heard evidence in a committee convened by Carl Hayden, the representative from Arizona, to consider a prohibition on 'anhalonium or peyote'[65] by attaching it to an existing bill criminalising the trafficking of liquor on Indian reservations, settlements, school lands and pueblos.

For a federal government committed to assimilating Indians into the mainstream of American society, the growth of the peyote religion since James Mooney's first reports of it in the early 1890s was alarming. Then it had been largely confined to the peoples with direct contact to Mexico and the Kiowa–Comanche–Apache reservations of southwest Oklahoma. By the end of the century it had spread across the state to tribes such as the Cheyenne, Oto, Osage and Winnebago and into the pueblos of the Southwest; over the following decade it was adopted from Kansas to Utah to Missouri, by members of the Arapaho, Ponca, Shawnee and Kickapoo and the Northern Plains Sioux groups.[66] Federal officials took firm measures to stamp it out. In 1909 the Bureau of Indian Affairs sent an officer, the ardent prohibitionist William 'Pussyfoot' Johnson, to Laredo, where he extracted a promise from the local *peyoteros* to curtail their trading, and burned 176,400 confiscated buttons. Walter Runke, superintendent of the Yankton Sioux agency in South Dakota, was typical in his response to its arrival in 1911: 'It will be much easier at this time to prevent the introduction [of peyote] than it will be later to stamp out its use. I have taken drastic measures with the ring-leaders of our new so-called Mescal Society and have them now lodged in the Agency jails.'[67]

The list of charges laid against peyote in the committee hearings was extensive. Missionaries and agency administrators had supported the formation of native Christian groups such as the Indian Rights Association and the Society of American Indians, who testified that addiction to peyote was spreading among the tribes with demoralising effect. Their reports, with titles such as 'The Ravages of Peyote'[68] and 'Mescal, a Menace to the Indians',[69] asked the government to step in to 'protect helpless, downtrodden people from the ruthless hand of the oppressor'.[70] Gertrude Bonnin, the secretary of the Society of American Indians, claimed to have witnessed a death by peyote overdose within 'a few minutes' of the victim swallowing it.[71] Dr Harvey Wiley, now retired from the Department of Agriculture, testified that the 'toxic principle' of peyote, like that of alcohol, produced rapid tolerance and dependence in its regular users.[72] He also maintained this principle was contained in its resins, like cannabis, a theory that had been debunked twenty years previously. He related his version of the now deceased Erving Ewell's experiment in 1895 which had, Wiley recalled, left him babbling about visions of 'angels in streets of gold' and making other 'wholly incoherent remarks' that 'showed an absence of events of a logical character'.[73]

The chief witness against peyote's prohibition was James Mooney, the acknowledged expert on the subject who had by now been called to its defence many times, notably in 1915 when he had testified in Washington to the Board of Indian Commissioners. Peyote, Mooney argued, was not a cause of degeneracy but a mark of progress. 'The Indians now are largely civilised,' he maintained; 'they are becoming citizens, they are educated'. It was this younger generation who had 'taken up the peyote cult and organised it as a regular religion'.[74] He described the ceremony in detail; questioned as to whether it was a true Christian religion, he replied, 'It is not a Christian religion, but it is a very close approximation . . . by a process of evolution the Indian has interwoven with this peyote religion the salient things of Christianity.' One will, for example, 'catch the name of Jesus constantly through the prayers'.

To attach peyote to a bill prohibiting alcohol, Mooney continued, was a gross misunderstanding. 'The peyote does not like whisky,' he explained, and 'no real peyote user touches whisky or continues to drink whisky after he has taken up the peyote religion.'[75] It had been the Indians' most potent weapon against the scourge of alcohol, a contrast made more pointedly by Francis La Flesche, an Omaha Indian employed by the Bureau of Indian Ethnology, who testified that the peyotists were 'decent, sober and kindly people' who had 'saved my people from the degradation that was produced by the fiery drinks white people manufacture'.[76]

Mooney turned the argument, as he usually did, to its medical virtues: a catalogue of scientific reports, he reminded the committee, 'warrant the general conclusion that it is a valuable medicine, for which we are indebted to the Indians, and that it is our business to utilize it'.[77] In response to Silas Weir Mitchell's warning of its 'perilous reign', which Wiley had highlighted, he presented a letter he had received from Mitchell in 1903 expressing his 'amazement' at the 'cruelty and injustice' of the attempts to prohibit peyote to the Oklahoma Indians. He quoted from a pamphlet in which Mitchell had written: 'I took the substance of nine buttons, and had an afternoon and evening in fairy-land . . . I wish you would tell me where I can find the law forbidding its use in the United States under penalties. It is really rather a harmless drug compared with most of the others which men use.'[78]

As the hearings went on, the rift that peyote exposed between the ethnographers and the Bureau of Indian Affairs became ugly. General R.H. Pratt, former superintendent of the Indian school at Carlisle, Pennsylvania and an old friend of Wiley, declared himself 'absolutely against peyote' and the 'nightly orgies that have been described so graphically by the Bureau of Ethnology itself'.[79] The country was misinformed by the 'large and expensive books that come from the Bureau of Ethnology', in which the descriptions of peyote meetings were slanted by the ideology of authors who 'always lead the Indian's mind back into the past'.[80] He alleged that Mooney had once, during a Sun Dance ceremony, tried to find an Indian 'who would submit to having his back slit, the skin lifted and thongs put in his back and . . . dragged around while this gentleman dashed around making photographs of it for this govenment publication'. 'I denounce that as an absolute falsehood,' Mooney responded, and questioned in turn the standing of the Indian Christian bodies presented by the committee. 'An Indian delegate from a sectarian body or alleged uplift organisation is not a delegate for his tribe.'[81] If the Representatives wished to learn about peyote, they should ask the tribal leaders themselves. He had brought several of them to Washington with him, and 'you can look at them and see whether they are physically or mentally degenerate'.[82]

✸　　✸　　✸

After the hearings concluded, the bill was passed by the House but rejected narrowly by the Senate, thanks to pressure from the senator from Oklahoma, who had been energetically lobbied by his Indian constituents. Mooney returned to continue his fieldwork in Oklahoma, where he was invited by the tall and imposing Comanche peyotist Post Oak Jim to a meeting to celebrate the legislative victory.[83] He circulated among the tribes, attending peyote meetings and dances with the Kiowa, the Arapaho and the Caddo, where the idea was mooted that the peyote religion needed to constitute itself officially in some form. As long as it was defined by others as a 'cult', it would lack legal rights and protections, and the ratchet of prohibition would continue to tighten around it.

Others had been considering this possibility, including the Oklahoma attorney Karl Cunningham. Growing up in the wide prairie lands of Cheyenne country to the north and west of Oklahoma City, as a young boy Cunningham had been struck with a life-threatening illness and in desperation his parents had begged the local Cheyenne people for their medicine. At first the medicine men refused, but the elders intervened and held a ceremony in which Cunningham was cured.[84] When he entered the legal world he was shocked by the state prosecutions of peyote meetings, for which terms of imprisonment were being handed down, and wrote to the superintendent of the Cheyenne and Arapaho agency at Darlington to protest the harassment of private worship in which the Indians 'did nothing which is disrespectful to the civilized Christian religion'.[85] He accompanied the Comanche peyotists Marcus Poco and James Waldo on a peyote-buying trip to Laredo for their legal protection, and became friendly with a young Cheyenne named Mack Haag, who had grown up speaking English with his German father and often acted as a spokesman for his people in dealings with the white community.

During his stay in Cheyenne country Mooney met frequently with Cunningham and Haag to discuss solutions to the legal problems of peyote worship, either at the shingle-roofed house Haag had recently built on his 160-acre land grant outside the small town of Calumet or at the nearby house of Bob Cook, a local farmer who was married to a Cheyenne woman. Cunningham stressed the need for an 'umbrella of protection' for their worship: an official structure of charter, membership and incorporation under the First Amendment of the US Consitution. By this time there were precedents for legally recognised Indian churches: a Native Christian Church had recently received its charter in Kansas and an Oto leader named Jonathan Koshiway was in the process of chartering a First Born Church of Christ for his people in Oklahoma.[86]

From the meetings between Mooney, Cunningham and Haag emerged the name Native American Church, disarming in its simplicity and radical in its implications. It was the first time the term 'Native American' had been used by Indians to describe themselves. It had previously been claimed by Anglo-Saxon pioneer descendants to differentiate themselves from more recent immigrants such as Germans, Italians and Irish. During the 1850s there had been an anti-immigrant political society who called themselves the Native American Party; they were commonly referred to as the 'Know-Nothings'. The new church's name reclaimed the term from internecine disputes between European factions, asserted there was only one truly native population in America and linked it confidently to an Indian future. US citizenship for all Indians was still some years away, but 'Native American' yoked together their indigenous heritage and their presumptive constitutional rights in a formulation that anticipated the Indian New Deal that John Collier would enshrine in the Indian Reorganization Act of 1934. Conjoined with the simple 'Church', which asserted its doctrine as a form of Christianity, it claimed its natural rights under the joint protection of God and the Constitution.

In August 1918 in El Reno, the nearest town to the Darlington agency, representatives of the Cheyenne, Oto, Ponca, Comanche, Kiowa and Apache tribes signed the charter of incorporation of the Native American Church (NAC), 'to foster and promote the religious belief of the several tribes of Indians in the State of Oklahoma, in the Christian religion'. For clarity and legal protection the text of the charter explicitly stated that worship would involve 'the practice of the Peyote sacrament'.[87] The NAC was officially incorporated, a status that automatically applied to all the states in which the possession of peyote was not a criminal offence (at this point Utah, Colorado and Nevada).

Of all the various attempts to place peyote at the centre of a twentieth-century religious practice, the NAC was the only one to thrive and endure. The charter of 1918 was by no means the end of its struggle for legitimacy, and in many respects only the beginning. The anti-peyotists redoubled their efforts and similar bills for peyote's federal prohibition were introduced to the House every year and, though none of them won another hearing until 1937, they continued until 1963. Even after that, state prosecutions continued and convictions were upheld on appeal before higher courts reversed them on First Amendment grounds. The most serious threat came in the 1990s, when years of litigation following the case of Alfred Leo Smith, who had been fired from his job as a substance abuse counsellor for refusing to stop attending NAC meetings, culminated in a Supreme Court judgement in which the church's First Amendment rights were rescinded, with Justice Antonin Scalia arguing that religious diversity had become a 'luxury' and there was no 'compelling state interest' to maintain it.[88] A concerted campaign to reinstate the NAC's rights led to the passing of a new law specifically to protect them, the American Indian Religious Freedom Act Amendments of 1994.

For Mooney the foundation of the Native American Church was the culmination of over twenty years of advocacy, but he paid a high personal price for his conspicuous role. While laying the groundwork for it with his travels around Oklahoma, he had written to the Smithsonian that 'on each occasion and in every tribe the Indians have made me the special guest of honour and their priests have voluntarily admitted me or invited me to be present at their most sacred mysteries'. He felt that 'I could live here from tribe to tribe for the rest of the year . . . we have won the Indian heart in all these tribes.'[89] In the reservation agencies, however, his presence was much less welcome. Without his knowledge, Cato Sells, the commissioner of Indian Affairs, wrote to the director of the Smithsonian requesting him to recall Mooney on the grounds that he was 'interfering' with the work of the Bureau.[90] Mooney was summoned back to Washington, and when he applied in 1920 to return to the Kiowa reservation, to finish his study of the peyote religion, he was refused.

Hoping to enlist the support of the Church of Latter-Day Saints, he wrote to Frederick Smith. 'My most important investigation,' he lamented, 'which promises to be of most value to the medical and scientific world, a research which I initiated and to which I have given a large part of thirty years, is blocked and killed . . . I am debarred from the field at the instance of Cato Sells, for declaring the scientific truth and defending the freedom of religion of our citizen Indians as guaranteed under charter and incorporation of the State of Oklahoma.'[91] The following year he suffered a fatal heart attack in Washington, his study of the peyote religion unwritten.

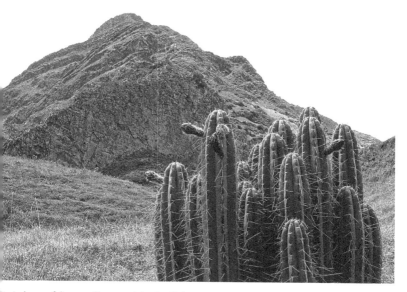

1. A cluster of the mescaline-containing San Pedro cactus growing at the temple site of Chavín de Huantar in the Peruvian Andes, where its ancient use is attested by a 3,000-year-old bas-relief.

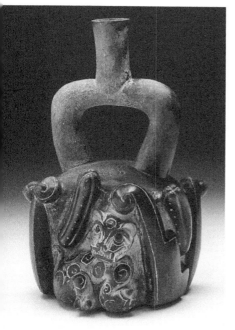

2. San Pedro was commonly depicted in the pre-Hispanic art of Peru's coastal cultures, such as this stirrup-spout vessel, on which the cactus stems are entwined with jaguar heads.

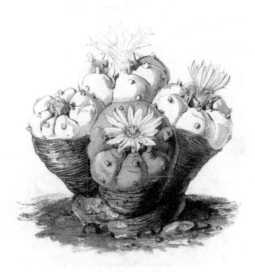

3. The first botanical drawing of the peyote cactus appeared in *Curtis' Botanical Magazine* in 1847. At this point its mind-altering properties were unknown to western science.

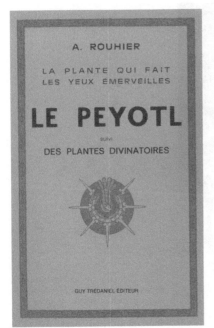

A. ROUHIER

LA PLANTE QUI FAIT
LES YEUX ÉMERVEILLES

LE PEYOTL

suivi

DES PLANTES DIVINATOIRES

GUY TRÉDANIEL ÉDITEUR

4. In *Le peyotl* (1926), the French pharmacist Alexandre Rouhier introduced European readers to peyote's botanical history and its ancient use in divination and healing. He cultivated the plant on the Côte d'Azur and marketed an extract, Panpeyotl, for 'psychological experimenters wishing to study the mental phenomena produced by powerful doses'.

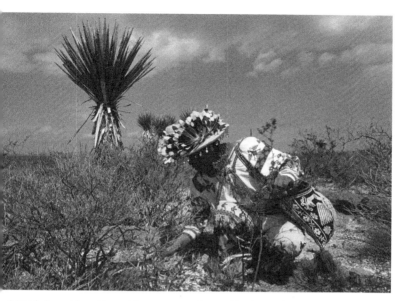

. A Huichol *mara'akame* (shaman) hunts peyote in the sacred landscape of Wirikuta, in the high esert of northern Mexico.

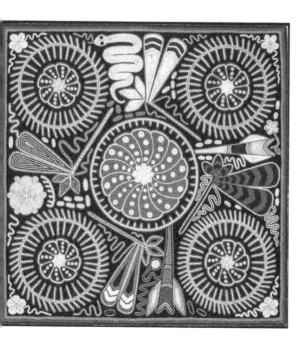

6. Peyote is a common motif in contemporary Huichol art, in which dazzling coloured yarn is pressed onto a wooden board with beeswax. This work by Alejandro Lopez Torres uses the form of the cactus to represent the five pillars that support the sky.

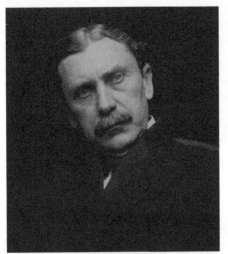

7 & 8. James Mooney (left), ethnologist with the Smithsonian Institution, and Quanah Parker (below), chief of the Comanches, were both powerful advocates for the peyote religion of the Plains tribes. In 1893 Quanah supplied Mooney with 50 pounds of dried peyote buttons, which Mooney brought back from Oklahoma to Washington. They were used in the first scientific trials, including self-experiments by the neurologist Weir Mitchell and the philosopher William James.

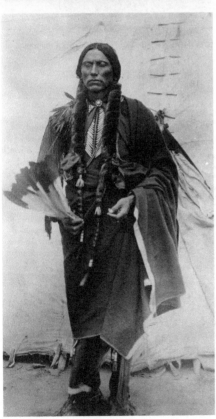

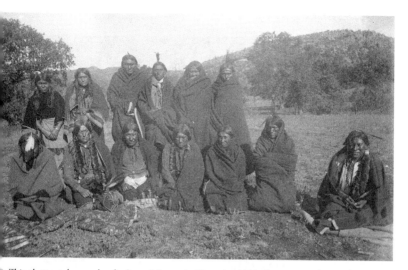

9. This photograph was taken by James Mooney in November 1893, the morning after an all-night peyote meeting with Quanah Parker (second from left, front row) and his Comanche band in the Wichita Mountains, Oklahoma.

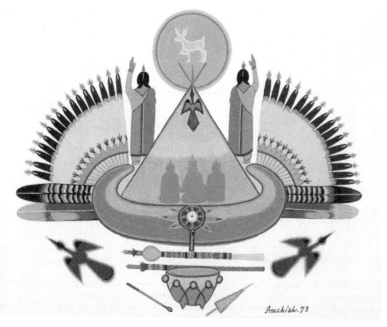

10. *Peyote Medicine Man* (1973), by the Kiowa artist James Auchiah, depicts the elements of the Plains peyote ceremony: the tipi, the rattle and drum that accompany the songs, the sacred eagle feathers, the carved altar of mounded earth and the peyote occupying its central place of power.

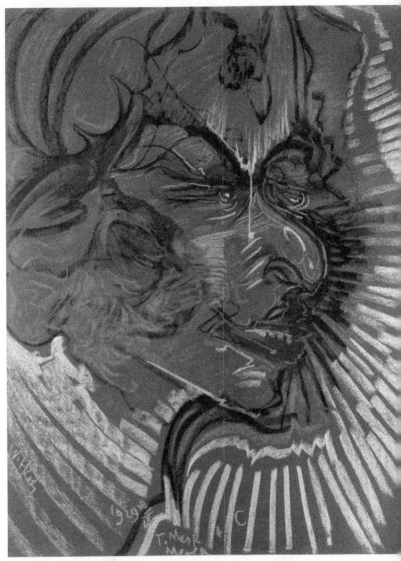

11. The Polish artist Stanisław Ignacy Witkiewicz experimented with both peyote and pharmaceutical mescaline, writing about them in his essay-memoir *Narcotics* (1932) and painting under their influence. He regarded these works as collaborations with the drug: this portrait from 1929 includes 'Mesk' (mescaline) and 'C' (alcohol) in the signature.

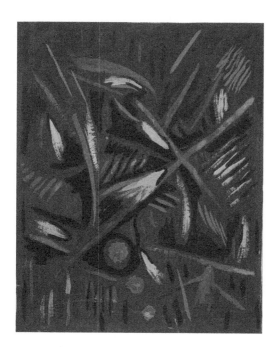

12 & 13. In 1936 two psychiatrists at London's Maudsley Hospital enlisted British Surrealist artists to paint under the influence of mescaline. The work above is anonymous; below is the painting by Basil Beaumont, who left a description of his nightmarish experience in which time 'went very wrong', his supervising psychiatrist took on the appearance of 'a most diabolical goat' and he ended up spending the night in a mental hospital ward.

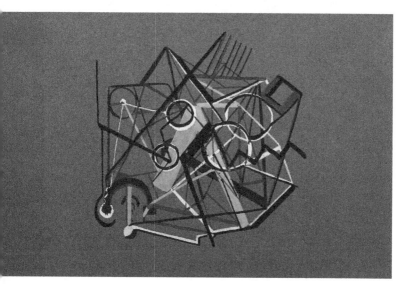

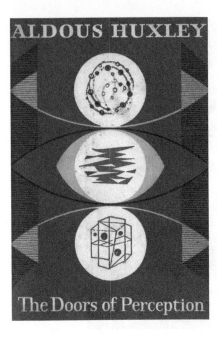

14. The publication of Aldous Huxley's *The Doors of Perception* in 1954 made mescaline world famous. John Woodcock's cover design for the British edition reflected Huxley's marriage of science and mysticism and anticipated the psychedelic style of the decade to come.

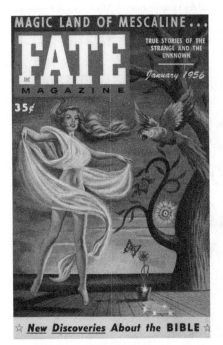

15. After Huxley, mescaline became a subject of fascination in popular culture, as seen in this 1956 cover story of *Fate* magazine, which concluded: 'science is probing into a fabulous new universe of the mind'.

CHAPTER SIX

DER MESKALINRAUSCH

1919–28

VIENNA, HEIDELBERG, CHICAGO, CÔTE D'AZUR

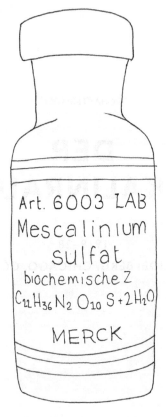

Merck's mescaline sulphate.

In 1919 the chemist Ernst Späth, a leading specialist in alkaloids, published a paper entitled 'Über die *Anhalonium*-alkaloide' in which he described the first chemical synthesis of mescaline in the laboratories of the university of Vienna.[1] He had taken 3,4,5-trimethoxybenzoic acid, an oil found in eucalyptus, transformed it into its corresponding aldehyde and, by a series of reactions with nitromethane, zinc, acetic acid and finally a sodium amalgam, reduced it to a solution containing 20 per cent pure mescaline.[2] In the process he determined that its chemical formula was 3,4,5-trimethoxyphenylethylamine, slightly different from that proposed by Arthur Heffter in 1901.[3] It was a derivative of phenethylamine, a molecule biosynthesised from the amino acid L-phenylalanine by many fungi, bacteria and animals, including humans. Phenethylamine had been detected in foods such as chocolate and would turn out to be present in the human nervous system and in trace amounts in the brain. Späth went on to synthesise ephedrine in 1920 and over the next twenty years worked his way through several of peyote's other alkaloids.

The 'total synthesis' of mescaline in the laboratory – as opposed to Heffter's extraction of it from the cactus – gave it a new scientific identity. It was reborn as a 'pure white drug', one among an ever-lengthening list at the disposal of the organic chemist. Its link to indigenous peyote use was severed, and the unruly complexities of its botany and biochemistry reduced to a footnote. This was a process that had repeated itself many times with the isolation of plant alkaloids by German chemists over the previous century, beginning with the extraction of morphine from opium by Friedrich Sertürner in 1817 and continuing with substances such as caffeine, nicotine and cocaine. The coca leaf first appeared in pharmacies in patent preparations that highlighted its provenance with exotic images of Incas, jungles and conquistadors, but once cocaine was isolated from the leaf it was sold in factory-milled white tablets with packaging that signalled its chemical purity. Similarly, from 1920 the German pharmacy giant Merck supplied 'Mescalinium-sulfat' in solution, in sterile vials suitable for injection, its chemical formula beneath its name in red block letters. Henceforth mescaline's natural form, from the scientific point of view, was the glittering white needles into which its sulphate and hydrochloride salts crystallised.

Mescaline arrived at an opportune moment for German scientific research, particularly in the rapidly transforming field of psychology. The discipline had been a German invention: Wilhelm Wundt had been the first person to call himself a psychologist in 1879, though his formal title was professor of inductive philosophy at the University of Zurich. That year he set up the first experimental psychology laboratory in Leipzig, where he used novel instruments such as fine chronometers, electrical meters and sensory mapping devices to measure human responses to various stimuli. With these he was able to tease apart the functions of perception, sensation and cognition, and to demonstrate that many of the processes involved occurred beneath the threshold of conscious awareness.

By the early twentieth century, however, researchers were looking to move beyond the 'brass instrument psychology' Wundt had developed and the limits of physically measurable data that it imposed. In the words of Heinrich Klüver, a psychologist of the generation that followed, 'It became apparent that empirical psychology, starting with "elements" of some kind in the laboratory, could not attain the promised insight into the higher processes of the mind, nor could it do justice to the fact that man is an historical being as well as a mammal.'[4] With the arrival of psychoanalysis and gestalt psychology, which aimed to study the mental processes that knitted perceptual data into a coherent consciousness, psychology took an inward turn, away from quantitative and analytic methods and towards subjective experience. Mescaline presented itself as a unique tool for accessing dimensions of mind that no brass instrument could measure.

Researches of this kind were already underway before Späth's synthesis. In 1913 Alwyn Knauer, professor of experimental medicine at Fordham University in New York, and William Maloney of the New

York Neurological Institute administered 'the sulphate of mescalin', the 'essential principle' that Arthur Heffter had extracted from a 'delusional Mexican drug . . . a favourite narcotic among Mexican Indians and dilettante drug habitués', to twenty-three volunteer subjects and 'several times to each of ourselves', in subcutaneous injections of around 200mg.[5]

Knauer had previously been assistant at the University of Munich to Emil Kraepelin, who had revolutionised clinical psychiatry with a taxonomic system that formalised the concept of psychosis and (in conjunction with his colleague Eugen Bleuler) developed the diagnosis of schizophrenia. Kraepelin had long been interested in the idea of experimentally induced psychoses and he and Knauer had pursued this with drugs including alcohol, morphine and bromides, but the states these produced turned out to have 'little similarity to actual insanities'.[6] Mescaline, however, appeared more promising. 'In the world of psychical things,' he and Maloney wrote, 'our experience is always confined within the narrow limits of what we call our own mind.'[7] Yet here was an 'intoxication of a curious and unique nature' that left conscious mental processes 'practically unclouded', while at the same time narrowing their focus and presenting mental events to the attention 'in a much more intense and exclusive manner than normal'.[8] The 'apperceptive faculties'[9] – Wundt's term for the process by which responses are brought into conscious awareness – were retained while the experimental subject was in the grip of 'subjective abnormal mental complexes',[10] symptoms of insanity that they were able to describe almost as external observers.

This peculiar property of mescaline intoxication – or 'poisoning', as Knauer and Maloney refer to it throughout their report – had been noted from the first, when Prentiss and Morgan described its ability to induce a 'sense of dual personality' or 'double consciousness' in which the external world coexisted with a private visionary theatre.[11] The phenomenon had been observed previously with hashish, and in 1845 theorised in some detail by the nineteenth-century French alienist

Jacques-Joseph Moreau in his major work on the subject, *Du hachisch et de l'aliénation mentale* (*Hashish and Mental Illness*). Moreau referred to hashish intoxication – taken orally, in very large doses – as an *état mixte*, a 'mixed state' that he compared to dreaming while awake. He argued that it offered unique insights into abnormal mental states: 'however misled one may be by delusions or hallucinations in the midst of a fantastic world of wild dreams . . . one still remains one's own master'. He believed on these grounds that hashish had great therapeutic potential, not so much for mental patients as for their doctors. 'To comprehend the ravings of a madman,' he wrote, 'it is necessary to have raved oneself, but without having lost the awareness of one's madness, without having lost the power to evaluate the psychic changes occurring in the mind.'[12]

During their experimental sessions Knauer and Maloney discovered that mescaline produced an *état mixte* similar to that of hashish in which their subjects could articulate a detailed commentary on the hallucinations they were experiencing. The visions unspooled relentlessly for hours, as fast as they could transcribe them:

> Immediately before my open eyes are a vast number of rings, apparently made of extremely fine steel wire, all constantly rotating . . . these circles are concentrically arranged, the innermost being infinitely small, almost point like, the outermost being about a meter and a half in diameter. The spaces between the wires seem brighter than the wires themselves. Now the wires shine like dim silver in parts. Now a beautiful light violet tint has developed in them . . .[13]

The data was mesmerising in its detail and staggering in its sheer volume, but it was unclear what kind of meaning could be extracted from it. The visions could on occasion be influenced by conscious control, but for the most part they 'came unsought, they were uncontrollable, and they were only remotely interfered with by the will'. In normal reveries, even in dreams, such visions might be connected to the subject's personal history, their personality or their mood; these, however, 'seemed to be something arising outside of and independent of the investigated person'.[14] They existed in a perceptual limbo, more solidly 'real' than figments of the imagination but never attaining a definite or final form. Knauer and Maloney attempted an analysis of their developmental stages – the initial visual idea gradually being clothed in shapes, perhaps modulated by retinal after-images – but their overriding conclusion was that 'our work has only served to show how complex is the question of hallucinations'.[15]

※　　※　　※

Once pure mescaline was readily available from Merck's manufactory in Darmstadt, the pace of such researches picked up. The largest and most high-profile study was conducted in the psychiatric clinic at Heidelberg University, where since 1914 Karl Jaspers had been teaching psychology in what had previously been Emil Kraepelin's department. Jaspers believed that abnormal mental pathologies were more than simply biological in nature and he developed the 'biographical method' in which patients were studied as individuals, with careful consideration given to their personalities, life situations and emotional states. Working alongside him as a psychiatrist and neurologist was Kurt Beringer, who in 1921 began a programme of mescaline experiments that ran for several years and culminated in his exhaustive report on its effects, *Der Meskalinrausch* (*Mescaline Intoxication*, 1927). Beringer administered mescaline to over sixty subjects, many of them more than once, injecting them with a starting dose of 200mg of mescaline salts doses but often raising it to 400, 500 or even 600mg.

Most of Beringer's subjects were doctors or medical students at the clinic. Fifty-four of the sixty were male. Some were given the drug under laboratory conditions but others took it during the course of their daily routine, including shifts on the psychiatric wards: Beringer, like Moreau, believed that experience of abnormal mental states would help them to become more insightful and empathetic clinicians. Rather than fixating on the visual hyperesthesia that had captivated scientific researchers thus far, he wanted to use mescaline as a tool for exploring the basis of personality and the workings of the pre-conscious mind. 'Here we have a method,' he put it in terms that echoed Moreau, 'by which abnormal symptoms can be manifested in normal people.'[16] Like Jaspers, he wanted not merely clinical descriptions or diagnoses but accounts by the subjects themselves that rendered up their individual personality structures. *Der Meskalinrausch* included the written (and occasionally sketched) experiences of thirty-two subjects across two hundred pages, an appendix twice as long as Beringer's main text.

The cumulative effect of all this reportage, however, was to bury the individual subjects. The only way to manage the data was to arrange them into general categories: distortions of time, mental confusion, 'cosmic emotions' and of course the torrent of visions.[17] Beringer recognised at an early stage, as Knauer and Maloney had, that there was no reliable link between personality type and the content of the visions. Even when informed by a close character study, the most that the hallucinations usually revealed was some obvious and trivial connection to the emotional state of the subject at the moment of the experience. What Beringer ended up with was, rather, a panoramic collage of what he termed the 'mescal psychosis': an endless cavalcade of sensory and perceptual illusions, cosmic insights and psychomotor distortions.

Beringer settled on a higher-order classification with three broad categories: abnormal sensory phenomena, changes in conscious attitudes and abnormal emotional states. In most of the individual reports, however, these bled constantly into one another. Beringer's colleague Wilhelm Mayer-Gross, for example, attempted to shape his account to Beringer's clinical template but his stream of consciousness failed to respect its boundaries. From the beginning of his report – 'a general feeling of pleasant carelessness with slight fatigue' and 'a background of sickness' – the physical phenomena carried an emotional substrate. The familiar next stage, shifting visual patterns on closed eyelids – 'Oriental tapestry, mosaic-like wallpapers, kaleidoscopic coloured geometric patterns, lines in brilliant luminescent colours or in black and white, etc.' – was accompanied by euphoric emotions: a 'feeling of superiority and joviality; I was ready to joke about everything, and especially to sneer at some psycho-physical tests and at the people trying to test me'. (Mayer-Gross confessed later that 'my remarks were objectively not at all as strikingly witty as I thought them at the time'.) Over the course of the afternoon his mood deepened into profundity, and the accompanying visions seemed more meaningful: a huge, imposing dome struck him as 'the perfect representation of my emotional condition, which was far away and completely detached from all the small idyllic things of the little-valley-with-mill type which I like so much in ordinary life'.[18] Laughter, sickness, mental superiority, visions and depth psychology jostled throughout, simultaneous and contradictory.

Beringer's term 'mescal psychosis' reflected the parallels he discerned between mescaline's effects and the onset of schizophrenia, which suggested to him that mescaline and the psychoses might share a common biological basis. He expressed the hope that further research might elucidate 'the disorders of intermediary metabolic processes' that underlay it.[19] But this path led in the opposite direction from the one he had set out to follow: away from normal subjects and into the pathological; away from individuals and into diagnostic categories; back into the biology from which he was attempting to escape. Wilhelm Mayer-Gross, however, developed this line of thought by enumerating the sensory distortions of mescaline and comparing them to the symptoms of psychotic disorders. Mayer-Gross would later introduce mescaline to British psychiatry, where studies of this kind became a staple of schizophrenia research in the post-war era.

＊　　＊　　＊

In the meantime, the most successful outcome of the Heidelberg researches was one that, on the face of it, seemed unpromising. It focused entirely on visual hallucinations, the aspect of mescaline researches that appeared to have been studied to death; it was essentially a review of the literature on the subject to date, though the author did undertake experiments on himself. Yet the psychologist Heinrich Klüver's *Mescal*, published as a slim monograph in London in 1928, made greater progress in bringing order to the chaos of its hallucinations than any of his sources had. It also introduced the German mescaline researches to the Anglophone world, where it was rediscovered in the 1960s and reprinted in psychedelic-jacketed paperback editions that vastly outsold the original.

Klüver studied at Hamburg and Berlin universities but by the time *Mescal* was published he had been in the United States for five years, teaching at the University of Minnesota before taking up a post in the psychology department at Chicago, where he became a professor in 1938 and remained throughout his long career. He refused to teach and worked mostly alone in an idiosyncratic laboratory designed to investigate the mechanics of the visual system constituted by eye and brain. For decades he worked ever deeper into the territory opened up by his mescaline studies using animal experiments, mostly on rhesus monkeys, to investigate the role of optic nerves, corneal secretions and capillaries in generating eidetic imagery (visual patterns on closed eyelids) and the causes of optical distortions such as polyopia (multiplied objects), micropsia (miniaturised images) and palinopsia (visual persistence and trails).

He began his study by taking a dose of powdered peyote buttons – easier to source in the USA than Merck's mescaline – feeling nauseous, vomiting and then recording the visual procession that ensued: 'Clouds from left to right through optical field. Tail of a pheasant (in centre of field) turns into bright yellow star; star into sparks. Moving scintillating screw; "hundreds" of screws. A sequence of rapidly changing objects in agreeable colours . . .'[20] After this he combed through the volumes of hallucinatory reportage collected by Prentiss and Morgan, Mitchell, Ellis, Knauer and Maloney, Beringer and Mayer-Gross with

fresh intent. Rather than attempting to match the visions to personality type or to correlate them with psychopathologies, he ignored their
content entirely. Instead he concentrated on their structures and
noticed that the thousands of objects and shapes described had a
tendency to cluster around a small number of recognisable visual forms
and motifs.

Klüver quoted Havelock Ellis's assertion that 'the chief character of
the visions is their indescribableness',[21] but he begged to differ. He
discerned, for example, a characteristic sequence of stages: beginning
with brightness and flashes of colour (the violet glow and green after-
image across the white notebook page), evolving into geometric or
kaleidoscopic shapes (the tapestries, Persian carpets and floral designs),
then the appearance of objects (buildings, vases, filigreed metal armour)
and finally – and only at higher doses – fantastical scenes and landscapes in which elements from all these stages meshed into a realistic
panorama.

There were also commonalities of visual tone and contrast. Some
subjects reported a preponderance of certain colours – often opposites,
such as red and green – but all seemed to experience a general colour
saturation and heightened illumination, captured by the analogy with
electric light. Objects were commonly described as surrounded by
haloes: this seemed to be part of a more general effect by which contrast
was enhanced. He recalled that, as far back as 1819, the Czech anato-
mist Jan Purkinje had compiled a table of 'subjective visual phenomena'
produced by physical means such as pressing on his closed eyelids or
staring at the sun. The hallucinations of mescaline, Klüver proposed,
must similarly reflect the organisation of the visual system: they were
comparable, as we might say today, to turning up the brightness, colour
and contrast dials on a TV screen.

There were further clues in the ways that the hallucinations moved.
Often a moving object was perceived as a succession of vivid snapshot
images. Klüver cites one of Beringer's subjects whose cigarette, when he
waved it, left a series of glowing balls in the air: 'Then these balls jumped

all of a sudden in a great hurry into the glowing end of the cigarette, but always along the path taken by the cigarette. They did not fade, but all of them went along the curve to the terminal point just as if they were connected by a rubber band.'[22] Other subjects described movements that in normal vision would have been smooth as 'jerky', 'automatic' or 'peristaltic'.[23] There were dozens of descriptions of polyopia, a symptom described by the philosopher Charles Bonnet in 1760 and witnessed in cases of brain lesion, in which hallucinated shapes or objects duplicate themselves into rows: 'suddenly a little man is standing there changing continually in appearance, sometimes he has a beard and sometimes not . . . now the little men increase again in number until there is a whole line of them . . . one of them twirls his moustache, and at once all of them twirl their moustaches with tremendous speed'.[24] These apparently nonsensical visions, Klüver suggested, pointed to glitches in the visual system, the normally seamless and invisible operations of eye and brain coming unstitched.

More complex underlying mechanisms were suggested by the visual motifs that Klüver called 'form-constants', his most enduring contribution to cognitive psychology.[25] He discerned one in the repeated use of words such as 'grating, lattice, fretwork, filigree, honeycomb or chessboard design':[26] the reticulated two-dimensional plane, often shimmering with contrasting highlights. A second was the tunnel ('funnel, alley, cone or vessel'),[27] which often seemed to be in gyratory motion, drawing the eye into its centre. A third was the spiral, often rotating or multiplied, or opening and closing like a concertina; a fourth was the cobweb, in which lines and forms radiated symmetrically from a central source. Like the intensification of colours and contrast, these form-constants seemed to be hardwired into the structure of the hallucinations: on a strong dose of mescaline, they pulsed and swirled across external objects just as they did with closed eyelids or in darkness. They never manifested in dreams following the intoxication, which suggested that they were physiological productions of the drug itself.

Klüver brought a precision to the analysis of mescaline hallucinations of the kind that Silas Weir Mitchell had glimpsed but not systematised a generation earlier. He was, however, aware of its limitations. The visions, he knew from his own experience, were more than simply optical illusions: they seemed full of wonder and significance that evaded capture by the rational mind. They had, as he put it, a sense of *presque vu*, suggesting a moment of clarity and completion that never arrived: 'the contour of a figure is almost complete, but it never is quite . . . the final and satisfying completion never takes place'.[28] They were in constant flux, on the cusp of revelation; the subject was suspended in awe, feeling that 'he is near grasping a "cosmic" truth, but that, unfortunately, he does not quite succeed'. This feeling, Klüver speculated, 'may become of central importance in the mescal psychosis', generating a sense of imminent epiphany in which the individual is becoming united with the universe at large.[29] 'One looks "beyond the horizon" of the normal world, and this "beyond" is often so impressive or even shocking that its after-effects linger for years in one's memory.'[30]

Klüver proved that the tools of twentieth-century psychology could impose some structure on mescaline's apparently chaotic visions, but their mystery nevertheless remained untouched. In the introduction he wrote for the new edition of *Mescal* in 1966 he felt that little had changed. Psychology had professionalised and systematised its methods, but its pursuit of objective and replicable results meant that 'the conceptual tools for coping with so-called "subjective" aspects are often inadequate or entirely lacking'. Mescaline's deeper mechanisms would only be revealed by some as yet unimagined combination of external observation and introspection, psychology and 'non-psychological tools'.[31] He recalled the memoirs of the pioneering neurologist Santiago Ramón y Cajal, in which he wrote that he had spent his life hunting 'in the flower garden of the grey matter' for 'the mysterious butterflies of the soul'.[32]

✸   ✸   ✸

Although Kurt Beringer's studies had no specific therapeutic intent, the structural similarities between 'mescal psychosis' and schizophrenia proposed by the Heidelberg researchers highlighted the fact that, thirty years after Parke, Davis had made their peyote tincture commercially available, the medical possibilities of mescaline were still no more than vaguely outlined. When Albert Hofmann synthesised LSD in 1943 he and his colleagues recognised the similarity of its action to mescaline; Hofmann recalled that 'in the 1920s, extensive experiments with mescaline were carried out on animals and human subjects, which were described comprehensively by K. Beringer in his *Der Meskalinrausch*'. In the received opinion of his generation of pharmacists, 'because these investigations failed to suggest any applications for mescaline in medicine, interest in this active substance soon waned'.[33]

The application of science to mescaline had, with the exception of Klüver's insights into the structures of optical perception, generated a procession of negative results. Beringer's work had demonstrated that mescaline hallucinations revealed little or nothing about the personality or mental state of its individual subjects. Klüver counted himself sceptical that the drug might ever become 'a tool in the hands of the psychoanalyst'.[34] Ever since Prentiss and Morgan's original trials, doctors and pharmacists had been unable to solve the problem of its unpredictability. Researchers called repeatedly for further trials, but they produced the same outcomes. In 1932 another study of peyote by Samuel Fernberger at Pennsylvania University on nine faculty members showed that apart from some physiological responses (greater or lesser degrees of nausea, for example) 'there were wide individual differences in the reports'.[35] Mescaline demonstrated mental and psychic benefits in individual cases but it was deleterious in others. The differences did not correspond in any straightforward way with dosage, nor with subjects who assessed themselves as good or poor visualisers.

In 1926 the French pharmacist Alexandre Rouhier approached the question from a different angle in his monograph *Le peyotl: la plante qui fait les yeux émerveillés* (*Peyote: The Plant That Fills the Eyes with Marvels*). Rouhier practised in Lyon and had for some years been growing peyote in the hills above the Côte d'Azur. His book drew together his extensive researches, many of them previously published, on peyote's botany, alkaloid chemistry, history, ethnography and medical properties. Stylishly written, handsomely illustrated and widely read, it introduced to mainstream Francophone culture the peyote rites of the Tarahumara and Huichol peoples, James Mooney's descriptions of the Kiowa ceremony and the pioneering self-experiments of Silas Weir Mitchell and Havelock Ellis. It rendered 'mescal psychosis' as '*l'ivresse peyotlique*' ('peyote drunkenness') and drew examples of it from Rouhier's own experiences, which he prefaced with Macbeth's lines to the witches: 'Were such things here as we do speak about? / Or have we eaten of the insane root / That takes the reason prisoner?'[36]

Rouhier drew further literary comparisons with Baudelaire's descriptions of synaesthesia and the uncanny fictions of E.T.A. Hoffman, and his frame of reference extended beyond medical science in other respects. In a separate paper he placed it at the head of a list of plants that gave its subjects clairvoyant powers: in his coinages a 'hierobotany' or 'divinatory palaeo-pharmacy' that drew together cannabis, opium, coca, *oloiluqui* [morning glory] and ayahuasca.[37] He also included *huachuma*, a 'beautiful arborescent cactus of South America', citing Bernabé Cobo's seventeenth-century account of its use in Peruvian sorcery, though he was unaware that it also contained mescaline.[38] All these plants, he observed, produced hallucinations that were believed in their native cultures to be prophetic glimpses of other times and places, and their healing powers were attributed to these supernatural properties. Rather than conceiving their native medical uses as rudimentary forms of pharmacy to be improved by western science, they should be understood in the context of their other uses, such as finding lost objects or bringing news of distant relatives. They were another form of clairvoyance, in which the distant and invisible causes of sickness were brought into the shaman's awareness.

This, Rouhier argued, was the root of the puzzling disjunction between Indian cultures in which peyote was a panacea and the modern clinic in which its therapeutic applications were so elusive. 'For the Indians of Mexico, and equally those of the prairie, illness does not have a physical cause.' It is caused by spirits, and 'only a divine power, or the magical qualities of a plant that contains one', can cure it.[39] Within Indian belief systems the therapeutic range of peyote was virtually limitless and it could indeed produce miraculous results: Rouhier cited Mooney's eyewitness testimony of Paul Setkopti's recovery from tuberculosis. But it was naïve to dismiss prophecy or divination as superstition and at the same time expect healing magic to translate obligingly into western medicine. Within the scientific model, peyote had no totalising spiritual power, only a scattering of possible applications in which it was obliged to compete with other established drugs. It might rival or complement, but it was doubtful whether it could replace, 'opium or hashish as a euphoric, or bromine, chloral and barbiturates as a nervous sedative, or digitalis as a cardiac medicine'.[40] Its medical virtues were not illusory: it did indeed have valuable actions on the nerves, in different contexts as stimulant and sedative, but none that were unique to it. At the same time, it was impossible to pick and choose from its unruly bundle of physical, mental and psychic effects.

Synthetic mescaline was also, in Rouhier's view, inferior to plant extracts. As Heffter had originally demonstrated, there were at least half a dozen alkaloids in the cactus with overlapping but distinct biochemical profiles, and he believed that the combination in their natural source had its own distinct virtues.[41] He produced and sold by mail order his own 'Panpeyotl' preparation, an alcohol and chloroform tincture of the alkaloids from dried buttons grown in his Côte d'Azur nursery, 'particularly for psychiatrists and psychological experimenters wishing to study the mental phenomena produced by powerful doses'.[42]

Writing at the time of the League of Nations' 1925 Geneva Opium Convention, in which the international traffic in hashish was being controlled for the first time, Rouhier strongly opposed similar controls being placed on peyote. By the 1930s, however, it was attracting the attention of pharmaceutical regulators. Rouhier's Panpeyotl now had competition from similar preparations including 'Peyotyl R.D.', supplied by a Geneva pharmacy that promoted it in trade catalogues and handbills. This was advertised, with a description that echoed Rouhier's subtitle, as containing 'all the marvellous properties of the peyotl (*Lophophora williamsii*)', and recommended as a stimulant and mental tonic for a long list of conditions including asthenia (weakness), overwork, nervous depression, insomnia, migraines, neuralgia, asthma, hysteria and neurasthenia. In 1936 these advertisements were brought to the attention of the League of Nations Advisory Committee on the Traffic in Opium and other Dangerous Drugs, set up by the 1925 Convention, which recommended that it should be restricted to medical prescription only. From this point on peyote and mescaline disappeared from general pharmacy catalogues, though they were still available to doctors and for scientific research.[43]

※　　※　　※

For its German researchers, mescaline's hallucinations posed, but were unable to answer, one of psychology's central questions. They were private, subjective and unique to the individual subject, and yet they seemed to have no basis in personal experience. Were they simply a mechanical product of human biology, or were they shaped in some inscrutable way by culture or the individual psyche? Questions of this kind were moving German psychology towards wider horizons. From his vantage point in Chicago Heinrich Klüver observed in 1929 that 'the main conceptions of present-day psychology assume a striking similarity to questions developed in fields of philosophical thought'.[44] The discipline had become more interested in dynamic processes than empirical measurements, the nature of experience rather than taxonomies of its constituent parts. Kurt Beringer developed friendships with holistic and mystically inclined thinkers such as Carl Jung and

Hermann Hesse; his Heidelberg mentor Karl Jaspers had already stepped back from clinical practice, his lecture topics evolving from psychology into philosophy as he grappled with the questions posed by the new disciplines of phenomenology and existentialism. The study of mescaline, always impossible to contain within a single frame, would follow the same trajectory.

CHAPTER SEVEN

PROFANE ILLUMINATIONS

1929–36

WARSAW, BUCHAREST, PARIS, BERLIN, MEXICO

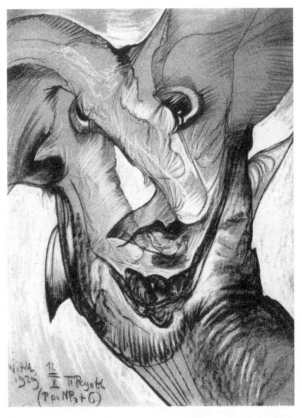

A portrait of Nena Stachurska by Stanisław Witkiewicz on peyote, 1929.

Der Meskalinrausch and *Le peyotl* brought mescaline and its marvellous visions from the specialist worlds of psychology and pharmacy to a wider European culture, particularly at the interface of the mind sciences and the arts. Psychiatrists were drawing on what Heinrich Klüver had called 'non-psychological tools' to advance their understanding of perception and cognition. New frameworks were advanced in works such as *The Art of Thought* (1926), in which the British social psychologist Graham Wallas teased out the mental faculties involved in different stages of the creative process: preparation, incubation, illumination and verification. Collaborations emerged such as that between the psychoanalyst Ernst Kris and the art historian Ernst Gombrich, who in 1931 began a joint project to elucidate the extent to which visual perception was created in the brain by constant iterations of guesswork, extrapolation and imagination. There was, in Gombrich's phrase, no such thing as an 'innocent eye' that received a 'true' image: vision was an act of subconscious creativity.[1]

A new generation of artists and writers, in turn, were exploring the insights of psychoanalysis, pursuing the creative derangement of the senses with intoxicants and channelling the unconscious through automatic writing and séances. Abnormal states of consciousness were congenial to the modernist urge to subvert conventional frames of reference and present the world from fractured and unfamiliar perspectives. Most of the well-documented mescaline experiments of the interwar era took the form of private one-on-one sessions in which a psychologist or psychiatrist administered the drug to a writer, painter or philosopher, presenting them with artistic or intellectual stimuli and recording their creative responses. In the process the mescaline experience was reconceived once more, in terms anticipated during the *fin de siècle* by Havelock Ellis and his Symbolist associates: neither as a spiritual epiphany nor a model psychosis, but as a zone of aesthetic, creative and existential possibility.

The negotiation between expectation, illusion and reality was a process with which artists were already intimately familiar and mescaline offered a new route for science to explore it in conjunction with them. The collaboration created freedoms and limitations for both parties. Drawing or painting in the throes of mescaline intoxication posed obvious challenges to the artist – physical tremors, impaired concentration and hand–eye coordination – and often left scientists struggling to interpret cursory dabs and squiggles. Some artists found these limitations exhilarating, others restricting. All were faced with the question of whether to employ their habitual style to capture mescaline's effects or to abandon their hard-won expertise and submit to its flow. Some found, as had Havelock Ellis before them, that it heightened their aesthetic sense and revealed previously hidden creative dimensions. Others felt that the drug, and the context of scientific experiment, made the process forced and mechanical, as if they were taking dictation or producing 'specimen' work in which their artistic agency was erased.

Mescaline's irrepressible visions had obvious affinities with the productions of the Surrealist movement, in its founder André Breton's definition 'pure psychic automatism . . . thought dictated in the absence of all control exerted by reason'.[2] Evidence of direct connections is elusive, however, as Breton summarily expelled from the movement anyone who confessed to using drugs. He had worked in neurology and psychiatry and was acutely sensitive to the dangers of exploring madness and the unconscious with anything less than a balanced mind (he banned all sorts of practices on these grounds, including homosexuality and Catholicism). The Surrealist approach, Breton insisted, allowed the artist to explore worlds previously accessible only to the mad, hysterical, delirious or drugged. Quoting Baudelaire, he asserted that 'like hashish, there is enough there to satisfy the most delicate systems'. Adherence to Surrealism was intoxication enough.[3]

Breton quarrelled with members such as Antonin Artaud and Robert Desnos over their open use of narcotics. Other surrealists did confess later to having used mescaline productively: Artaud's psychiatrist Gaston Ferdière, a close ally of the movement in 1920s Paris, remembered that 'the Surrealists especially appreciated mescaline' above other drugs.[4] None, however, acknowledged it at the time, and explicit links were only made by artists who worked in milieux far removed from Breton and Paris. The era's most dedicated explorer of mescaline was the prodigious Polish writer-artist Stanisław Ignacy Witkiewicz, known as Witkacy, who recorded his experiences in both art and writing: in his essay collection *Narcotics: Nicotine, Alcohol, Cocaine, Peyote, Morphine and Ether* (1932), under the guise of a fictitous hallucinogenic drug in his novel *Insatiability* (1930), and in a series of drawings and pastel paintings made under the influence of both peyote and mescaline between 1928 and 1930.

Witkacy – he had taken this *nom de guerre* in order to distinguish himself from his father, also Stanisław, a celebrated Impressionist painter – began painting and writing plays at an early age and careened out of control in his early twenties with a series of self-destructive love affairs and a mysterious illness, possibly venereal. He began painting his friends as deformed monsters, dabbled in demonology and drifted to the far edges of sanity. In 1914, after his fiancée shot herself over an affair with one of his friends, his father arranged for him to accompany Bronisław Malinowski, Poland's leading anthropologist, to a scientific convention in Sydney, travelling via Ceylon. Witkacy was swallowed whole by the beauty of the tropics and proclaimed himself at war with western rationalism (and with Malinoswski, whom he saw as its ambassador). His plays took on the quality of magic rites, steeped in the dark allure of the primitive.

When he returned to Europe in September 1914 he was sent to Saint Petersburg for officer training, after which he spent much of the Great War in action. He was wounded at the front and present for the revolution in 1917, in which he was elected political commissar by his regiment. After the war he returned to Poland and spent the next twenty years writing over two hundred literary works and producing thousands of paintings. His abstract plays, conceived according to his theory of 'Pure Form', were derided by critics: one was reviewed as 'the ravings of a siphylitic in the last stages of creeping paralysis . . . a total absurdity from which nothing can ever arise', which 'should be put in alcohol and studied by psychopaths'.[5] In 1924 Witkacy abandoned his tropic-inspired art in favour of portraiture and experimental fiction, declaring that 'art is the sole crack through which it is possible to get a glimpse of the horrible, painful monstrosity' of western civilisation.[6] He made his living from commercial portraits of fashionable society figures dashed off at top speed to strictly defined, numbered and priced standards of workmanship. In the time these bought him, he painted hallucinatory scenes and self-portraits, wrote unclassifiable prose and drama and experimented with mescaline, along with every other drug he could get hold of.[7]

Witkacy was no cheerleader for drugs, which he saw as symptoms of cultural decadence and predators on human weakness. They were a symbol, above all, of the theme he took for the title of his drug novel, insatiability. This blind, self-destructive force was the root of all evil, he wrote in *Narcotics*, and 'if it is not eradicated by excessive satiation of real-life feelings, by work, by the exercise of power, by creativity etc., can be appeased solely with the aid of narcotics'.[8] He placed nicotine and alcohol at the head of this list, the most self-destructive and naturally the most popular; it was only later that he came to peyote and mescaline. 'Of course, since first hearing about peyote and the visions it produces, my dream was to try that marvellous drug.' But it appeared to be a great rarity in Europe and 'I despaired of ever having the opportunity.' Eventually Prosper Smurzło, a friend from his army days in Saint Petersburg who had subsequently become devoted to spiritualism and parapsychology, passed on some small dried buttons from Mexico, obtained via the International Society for Metaphysical Research.[9] Witkacy later managed to order some of Alexandre Rouhier's Panpeyotl extract in pill form, but was not impressed: it was 'far less potent in summoning visions and had many more negative side effects'.[10] He also experimented with pure mescaline from 'the splendid firm Merck', making him perhaps the first person able to make an informed comparison of its natural, processed and synthetic forms (his favourite was the dried peyote from Mexico).[11] On occasion he took mescaline under the supervision of doctors, including Stefan Szuman, director of the educational psychology department at Kraków's Jagiellonian University, a specialist in the study of children's drawing who probably supplied him with Merck's mescaline.

Of all drugs Witkacy found peyote the hardest to write about, 'as difficult to reconstruct as certain dreams in which it is impossible to tell what it is all about'. As Beringer's subjects had, he found visions, sensations and emotions 'forming strange tangles, the images interlock with the muscular feelings and the sensations of the internal organs'. Unlike alcohol and cocaine, 'the *realistic* poisons' which heighten sensation without greatly altering it, mescaline is 'a *metaphysical* drug, producing a sense of the strangeness of existence'.[12] It dilates the pupils until the subject's 'peyote eyes seem about to explode from the inexpressible intensity of the feelings and thoughts packed into them'. These shining black eyes are 'the true mirrors of the soul – diabolical mirrors with which the demon of peyote denudes us, making us believe that even in this life it may be possible to know another being's psyche'. The visions that danced in peyote-dilated pupils were, he suggested, 'created by the Aztec God of Light'.[13]

During his first and most potent experiment with dried peyote, Witkacy attempted some clairvoyance but found concentration exhausting: 'I was hit by a great lethargy, and my movements were so slow that eating a few tomatoes took over half an hour.'[14] In his attempt to record the visions that flowed far faster than he could write, he asked his wife to transcribe them as he spoke. After he had taken six of Rouhier's Panpeyotl pills, she scribbled pages of staccato reportage in the third person:

> Various sculptures in sharp relief, tiny faces, feels 'weird' but good. Sees rainbow stripes, but incomplete – the following colours predominate: dirty-red and lemon-yellow. Desire to forget reality.

Huge building, the bricks turn into gargoyle faces, like on the cathedral of Nôtre-Dame in Paris. Monsters similar to plesiosauruses made out of luminous filaments. The trees turned into ostriches. A corpse's brain, abscesses, sheaves of sparks bursting out of them . . .[15]

Like the productions of trance mediumship, hypnosis or automatism, the notes have the raw, unmediated quality of subconscious transmissions, inflected with Witkacy's saturnine aesthetic yet beyond his control, simultaneously impressive, meaningless and maddening. 'I only fear that readers will soon have had their fill,' he concluded, 'much as I had myself around five o'clock the next morning, when I begged those mysterious forces to clear my weary brain of the ruthless procession of monsters and monstrous events.'[16]

Witkacy's drawings and paintings have the same freeform virtuosity as his writings; they are simultaneously artistic and scientific experiments, referenced today both in modernist art histories and the clinical literature on hallucinations.[17] With the exception of a few sketchy line drawings by Beringer's subjects, reproduced in *Der Meskalinrausch*, Witkacy's peyote and mescaline canvasses are probably the first examples of western art produced under the influence of a major psychedelic. His professional facility with high-speed portraiture, in pastels as well as pencil, allowed him to work deftly while still under the drug's influence, and his dynamic compositions capture its pulsating visual distortions. Witkacy did not regard narcotics as creative forces in their own right, nor did he feel dictated to by them: he regarded his works under the influence of mescaline as collaborations with the drug and included 'Peyotl' or 'Mesk. Merck' in the signature. All are to some degree monstrous: in one the realistically rendered head of a middle-aged man is appended to a worm-like reptilian tail; in another a female subject is surrounded by distorted semi-Cubist spectres; in another a face, rendered in livid reds and oranges, is folded across itself into the head of a demonic goat.

Despite the nightmare quality of his productions under its influence, Witkacy's summation of peyote and mescaline was highly positive. He saw it as the 'anti-drug', a remedy for the insatiability that all
the others fed. He noted that it produced a 'strong physical and moral
revulsion to alcohol and tobacco, a revulsion that lingers long after
the trance is over', and recommended that it should be 'administered
to addicts during rehabilitation and detox'.[18] 'Smokers, drinkers and
other addicts, arouse yourselves while there is still time!' he urged.
'Down with nicotine, alcohol and all forms of "white lunacy"! If peyote
turns out to be an antidote to all those filthy poisons, then in that case
and only in that case: long live peyote!'[19]

Witkacy's mescaline and peyote art was first published in 1930 by Dr
Szuman and over the next decade there were more mescaline experiments, more or less formal, in which the agendas of art and science
blended. Among the earliest and most fully documented was a collaboration in 1932 between Romania's most distinguished neurologist and
its leading avant-garde painter. Gheorghe Marinescu had begun his
career, like Sigmund Freud, studying under Jean-Martin Charcot at the
Salpêtrière Hospital in Paris. In 1897 he returned to Romania where a
chair of clinical neurology was created for him at the University of
Bucharest, which he held until he retired. In 1898 he had been the first
scientist to use the new technology of cinema, producing short films
that recorded the symptoms of neurological disorders such as paraplegia
and locomotion ataxia and were hailed by the Lumière brothers as
groundbreaking applications of their invention. He was seventy when
mescaline presented itself to him as another new technology with the
potential to open the workings of the brain to visible scrutiny.

Marinescu invited several artists with contrasting styles to participate in his experiment.[20] The first was Corneliu Michailescu, who
occupied a comparable status in Romanian art to Marinescu's own in

neurology. Michailescu had also travelled to begin his career, in his case to Zurich where he had worked with Dadaists such as Tristan Tzara. On his return he became the first Romanian artist to experiment with Cubism, though he never attached himself to a movement and his style, though it included elements of Expressionism and Surrealism, remained idiosyncratic. He was forty-five and at the peak of his career when Marinescu injected him with 330mg of mescaline sulphate and asked him to speak and draw in response to a series of prepared stimuli.

Marinescu waited two hours until the drug had fully taken hold, at which point he produced a gramophone; Michailescu reported, in response to music, 'dynamic visions, arabesques, rising out of semi-darkness'. A piece by the Russian Romantic composer Mikhail Glinka stimulated a vision of 'vague forms, opal tones, a waterfall and a rock', which he captured in swift dabs of watercolour. A minuet by Ignacy Jan Paderewski produced arabesques and disagreeable sensations of shivering and nausea; a rumba conjured up 'African art, flowers and exotic animals'.[21] The smell of creosote gave him brown visions, a whiff of alcohol produced a sensation of travelling. Another doctor who was observing him reminded him of a chimpanzee. By now music was prompting electric-blue flashes and explosive laughter. The scent of lily of the valley gave him voluptuous sensations. As the visions faded he began to paint them; ochre looked to him like mother of pearl. 'Throughout the experiment,' Marinescu wrote, 'the subject showed a marked tendency to introspection. He was aware he was intoxicated but could not banish the phenomena the intoxication produced . . . His will was almost non-existent, and he became highly suggestible.'[22]

Another artist, whose name Marinescu withheld, underwent a similar course of stimuli. In this case he was able to manifest a purer synaesthesia, with single notes played on the violin producing visions of ornaments coloured violet, yellow, green and red. The artist painted in a quite different style from Michailescu, overlaying geometric forms in different planes and superimposing stylised objects – a lion's head, an acanthus flower, a cluster of domed buildings – over a dark ground to produce a strikingly authentic representation of mescaline's closed-eye visions. In both cases, Marinescu concluded, 'the hallucinations were generally pleasant and at times quite marvellous. The painters we studied were enchanted by the richness, the beauty and the radiance of the colour visions'.[23] He speculated on the interplay between the automatic quality of the visions, the personality of the subject and their artistic style.

Marinescu presented his findings and the paintings at a conference in Bucharest in November 1932, writing them up for a French medical journal the following year. But for Corneliu Michailescu the outcome was more enduring. His style was permanently altered: his work now exploded with colour, strange geometries and futuristic shapes. It was a transformation that drew parallels with *Stilwandel*, a term used by German psychiatrists to denote the radical change in artistic expression that sometimes accompanied the onset of psychosis.[24] He painted less and less, however, and in 1935 retired to a village on the shores of Lake Cernica in the south of Romania, where he turned to writing Surrealist novels.

♣   ♣   ♣

Beyond their visual qualities, mescaline's hallucinations posed profound philosophical questions. During the mid-1930s three prominent writers and thinkers left records of their experiments with it. In 1934 and 1935 respectively, Walter Benjamin and Jean-Paul Sartre participated in the now-familiar modus operandi of private session between psychiatrist and artist, with the scientific gaze and the philosopher's insights informing – or, more often, pitted against – one another. And in 1936, Antonin Artaud, cut loose by Breton from the Surrealist movement and having abjured scientific materialism, abandoned the Old World for the New and the narcotics of western pharmacy for the ancient sacrament of the cactus, and launched himself into a self-experiment without limits.

Sartre was injected with mescaline by his old school friend, the psychiatrist Daniel Lagache, at Saint-Anne Hospital in Paris in January 1935 in the course of his researches into phenomenology, Edmund Husserl's radically reconceived form of philosophy which Sartre had encountered in 1933 and relocated to Berlin over that summer to study more deeply. Mescaline was a tool of obvious relevance to Husserl's injunction that 'a new way of looking at things is necessary'. Phenomenology aimed to describe reality purely as it was perceived, stripped of all theories, categories and definitions: turning attention exclusively, in Husserl's famous dictum, 'to the things themselves'.[25] Much of the mescaline literature to date, from the early peyote reportage of Silas Weir Mitchell and Havelock Ellis to the stream of consciousness dictated by Witkacy, had tended in this direction: in aiming simply to describe its visions and sensations without imposing definition or meaning on them, it had in a sense been phenomenology *avant la lettre*.

Sartre wrote little directly about his experience, describing it briefly in notes that later found a place in *L'imaginaire*, his 1940 study of the phenomenology of the imagination. He found its effects elusive and sinister. 'It could only exist *by stealth*,' he wrote; it distorted every sensation, yet whenever he attempted to perceive it directly it withdrew into the background or shifted shape. Its action on the mind was 'inconsistent and mysterious', offering no solid vantage point from which to observe it.[26] In contrast to previous descriptions of the 'double consciousness' or *état mixte*, in which the normal self was able to observe its hallucinations dispassionately, Sartre found it impossible to be a spectator of his own experience. On the contrary, he felt submerged against his will in a miasma of sensations that assailed him viscerally at every turn, a world of grotesque extreme close-ups in which everything disgusted him.

The best-known detail of Sartre's bad trip is Simone de Beauvoir's anecdote of him being haunted for weeks after by lobster-like creatures scuttling just beyond his field of vision. Sartre, like Aldous Huxley, was partially sighted – a curious coincidence linking two of the most cele-brated intellectuals to have taken the vision-producing drug – and his poor vision may have exacerbated his anxieties about shapes lurking just beyond its reach. Later in life he claimed that it had driven him to a nervous breakdown. 'After I took mescaline, I started seeing crabs around me all the time,' he recalled in 1971; 'I mean they followed me into the street, into class.' Even though he knew they were imaginary he spoke to them, requesting them to be quiet during his lectures. Eventually he sought psychotherapeutic help from a young Jacques Lacan, which generated 'nothing that he or I valued very much', though 'with the crabs, we sort of concluded that it was fear of becoming alone'.

'The crabs really began when my adolescence ended,' he added, raising the question of whether they were entirely the product of a mescaline trip at the age of thirty.[27] They made a cameo appearance years later in his play *The Condemned of Altona* (1959), in which a race of monstrous crabs sits in judgement of future humanity. Mescaline is a less explicit but more pervasive influence on *Nausea* (1938), in which mundane objects continually reveal hideous aspects or dissolve into viscous masses, and a closer look at reality always risks an unwelcome surprise. In 1972, however, later in his series of conversations with the scholar John Gerassi, he recalled that 'I liked mescaline a lot.' He recalled taking it in the Pyrenees: 'as you know I am not a nature lover. I much prefer to sit four hours in a café' – but on mescaline the moun-tains 'take on so many colours, it's really art'.[28]

Ten years after Sartre's first experiment the phenomenologist Maurice Merleau-Ponty quoted some of his previously unpublished self-observations on the drug: 'Everything seemed at once clammy and scaly, like some of the large serpents I have seen uncoiling themsleves at Berlin zoo. Then I was seized with the fear of being on a small island surrounded by serpents.'[29] Merleau-Ponty himself took mescaline in a dose much smaller than Sartre's and found it more philosophically useful. He observed that hallucinations pose a particular problem for the scientific method, which tries to explain them as 'an event in the chain of events running from the stimulus to the state of conscious-ness',[30] and thereby struggles to formulate their difference from reality. He offered an alternative explanation, located not in brain activity but in the subject's relations with the wider world. 'When the victim of hallucination declares that he sees and hears' we cannot contradict him, but at the same time 'we must not believe him',[31] since to call something a hallucination is also a statement that the sight and sound are not real. The phenomena are not purely intellectual: 'all hallucina-tion bears initially on one's own body',[32] as a physical product of the senses. A hallucination is presented to the observer alone, and 'the normal person does not find satisfaction in subjectivity . . . he is genu-inely concerned with being in the world'.[33] Hallucinogenic drugs such as mescaline show that perception and consciousness are more than private cerebral activities. They are irreducibly embodied and social.

On 22 May 1934, eight months before Sartre's experiment in Paris, the critic and philosopher Walter Benjamin was administered mescaline in Berlin, also via an old friend turned psychiatrist. Benjamin had known Ernst Joël since college days, after which Joël served as a doctor during the Great War. On his return to Weimar Berlin he turned to what he called 'social psychiatry', abandoning the world of private clinics and their wealthy clientele to practise among the poor in their homes. With his colleague Fritz Fränkel he was conducting an extensive series of drug experiments that generated clinical papers on the psychology of addiction, a book on cocaine dependency and a 1926 study of *Der Haschischrausch*. The pair approached Benjamin, well known at this time as a newspaper columnist and public intellectual, as an exper-imental subject, first with hashish and later with mescaline. The sessions were non-clinical and loosely supervised: sometimes Benjamin was hosted in Joël's Berlin apartment, at other times he wandered the streets and filed his report later. The mescaline session was supervised

by Fritz Fränkel in Joël's apartment and was largely unstructured, though Benjamin was presented with a few standard psychological tests. As was their protocol, doctor and subject filed parallel reports.

Benjamin's interest in drugs developed early in his career, after he read Charles Baudelaire's *Les Paradises artificiels*; in 1919 he had written to a friend, 'it will be necessary to repeat this attempt independently of this book'.[34] The year 1927, when he first took hashish, was also the year he began his *Arcades Project*, a series of excursions and excavations into the Baudelairean street life of nineteenth-century Paris; it remained unfinished (as did the book about hashish itself that he decided to write in 1932). The many notes, text fragments and experimental protocols that survive are a blurred composite of drug experiences and wanderings as a *flâneur* through cities past and present, real and imagined. His recollections of hashish and mescaline similarly blur into one another, and into the broader tapestry of his researches.[35]

Throughout his writing on drugs Benjamin circled around the German term *Rausch*, usually rendered in English as 'intoxication' but with deeper resonances: its underlying literal meaning of rush, roar or thunder and, prominent for Benjamin, Nietzsche's use of it to denote Dionysian ecstasy, the rending of the veil of appearances to reveal the primal life force. In its grip, as Benjamin wrote in his wanderings around Marseille on hashish, 'images and chains of images, long-submerged memories appear'; the borders between subject and object weaken, imagination bleeds into reality, the world comes to life in new ways. It is not purely a dream or a fantasy but 'a continual alternation of dreaming and waking states, a constant and finally exhausting oscillation between totally different worlds of consciousness'.[36] 'Intoxication' suggests a transient state of impairment, but *Rausch* describes an 'ecstasy of trance'[37] that holds out the possibility of re-enchanting the world without demanding a romantic or religious leap of faith. It is not an effect of the drug per se but 'a *profane illumination*, a materialistic, anthropological inspiration, to which hashish, opium or whatever else can give an introductory lesson'.[38]

The mescaline experiment of 1934 began with Fränkel giving Benjamin an injection and then leaving the room. On his return a few minutes later, his subject seemed in a bad mood. He was irritable and fidgety, and described the onset of the drug's symptoms as 'an impertinence'.[39] He complained that this was the wrong setting: the experiment should be taking place in a palm grove. He shivered, and in his own notes recorded: 'In shuddering, the skin imitates the meshwork of a net. But the net is the world net: the whole universe is caught in it.'[40] When he closed his eyes he described not coloured images but ornamental figures which he compared to those carved on Polynesian oars. He observed that the ornamental tendency could equally be applied to words, and doodled some repeated phrases in decorative shapes. When presented with Rorschach inkblots he complained – 'the peevishness, the mood of discontent keeps returning',[41] noted Fränkel – before concentrating and tossing out a quick series of associations: two Siberian women, two poodles, a little woollen sheep, two embryos. He returned frequently to the subject of Nietzsche's sister, Elisabeth Förster, and her attempts to control and pervert the meaning of her late brother's archive. He announced several times that he had discovered the secret of *Struwwelpeter*, the nightmarish children's book, but would not reveal it. Finally he pronounced: 'A child must get presents, or else he will die or break into pieces or fly away, like the children in *Struwwelpeter*. That is the secret of *Struwwelpeter*.'[42]

Benjamin's elliptical notes on mescaline are similar in texture to his jottings on hashish, and not much different from those he habitually made while sober. His ambivalence is also characteristic. The sensation of *Rausch* was never for him entirely comfortable: it was a dialectic in which one had to guard against being swallowed by 'the romantic turn of mind'.[43] Like Sartre, part of him sought a detachment from the experience, while another part sought immersion. There was also a political dimension to consider: 'The solitude of such intoxication has its dark side,'[44] as he wrote elsewhere. In Berlin in 1934 there were good grounds for being suspicious of the surrender to the irrational.

His nagging anxiety about the perversion of Nietzsche's legacy by his anti-Semitic sister perhaps reflects the intrusion of the political into his stream of thought.

Rausch was an awkward phenomenon in this context. To indulge in 'hours of hashish eating, or opium smoking'[45] was, from one angle, an act of escapism, a retreat from the communal and a betrayal of political responsibilities. At the same time the 1929 Opium Law had made the drug-taker a criminal and, as the Third Reich tightened its grip, a degenerate and an enemy of society; this made drug-taking a form of private revolt and a potential tool of liberation. The relation between *Rausch* and rebellion was fraught and paradoxical, and perhaps a clue to Benjamin's final insight about *Struwwelpeter*. Returning to his first reaction to mescaline at the end of his notes, he added: 'Impertinence is the child's chagrin at not being capable of magic.'[46] This is why 'a child must get presents': it is too harsh to expect children to endure a life of struggle without some gratuitous gifts. In *Rausch*, as he wrote at the end of his evening on hashish in Marseilles, 'our existence runs through Nature's fingers like gold coins that she cannot hold and lets fall so they can thus purchase new birth'.[47] Throughout his mescaline session Benjamin expressed to Fränkel his discontent with the drug, but at the same time complained he hadn't been given enough. When he repeatedly refused to tell Fränkel his revelation about *Struwwelpeter*, the doctor speculated: 'Punishment for the insufficient dosage'.[48] In the final jotted phrases of his notes, Benjamin wrote 'Wisdom of impertinence'.[49]

※　※　※

Sartre and Benjamin both approached mescaline with ambivalence, looking for a detached viewpoint from which they could observe its phenomena without drowning in them. Not so the poet, dramatist and Surrealist *manqué* Antonin Artaud. His journey to Mexico in January 1936 to take peyote was a leap into the void. He wanted an experience that would immolate all traces of western civilisation: as he put it, 'to throw off this abominable enslavement which I knew very well did not come from me'.[50] His journey took him to the brink of madness, or perhaps beyond; it's hard to tell as he never fully returned to sanity. Nevertheless, the 'two or three days' of his peyote trip seemed to him at the time 'the happiest days of my life'.[51]

Artaud conceived his journey during the dark days after the failure of his play *Les Censi*, his first and last attempt to put his theory of the Theatre of Cruelty into practice, which had closed in Paris after seventeen days. 'The French public,' he concluded, 'is not ripe enough for a feast fit for the gods.'[52] He embarked for Mexico under the impression that its revolution had returned it to the pre-Hispanic culture that prevailed before the arrival of Cortés. He was captivated by ethnographic descriptions of the Tarahumara, whom he conceived as a 'race of lost men' who stood apart from modernity and who 'live as if they were already dead. They do not see reality and they draw magical powers from the contempt they have for civilisation.'[53]

The source of their power, he learned from his reading, was the peyote rite, the 'mystery of mysteries', through which participants became 'immersed in the original mythic arcana'.[54] To be possessed, dismembered and reborn in this way was unthinkable to the modern European, who 'would believe himself mad and people would probably say that he had become a lunatic'.[55] But this was precisely because the rite struck at the root of modernity's sickness, 'that infernal coalition of creatures who have taken over and are polluting our consciousness just as they are disordering Reality'.[56] Peyote, Artaud intuited, marked a deep racial and cultural divide between the savage world of the Indian and the civilised west. As such it offered him 'a way of no longer being "white", that is, one whom the spirits have abandoned'.[57]

Artaud arrived in Mexico City armed for magical protection with a stiletto he had bought en route from an African sorcerer in Havana. He was distraught to discover that the revolution had not ushered in a return to the Aztec world but merely another form of modernity.

'There is no Mexican art in Mexico,' he declared.[58] Local contacts he had met in Paris arranged for him to give a series of paid lectures at the university – 'Surrealism and Revolution', 'Man against Destiny', 'The Theatre and the Gods' – and he acquired a permit to travel to the northern deserts. On his arrival there he discovered that peyote was still regarded by the revolutionary administration as the Devil's root. The mestizo director of the native school where he stayed was convinced that Indian culture had to be dismantled, and government officers were constantly occupied in destroying the peyote fields. Artaud pleaded with him that 'they will never forgive you for this destruction, but you can show them by an opposite action that you are not an enemy of God'.[59] 'The trouble,' the director replied, 'is that when they have taken Peyote, they no longer obey us.'[60]

The ancient mysteries began to reveal themselves to Artaud as soon as he entered Tarahumara country, before he had even met its human inhabitants. 'This Sierra,' he wrote, 'the Tarahumara have covered with signs, signs that are completely conscious, intelligent and purposeful.' He saw the high desert landscape filled with shaped and sculpted rock formations: tortured human figures, a naked man leaning out of a window, the figure of Death with an infant in its hand. Trees were burned into the shape of the cross, or of doubled creatures facing one another: 'the landscape exhales a metaphysical thinking in its rocks'.[61] Well before he took any peyote, the mundane reality of Artaud's journey is impossible to disentangle from his visions. He was undergoing withdrawal from heroin at this point, and opiate deprivation made the strangeness of his journey and the painful ecstasy of his anticipated transfiguration even more acute. Yet this section of his narrative, composed in fine lapidary style, is a model of clarity compared to most of the texts that made up his eventual travelogue, *The Peyote Dance*. Its fragments were written over several years in an array of ever more extreme circumstances: in Mexico, on his chaotic return passage to Europe, in the grip of a quasi-religious epiphany in Ireland and after being subjected to electroshock treatment in a French asylum.

When he finally arrived at the remote Tarahumara village of Norogachic he discovered that a peyote rite was scheduled to take place that very night. After dark a priest arrived with two assistants, drew a semicircle in the dirt and poured some dried and powdered peyote into the hands of the villagers. They took it and began to dance; as he watched the weave of their motion, Artaud 'thought [he] could see the point where the universal unconscious is sick'.[62] Afterwards he questioned the priest, who told him 'everything I say comes from Ciguri' – the Tarahumara term for peyote first recorded by Carl Lumholtz – and poured a heap of powder 'the size of a ripe almond' into Artaud's hand. This would be 'enough', he told him, 'to see God two or three times'.[63]

What Artaud saw was not God but himself. 'Peyote leads the self back to its true sources,' he wrote. In this sense it was a profane illumination, one in which all cosmic systems and higher powers were exposed as empty: 'with peyote man is alone, desperately scraping out the music of his own skeleton'. Yet it revealed to him that 'there is in consciousness a Magic that can go beyond things. And Peyote tells us where this Magic is.'[64] It sifts reality from illusion; it 'fixes the mind and prevents it from wandering, from surrendering to false impressions'.[65]

After this point Artaud's reportage becomes a palimpsest in which realities and timelines double and merge. A second narrative talks of twenty-eight days of waiting in the desolate village, of inscrutable preparations for the great annual peyote rite that echo Lumholtz's frustrating experience with the Huichol. Sorcerors and their messengers scurried up and down the mountains, neutralising the evil spirits, assembling the priests and ritual objects: 'the alcohol, the crosses, the mirrors, the rasping sticks, the jars'.[66] Finally, one day the commotion died down: 'I had suffered enough, it seems to me, to be rewarded with a little reality.'[67] The ceremony was about to begin. As dusk fell, he had a vision of Hieronymus Bosch's *Nativity*,[68] and the sorcerers processed down the mountain 'leaning on huge staffs, their women carrying huge baskets, the servants armed with bundles of crosses like firewood, and mirrors that glittered like segments of sky'.[69] Fires were lit, dancing commenced, ten crosses were driven into the ground. A magic circle was drawn, and within it the great peyote dance began.

From his reading Artaud had gleaned that the Great Feast of Ciguri was held once a year 'according to the age-old traditional rites'.[70] The shattering visionary experience that follows is a fantasia in which ethnography merges with his ideal for the Theatre of Cruelty: a dance of creation that dissolves the boundaries between participant and spectator, performance and reality.[71] The dancer leaps 'with his army of bells, like an agglomeration of dazed bees caked together in a crackling and tempestuous disorder' around the circle in which are contained ten crosses and ten mirrors, 'the epileptic dancer and myself, for whom the rite was being performed'. The dance weaves together the two principles that animate the globe of the world, 'represented by the hermaphroditic roots of the peyote plant'.[72] All drink a 'muddy gruel' of ground-up peyote, and Artaud is told to spit it deep into the ground. He suffers 'the rite of blows on the skull'[73] and the priests sprinkle water over his head. The peyote and maize liquor take hold, driving the participants to savagery, and the dance climaxes with his crucifixion.

Artaud wrote later that from this point on his life was guided by 'the Invisible'.[74] He was in freefall, his previous identity flayed away, suspended in 'a multitudinous abyss of possibility'[75] and vulnerable at all times to unknown forces. He was surrounded by demons; he constantly made the sign of the cross and scribbled incantations. He was being persecuted, he knew, because peyote 'was not made for whites' and 'it was necessary at all costs to prevent me from obtaining a cure by this rite.'[76] On his return to Europe in 1937 he gave every sign of having lapsed into madness. He harangued his audiences at lectures, became convinced the world would end on 3 November of that year, and made an impromptu trip to Ireland to return a knotted wooden stick he believed belonged to Saint Patrick. He was thrown out of a Jesuit community in Dublin and briefly imprisoned before being deported to France as a destitute and undesirable alien. On the ferry he attacked two men who threatened him with a monkey wrench, and on arrival at Le Havre he was straitjacketed and taken to an asylum.

During the Nazi occupation Artaud was discovered by his friends near-starving and neglected in a Paris hospital and was transferred to the mental asylum at Rodez, near Toulouse. Here he was subjected to electroshock therapy by doctors who treated his obsession with magic spells and protective sigils as symptoms of schizophrenia. For his part, he described electroshock as a new form of black magic, the ultimate destruction of the individual by modernity's sorcerers. The peyote dance had led him beyond the comprehension of his own society, which could only make sense of his transfiguration through the lens of psychopathology. Over the decade to come, as the biological sciences extended psychiatry's reach, mescaline itself would be reconceived in the same way.

CHAPTER EIGHT

M-SUBSTANCE

1936–52

OKLAHOMA, TAOS, LONDON, HAMBURG,
BASEL, SASKATCHEWAN

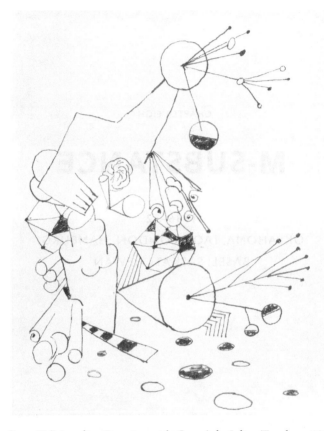

Stage II (Mescaline Drawing with Cones) *by Julian Trevelyan, 1936.*

As Artaud underwent his spiritual dismemberment in Mexico, peyote religion in the USA faced another high-level challenge to its legitimacy. The Federal Bureau of Narcotics, created in 1930 and expanded after the collapse of alcohol prohibition in 1933, was intent on extending its remit beyond those drugs – opiates and cocaine – controlled by the 1914 Harrison Act. In 1937 the Marijuana Tax Act was passed, effectively banning its sale, and despite the Native American Church's constitutional status the federal government once more had peyote in its sights. That year the New Mexico senator Dennis Chavéz submitted a bill to the Senate calling for the prohibition of peyote traffic across state lines, which would effectively constitute a ban in all states but Texas.

Peyote retained many sworn enemies, prominent among them Mabel Dodge Luhan (as she was known after marrying Tony). A series of letters from her prefaced a thick file of documents submitted to the Senate, most of which was the same anti-peyote testimony presented at the 1918 House of Representatives hearings. The bulk of the new material related to recent disputes at Taos pueblo between the peyotists and the traditional kiva worshippers, during which Dodge Luhan had urged the elders to arrest those who participated in peyote meetings. In February 1936 fifteen worshippers were charged with public disturbance, convicted and fined $100 each. They appealed to John Collier, now commissioner at the Bureau of Indian Affairs, who supported their case on grounds of freedom of religious practice. Dodge Luhan, whose friendship with Collier had cooled over the years, complained over his head to Harold Ickes, Roosevelt's secretary of the interior, the man who had recommended Collier's appointment. 'Do you really mean that you are defending *self-government* when you take the side of a few drug addicts against the efforts of the pueblo officers?' she wrote. 'Would you stand for hashish, cocaine, or morphine and defend them on the grounds of religious liberty?'[1]

By this time, however, the assimilationist policies that had driven the suppression of peyote were in retreat. In 1924 Congress had granted full US citizenship to all American Indians, and under Roosevelt and Collier the priorities of the Bureau of Indian Affairs were comprehensively reset. In 1934, after the Indian Reorganization Act, Collier published an executive order entitled 'Indian Religious Freedom and Indian Culture' that explicitly rejected assimilation in favour of cultural pluralism. Indians were to be given full access to modern knowledge and education, but they were not to be coerced into Christianity. Collier curtailed missionary activities, prohibited compulsory religious services at boarding schools and retired the Bureau's hostile pamphlets against peyote. They were replaced with a circular that enshrined the principles he had defended consistently since his early days of activism on behalf of the immigrant cultures of New York: 'no interference with Indian religious life or ceremonial expression will hereafter be tolerated'.[2]

Collier rallied a wealth of expert opinion against the bill including the most thorough fieldwork to date, which the young anthropologist Weston La Barre was in the process of writing up for his doctorate at Yale University. La Barre's study was published in 1938 as *The Peyote Cult* and over the course of many subsequent editions it became the definitive text on Native American peyote religion. Many of the tribal groups who adopted peyote over the following decades used it as their ritual handbook and bible, and in many respects it was the work that James Mooney had left unwritten at his death. Mooney, La Barre acknowledged, was 'undoubtedly the expert of the subject' but in the end had published little about it. His engagement had far exceeded that of his contemporaries, who were 'in general concerned with preserving complete records of older native cultures, and ignored or paid scant attention to the modern cult of peyote'.[3] Under the tutelage of Edward Sapir at Yale, La Barre represented a new generation of anthropologists who aimed to broaden the discipline beyond collecting artefacts and recording traditions, and drew on linguistics and psychoanalysis to elucidate the cultures and mental worlds of their subjects in their own terms.

The Peyote Cult disentangled the persistent linguistic confusions and botanical identifications surrounding the cactus, and used a combination of written records and oral tradition to track the historical diffusion of the ceremony from Mexico to Oklahoma and beyond. La Barre outlined a progression of ritual forms from the Huichol and the Tarahumara through the Mescalero Apache to the Plains ceremony, which he identified as Kiowa–Comanche, 'historically considered . . . the centre of this diffusion'.[4] In Mexico, he proposed, peyote had an essentially 'tribal' function, associated with hunting and gathering and with a ritual focus on witchcraft, divination and healing. In the American Plains it had become 'societal', a communal bonding drawing on forms of Christian worship, in which individuals were strengthened by their personal visions and confessions in the presence of their peers.[5]

While participating in ceremonies among the Kiowa in Oklahoma, La Barre noted how they were designed to incorporate and manage the spectrum of peyote's effects. Its stimulant qualities banished sleep and made all-night sessions possible, and its suppression of hunger made fasting natural. Many of the best-known songs were said to have been elaborated from the auditory hallucinations it induced. A taboo on salt during the ceremony stopped participants from becoming thirsty, and the sweetened ritual breakfast relieved the effects of low blood sugar. The sense of lassitude that characterised the early stages of intoxication was counteracted by the pounding rhythm of drum and rattle; it was after midnight, when these sensations faded and water was passed round, that, as Mooney had observed, 'the songs of those present are more vigorous',[6] lifting the participants through the hours of darkness.

'Every student of peyote,' La Barre wrote, 'has been met with a sometimes odd mixture of suspiciousness and candor.' In his experience, a sincere interest was generously rewarded and 'there is no very great difficulty in a sympathetic white man's attending a peyote meeting nowadays'.[7] The peyotists believed that the cactus had powers that protected it and its adherents against the hostility of the white man, just as in older times it had given advance visions of an enemy's approach and offered protection in battle. In many ways, La Barre observed, the federal policy of Indian assimilation had strengthened peyote's power and prestige, making it a touchstone for the lifeways the tribes were struggling to preserve. Education and resettlement policies intended to destroy Indian culture 'weakened the tradition of the older tribal religions without basically altering typical Plains religious attitudes, and multiplied friendly contacts between members of different tribes'.[8] The Native American Church was an authentically Indian response to the conditions the white man had created.

On La Barre's second visit to Oklahoma in 1936 he was joined by a twenty-one-year-old Harvard student, Richard Evans Schultes; this was to be the latter's first field trip of a sixty-year career during which he would open up a vast field of psychedelic ethnobotany, from the hallucinogenic mushrooms and morning glory seeds of Mexico to the DMT-containing snuffs and ayahuasca potions of the Amazon. Schultes had initially been inspired to study plant intoxicants by reading Heinrich Klüver's *Mescal* in the library of the Harvard Botanical Museum, and its director Oakes Ames had encouraged him to join La Barre and witness its traditional use.[9] La Barre and Schultes's grandly billed 'Harvard–Yale expedition' amounted in practice to the pair bumping across the hot and dusty Southern Plains from Philadelphia to Oklahoma in an old Studebaker. Their host and interpreter among the Kiowa was Charlie Apekaum, a game warden and navy veteran whose family had also hosted James Mooney.

Schultes's later celebrated discoveries would draw on pharmacology to identify the psychoactive agents in healing plants, particularly the combination of DMT and beta-carbolines that give the ayahuasca brew its prodigious visionary power.[10] In his report on peyote for the Harvard Botanical Museum he was working with a plant whose chemistry was already established, but he demonstrated the attention to ethnographic and ritual detail that would underlie his future discoveries. He noted that among the many plants involved in the ceremony – cedar and sage incense, mescal beans, fruits, Bull Durham tobacco rolled in corn shucks, sumac leaves, cottonwood smoke sticks – peyote was the only one that was new to Plains tradition.[11] It might be a new religion, but the ethnobotany of the ritual revealed deep roots in an extensive complex of traditions and practices. Peyote was now a significant article of commerce: arriving regularly in trailers from southern Texas and Mexico, it sold for $2.50 per thousand buttons.

Schultes joined La Barre for several peyote ceremonies, which he attended in his customary outfit of neatly buttoned shirt, pressed slacks and Harvard tie. But, as they would throughout his long career, the full-blown visionary effects of the cactus failed to materialise for him. 'I get colours,' he wrote later, 'lightninglike flashes, little stars like when you break a glass, sometimes colored smoke going by like clouds. I wish I could see visions. La Barre has tried to explain it to me, but I don't understand what he is talking about.'[12]

Both La Barre and Schultes submitted reports for the Senate Committee on Indian Affairs, along with a roster of distinguished anthropologists that included Franz Boas and Raymond Harrington, who had convened the disastrous peyote ceremony in Mabel Dodge's Greenwich Village home twenty years previously and was now curator of archaeology at the Southwest Museum in Los Angeles. Their testimony, published by the Department of the Interior as *Documents on Peyote* (1937), recommended firmly that Senator Chavéz's bill should not be enacted. It was voted down by a comfortable margin.

* * *

La Barre and Schultes were not alone among their generation in finding peyote more intriguing and significant than the bohemians of the Progressive Era had. Some of the visitors to the Luhan commune at Taos adopted it, such as Jaime de Angulo, an ethnomusicologist who spoke seventeen native American languages. De Angulo was Carl Jung's guide on his visit to Taos pueblo in 1925, acting as interpreter for Jung's conversation with the pueblo chief Ochwiay Bianco that Jung would recall at length in his 1963 *Memories, Dreams, Reflections*: de Angulo was astonished to discover that this was the first time Jung had ever spoken with a non-European. Originally a linguist at the University of California in Berkeley, he had abandoned the academy to immerse himself in shamanism, spiritual exploration and fiction written in the form of native myths, published posthumously as the bestselling *Indian Tales* (1953). De Angulo never wrote about peyote but brought its lore back with him when he returned to Berkeley where he remained, in the words of the beat poet Gary Snyder, 'a great culture hero on the West Coast' until his death in 1950. 'He never had a regular appointment,' Snyder recalled in 1970, 'he was just too wild. Burned a house down one night when drunk, rode about naked on a horse at Big Sur, member of the Native American Church.'[13]

In Southern California peyote was adopted by the flamboyant rocket scientist and occultist Jack Parsons, a founder of what is now the Jet Propulsion Laboratory in Pasadena and the resident magus of a commune he formed in the city in 1941 that centred around the Agape Lodge, a branch of Aleister Crowley's Ordo Templi Orientis. As with Crowley, it is hard to determine whether and how Parsons used peyote in his magickal workings, but it was part of an extensive phar-macopoeia, along with cocaine, marijuana and the amphetamines that Parsons synthesised in his rocket lab, that fuelled the Agape's orgiastic parties. He placed it in the opening line of the poem he contributed to the first issue of the occult lodge's journal in 1943: 'I hight Don Quixote, I live on peyote, / marijuana, morphine and cocaine, / I never knew sadness but only a madness / that burns at the heart and the brain.'[14]

This conspicuous advertisement succeeded in scandalising the ageing Aleister Crowley himself, who wrote to Jane Wolfe, an old associate from his days in Sicily, 'What could have been better calculated to revive the ancient stories about drug-traffic and so on?'[15]

The figure who pointed most clearly to the next generation's romance with peyote was Frank Waters, who met Tony Luhan on his first visit to Taos pueblo in the summer of 1937 and lived with him and Mabel on the Luhan estate while writing his best known novel, *The Man Who Killed the Deer* (1942), which he dedicated to them both.[16] Waters, who was himself part Indian, fictionalised a real-life incident from the pueblo into a drama of a young man caught between two worlds, returning to his village after education in government boarding school having fallen foul of the law by unwittingly killing a deer out of season. His journey to redemption takes in a peyote ceremony, which is introduced to him and the reader much as Tony presented it to Mabel: 'This I learned from the Cheyennes and Arapahoes,' the roadman tells him, 'and they learned it from the Kiowas . . . but the Kiowas learned it from the tribes of Mexico.'[17] During the ceremony the young man receives a vision of the peyote road, which makes him flee into the pines and mountains where he encounters the deer he killed; 'and he knew that he was an intruding stranger who had not stopped to consider this strange peace, this universal brotherhood between deer and pines and birds'.[18] He returns to the ceremony, where he learns that 'The Road leads to spiritual unity with the Great Father Peyote who in himself contains all.'[19]

Waters revered Tony Luhan as an 'older brother' and 'ceremonial uncle'[20] and this section of the novel bears his imprint, but he was also heavily influenced by Mabel, in particular her reverence for eastern religions and philosophies. She introduced him to the *I Ching* and the ideas of George Gurdjieff, whom she had met in Paris, after which Waters' explication of native American beliefs took on a universalist cast in which they merged with Hindu tantra, Jungian mythography, Robert Graves' *The White Goddess* (1948) and Walter Evans-Wentz's edition of the *Tibetan Book of the Dead* (1927). Waters' bestselling account of native spirituality, *The Book of the Hopi* (1963), was regarded by anthropologists as wildly inauthentic but became a founding text for the 1960s counterculture.

❀   ❀   ❀

By 1940 mescaline experiments were becoming widespread across psychiatry. The field was more systematically oriented around research, with the creation of university departments, professorships and large-scale clinical trials. Research was driven by new sources of funding, particularly the Rockefeller Foundation, which was drawn in by Adolf Meyer, professor at John Hopkins Medical School, and his mission to build links between practising psychiatrists, teaching hospitals and university researchers.

The Rockefeller Foundation extended its programme to Europe, taking as its base the Maudsley Hospital in London, Britain's leading centre for psychiatric research. In 1937 it funded the Maudsley's clinical director, Aubrey Lewis, to undertake a fact-finding trip around Europe's psychiatric institutions and report on the state of scientific knowledge. Lewis interviewed the staff of a clinic in Amsterdam where EEG readings were being taken from monkeys dosed with mescaline, pharmacologists in Kraków who had been trialling its use as a psychiatric medication, and doctors at the Military Academy in Leningrad who had been using it to study hallucinations. In Finland he met a professor working with the eyes of decapitated frogs, to whom he recommended that 'this was a field in which investigation into the effects of such drugs as mescaline, and also the changes that accompany visual hallucinations might be studied with profit'.[21]

At this moment a major research project using mescaline was under way at the Maudsley Hospital itself. From 1933 onwards, Jewish psychiatrists removed from posts in Germany by the Nazi regime were sponsored by the Rockefeller Foundation to relocate to Britain and several were offered scholarships at the Maudsley. These included Kurt Beringer's colleague Wilhelm Mayer-Gross, who had become a professor at Heidelberg in 1929, and a fellow psychiatrist from Breslau, Eric Guttman. Guttman teamed up with a Scottish psychiatrist, Walter Maclay, and secured Rockefeller funding for a project testing mescaline on the hospital's psychiatric patients. Karl Heinrich Slotta, another European émigré and a biochemist at the Maudsley's neurosurgical unit, provided the mescaline, following the synthesis described by Ernst Späth in his paper of 1919.

Guttman and Maclay were particularly interested in depersonalisation, the state in which a subject's sense of their body becomes lost and their thoughts seem beyond conscious control. This syndrome was often observed in patients diagnosed with schizophrenia and also reported experimentally under mescaline. They considered that the 300mg typically used to generate visions might produce unnecessary distress in mental patients, as might the method of injection, and consequently administered mescaline to their subjects in smaller doses dissolved in water. They noted changes in mood and emotional tone, but even at this mild dose they were highly inconsistent. In Beringer's subjects euphoria had predominated, but he had been working with healthy, excited and curious medical students. Among mental patients, Guttman and Maclay recorded a few cheerful responses but more who were 'bewildered' or 'depressed and anxious', and some curious emotional arcs including 'contented, later depressed' and 'depressed, later slightly euphoric'.[22] In some cases, they concluded, mescaline seemed to allow patients some insight into their feelings of depersonalisation, with one announcing 'I have seen that I can be as I used to be before.'[23] In most, however, there was no therapeutic consequence and patients were easily able to distinguish the effects of the drug from their habitual sense of depersonalisation.

The parallels between the effects of mescaline and the symptoms of schizophrenia, Guttman and Maclay decided, might be better explored through the medium of art. Studying drawings produced by psychotic patients at the Maudsley and the Royal Bethlem Hospital, the larger mental hospital with which it was associated, they suggested that 'the character of these hallucinations is very similar to what people describe as their experience during mescalin [*sic*] intoxication, especially the intensification of colours, the distortion of shapes, the apparent movements and the repetition of lines and patterns'.[24] They studied the work of artists-turned-patients such as Louis Wain, who had been a popular illustrator specialising in cartoon cats before being confined to a series of mental hospitals including Bethlem, and whose work included some dazzlingly colourful and abstract compositions.[25] They also studied spontaneous drawings – in the recently popularised slang term, 'doodles' – and persuaded a newspaper to solicit them from its readers for a competition. This generated some nine thousand entries which filled two sacks, each of which took two men to lift.[26]

In the course of their researches Guttman and Maclay came to recognise that 'only a minority of patients have the capacity and drive' to turn their mental landscapes into art, 'especially while they are under the fascinating impression of the acute psychotic experience'.[27] This suggested to them a new project: mescaline experiments with professional artists whose work under the influence of the drug could be compared with that of psychotic patients. They decided that Surrealist artists might be fruitful collaborators as many of them had an existing interest in Freud and theories of the unconscious, and used techniques such as dream diaries and automatic drawing in their work. They made enquiries via Lionel Penrose, professor of psychology at University College London, whose brother Roland was a member of the small and tightly knit group of British Surrealists. They succeeded in recruiting several participants including Julian Trevelyan, who had begun his career in Paris working alongside Max Ernst, Joan Miró and Picasso and was one of the organisers of London's International Surrealist Exhibition of 1936, and Basil Beaumont, who had also studied in Paris at the modernist Académie de la Grande Chaumière and subsequently established the Society for Creative Psychology in London.[28]

The experiences of the artists turned out to be as unpredictable as those of the patients. Trevelyan recalled being driven to the hospital in the morning and injected with mescaline crystals in solution at around 10 o'clock; after an hour of slight nausea, 'suddenly the fireworks started, with their magical transfiguration of everything I looked at'.[29] His hand shook as he attempted to draw what he was seeing, 'yet while it lasted I could not put a line wrong; the line was no longer on the surface of the paper but quivering in space like a wire. Perspectives and recessions dripped off my pencil.' When he shut his eyes 'a world of cosmic imagery, a sort of mechanical ballet, became visible'. After a couple of hours he was taken to lunch in the hospital canteen, where 'I remember sitting at a table amongst white-coated doctors, with a plate of spaghetti and cauliflower in front of me, whose intricate forms fascinated me beyond belief.'

Trevelyan took mescaline on two subsequent occasions and felt, much as Havelock Ellis had, that its primary effect was 'the hyper-awareness of the beauty of things'. This heightened sensation endured long after the experiment was over, and instilled in him the truth of Constable's statement that 'I never saw an ugly thing in my life'.[30] 'Under Mescalin [*sic*],' he wrote, 'I have fallen in love with a sausage roll . . . I have also looked at pictures by Picasso, Van Gogh, Michelangelo, and others, and have rejected them all as "ready-mades".' Some of his productions under the influence are labelled 'Stage 1' and others 'Stage 2', denoting those produced under the influence and after it had worn off: they are surprisingly similar to one another, and not very different from the geometrical clusters of cones and branches that he had produced on occasion before the experiment. He felt 'they have remained valid, though I know they are not great works of art', but 'only the traveller's sketches from that surprising region of the mind, from which, without Mescalin, I am forever debarred'.[31]

Basil Beaumont's experiment began identically with an injection at 10 o'clock but unfolded quite differently. He felt sick, cold and shivery, afflicted with twitching feet and hands and a feeling of paralysis around the injection site. The trees outside the window 'became waving, serpentine forms like octopuses',[32] and the walls of the room filled with Aztec designs that put him in mind of human sacrifices. Colour formations unfurled, 'never reaching a climax; pure colour and sound without orchestration, rest or pause – almost unendurable'. 'Excruciating pain and fear' blended with 'exquisite beauty of form and sound' in ways that he found impossible to communicate: 'it was too painful and too wonderful'. Time 'went very wrong', expanding and contracting; doctors came in and out, asking him questions. Dr Guttman appeared as 'a most diabolical goat', though Beaumont was keenly aware that he remained his only connection to sanity.

At Guttman's insistence, over Beaumont's objections, they went for lunch. The walk to the canteen was interminably long, through undulating corridors; Beaumont was seated at a table with Guttman and another experimental subject who kept asking, 'And is this the state actually known as the psychosis, doctor?' Other doctors arrived; Beaumont recalled that 'I thought they were making fun of me, then I thought they were mental patients; finally I decided that they had all been injected with the drug.' Tea in the clubroom, amid conversation about 'Fascism, Communism and the Jews', was an excruciating ordeal that Beaumont decided must be some sort of psychological test. Then somehow it was dusk and Guttman led him into the garden, where 'suddenly I believed that I was to be offered as a sacrifice'. The doctor hoped that fresh air would bring him round, but he was constantly being drawn 'miles and miles away into the world of illusions'.

As night fell a taxi was summoned and Beaumont, in the company of another experimental subject, was driven to the home of his psychoanalyst, Dr Karin Stephen, in Bloomsbury. When he arrived there he was convinced it was a simulacrum or stage set (he later discovered that it had, in fact, been recently redecorated). After he told Stephen that he believed her to be an impostor, 'it was decided that I should be better spending the night in the M. [Maudsley] hospital'. When he arrived back he was led to a general ward of mental patients; he 'could not take my gaze off the locks on the doors' and 'could not believe that Dr. G. was going to leave me there'. After a terrifying night of hallucinations, he was given breakfast and conversed with a nurse who 'gave me the impression I should be there for at least two weeks'.[33] Finally Guttman arrived, discussed the experiment and made notes, and Beaumont was released.

Karin Stephen was appalled by Guttman's conduct. He had inflicted on his subject, she wrote to him, 'an experience so hideous that no human being ought to undergo it without the very gravest necessity'.[34] He had at different points during the ordeal had murderous delusions and suicidal thoughts. Guttman assured her that 'I did not start giving Mescalin light heartedly or without adequate preliminary investigation,'[35] although he confessed he had been unaware that Beaumont was undergoing psychoanalysis. He had 'myself taken it in larger doses than I gave to Mr. Beaumont', and had taken precautions against 'suicidal or homicidal ideas which come up to the surface of consciousness during such an intoxication just as they do during psychotherapy'. He had subsequently received a note from Beaumont which described a much more rewarding experience. Generally, Guttman assured her, 'the anxiety is forgotten and there remains the recollection of a most interesting and fascinating experiment'.[36]

Beaumont's short note to Guttman made no mention of his trauma, apart from thanking him 'for all the trouble you took with me that night. I must have been very tiresome I am sure.' He went on to write that 'My appreciation of beauty, particularly flowers, is still enhanced greatly. My painting is becoming more brilliant in colour I think.'[37] Trevelyan was probably referring to Beaumont when he wrote later, 'There were other members of our little surrealist group who lent themselves to Mescalin; some had interesting hallucinations, but others who suffered from secret griefs were reduced to a state of acute hysteria; for Mescalin transports only those who are carefree travellers.'[38]

Guttman and Maclay's experiments inspired another clinical study at Warlingham Park Mental Hospital in nearby Croydon, where an assistant medical officer, G. Tayleur Stockings, had been administering the sedative sodium amytal to patients diagnosed with schizophrenia, after which he found them more able to give coherent accounts of their mental states. Reading Guttman and Maclay's work suggested to Stockings that mescaline might achieve similar results. He began by acquiring some from the London office of the pharmacy giant Burroughs Wellcome and administered it to 'a group of normal adults of ages from twenty to thirty years' and to himself. He noted that the drug produced some of the same physical symptoms, such as dry lips and tongue, flushed complexion and unnaturally bright eyes, as 'an acute toxic confusional psychosis or acute schizophrenic episode'.[39] He enumerated the similarities – hallucinations, delusions, disturbances of the intellect and the will – as many had before him, and much as Jacques-Joseph Moreau had with hashish a century earlier. He detected a 'close similarity of the art-forms and symbolism of the ancient Mexicans and Central Americans, who use mescaline freely in their religious rites, to the symbolic drawings of schizophrenic patients'.[40]

From these findings, however, he reached a novel conclusion: that the similarities might point to a shared chemical cause, 'probably a toxic amine with chemical and pharmacological properties similar to those of mescaline, and having a selective action on the various higher centres of the brain'.[41] Mescaline might achieve its hallucinatory effects, in other words, because of its chemical similarity to an organically occurring toxin that causes psychosis. This was the theory that launched psychiatry on the path that would, on that bright May morning in 1953, introduce mescaline to Aldous Huxley.

🌿   🌿   🌿

During the 1930s mescaline had occasionally been considered, along with more or less every other psychoactive drug, as a potential 'truth serum',[42] with the potential to elicit private and sensitive information from subjects under its influence. Across Europe and the US, experiments along these lines gained pace with the arrival of the Second World War and the loosening of peacetime codes of patient consent and safety. Though they came to focus on scopolamine, barbiturates, methedrine and the sodium compounds pentothal and amytal, mescaline was the first drug trialled in Washington, DC, in 1942 by a 'Truth Drug Committee' established by the recently formed Office of Strategic Services, the forerunner of the CIA, under the supervision of Dr Winfred Overhoser, director of the federally operated St Elizabeth's Mental Hospital. It was quickly rejected on the grounds that it made subjects too nauseous to trust their interrogators, and the committee proceeded to try marijuana instead.[43]

By this time there were suspicions that the Germans were using mescaline as a truth serum. A communication intercepted by British code-breakers at Bletchley Park indicated that injecting parachutists with scopolamine had shown some success and 'therefore experiments with mescaline are to be undertaken'.[44] But the full atrocity of such experiments only became clear after the war, when they were described to the US Naval Technical Mission in Europe by medical officers at Auschwitz and Dachau.[45] The appalling 'aviation tests' in Block 5 at Dachau, in which captive subjects were crushed and frozen to death, also included attempts to 'eliminate the will of the person examined' with drugs including mescaline, 'a Mexican drug that has been reputed to dissolve repressions and encourage talkativeness'.[46] Thirty subjects, mostly Jewish, Romani or Russian, were given mescaline in coffee. It turned out to be a disappointing truth serum. Responses were unpredictable: some prisoners became 'furious, in other cases very gay or melancholy'.[47] The nausea was distracting, as were the hallucinations. The only consistency was in the prisoners' attitude to their captors, where 'sentiments of hatred and revenge were exposed in every case'.[48]

The tests were run by Dr Kurt Plötner, a lecturer at the University of Leipzig, who after the war was promptly recruited by the CIA and in 1950 began work with them on Project BLUEBIRD, a secret programme of research into behaviour modification and mind control that would later develop into the notorious MK-ULTRA project. Other German doctors, however, were exploring mescaline's potential for therapy. In 1938 the Hamburg psychiatrist Walter Frederking had begun to administer it in mild doses to produce 'drug-induced dream-like states'[49] in which the patient's childhood memories and symbolic associations could be explored more rapidly and deeply than by talk therapy alone. Mescaline made patients easy to direct in conversation, and was especially conducive to approaching delicate subjects such as marital relations or impotence. At larger doses of 300–500mg his patients 'found the mescaline effect to be overpowering, deeply moving, elemental, spacious'.[50] There was a risk of abrupt and intense mood changes, but also the potential for profound insights that could radically shorten the course of treatment.

After the war Frederking became acquainted with the author Ernst Jünger, who had moved in 1939 to the village of Kirchhorst, between Hanover and Hamburg, where he was attempting to recapture his pre-war life of 'meditations, prolonged reading, walks on the moors and the wooded plains, little get-togethers with a small circle of intimate friends',[51] while sitting out the four years during which he was banned from publishing by the occupying British forces for refusing to submit to their 'Denazification' process. Jünger had spent much of his life experimenting with drugs, though he would not write about them directly until the late 1960s. Before the First World War he had been initiated into the rites of Bacchus – or, as he preferred, Gambrinus, descendent of 'the Æsir, the eight Nordic gods, those prodigious drinkers of mead'[52] – in youthful camping trips to the mountains as part of the back-to-nature *Wandervögel* movement. The Great War had been the making of him both as a soldier and an author with his powerful memoir of the Western Front, *Storm of Steel* (1920). 'After the First World War,' he later wrote, 'something supervened . . . a sense of claustrophobia, or suffocation.'[53] Having tested himself to the limit and stared death in the face, he found the ignoble compromises of Weimar democracy and the regimented utopias of totalitarianism equally unappealing. Drugs became for him the continuation of war by other means. In hospital in 1918 after narrowly surviving an artillery attack he experimented extensively with ether, and in 1920s Berlin with cocaine. Subsequently he moved on to opium and hashish. He knew of mescaline at that time but never encountered it, and consequently when he met Frederking the possibility 'excited my imagination with the prospect of all kinds of fabulous adventures'.[54]

Like Walter Benjamin, Jünger was in thrall to the drug writings of Baudelaire, but he read them very differently. Where Benjamin saw the potential for political resistance in expanded consciousness, Jünger saw a weapon of the individual against society. He had by this point elaborated an expansive cultural history around drugs and the pursuit of *Rausch*.[55] In his scheme the New World had a different historical trajectory from the Old. In the traditional cultures of the Americas, *Rausch* had never been overthrown, and ecstatic intoxication had remained at its cultural core. He resisted the term 'psychedelic' when it emerged, preferring his own coinage 'Mexican drugs' to descibe mescaline, LSD and psilocybin, reflecting what he regarded as their botanical and cultural homeland.

Jünger traced the culture of *Rausch* in western civilisation back to the mystery religions of classical antiquity, after which the cult of intoxication had been overthrown by Christianity. It had been rediscovered in the nineteenth century by the likes of Baudelaire and Thomas De Quincey and 'around their trunk a whole new literature grew like a vine'. But the Romantics and the *fin-de-siècle* Decadents conceived themselves as outcasts and their ecstatic pursuit of *Rausch* was rejected by the masses as 'a theft from society'.[56] Jünger, raised on Nietzschean individualism and, as a friend of Martin Heidegger, on phenomenology ('philosophy in the virgin jungle', as he called it),[57] was the avatar of a new culture that would embrace it wholeheartedly. When he met Walter Frederking he was working on his futuristic novel *Heliopolis* (1949), which featured a drugs researcher who 'captured dreams, just as others seem to pursue butterflies with nets' and 'went on voyages of discovery in the universe of his brain'.[58] Jünger would later coin the enduring term 'psychonaut' to describe such inner explorers.

Jünger hosted Frederking at his cottage on several occasions, and in January 1950 Frederking arranged for them to take mescaline together at a spacious private house on the edge of Stuttgart. They took the initial dose at about three in the afternoon, and another an hour later. After some mild nausea Jünger was 'immersed in visions, meditations, visual and auditory perceptions' until early evening. When 'the flow of images was no longer sufficient', he insisted on a third, stronger dose.[59]

Frederking performed a Chinese dance wearing 'a lampshade on his head, as if it was a conical straw hat worn by the peasants of the rice paddies'. Jünger felt that Frederking's abilities 'embraced much more than psychologists could offer, in general': he had 'the artistic substance', without which knowledge 'turns insipid, as if it lacked salt'.[60] Under mescaline, he pronounced, 'the therapist enters the domains of the priest . . . only they can lead us by the hand, far away, towards the nameless and even a little further'.[61]

Jünger took mescaline several more times but 'did not succeed in re-experiencing the intensity of the first trip' with Frederking in Stuttgart. During a solitary experiment at home looking at a snow-covered field, with a dog howling in the distance, 'the sinister predominated'. He gazed at his bookshelf and sensed acutely the folly of believing that authorship was a form of immortality; rather, it is 'a minor loan limited in time'. This was a painful realisation and 'it is good that our perception filters it'. But for the modern individual 'only thus does the mask fall and we recognise that the sinister is in reality our home – only by passing through estrangement can we recover the confidence in what is normal'.[62]

🌲   🌲   🌲

By this time Jünger was in correspondence with an avid fan named Albert Hofmann, a research chemist working for Sandoz Pharmaceuticals in Basel, Switzerland, who had recently developed the chemical that would within a few years eclipse mescaline. 'My first correspondence with Ernst Jünger,' Hofmann recalled, 'had nothing to do with drugs; rather I once wrote to him on his birthday, simply as a grateful reader.'[63] The correspondence quickly turned to LSD, which Hofmann had first synthesised at the Sandoz laboratory in 1938 while testing derivatives of ergotamine, an alkaloid derived from the ergot fungus, in the search for a vasoconstrictor to treat haemorrhages. By chemical cleavage he produced lysergic acid, a rather unstable compound that he combined with a sequence of different amines. The twenty-fifth in this series, lysergic acid diethyla-mide, was labelled LSD-25. In 1943 – on the strength, according to his later memoir, of 'a peculiar presentiment' – he resynthesised it, after which he felt a slight dizziness and 'dream-like state'.[64] At 4.20 p.m. on 19 April he took 'the smallest quantity that could be expected to produce some effect',[65] a quarter of a milligram, and set off home on his bicycle. That afternoon and evening, during which (by his later account) his world dissolved into a galaxy of kaleidoscopic spirals and fountains, stands together with Aldous Huxley's bright May morning as the origin myth of the psychedelic era.

Hofmann recognised that the action of LSD on the mind 'was not new to science. It largely matched the commonly held view of mesca-line.'[66] He recalled the work of Beringer and Klüver a generation previ-ously, and the fact that mescaline had demonstrated no medical applications. The significant difference between them was LSD's extraor-dinary potency: what he had expected to be a barely perceptible threshold dose had turned out to be a full-blown psychedelic ordeal. 'The active dose of mescaline, 0.2 to 0.5g,' he realised, 'is comparable to 0.00002 to 0.0001g of LSD; in other words, LSD is some 5000 to 10,000 times more active than mescaline!'[67] By 1943 Sandoz were breeding new strains of barley and ergot to extract ergotamine in bulk, and they moved swiftly into production of LSD under the brand name Delysid. Unsure of the appropriate dosage or medical applications, they made it available to research institutes and psychiatrists as an experimental drug, offering it free in return for clinical feedback.

In February 1951 Hofmann had the 'great adventure' of an LSD experiment with Jünger, who became his mentor in the programme of inner exploration that had unexpectedly been thrust upon him. It was the first LSD trip ever undertaken outside the context of clinical research and Hofmann set the stage with aesthetic stimuli: red-violet roses, and Mozart's concerto for flute and harp. 'In mutual astonish-ment' the pair contemplated 'the haze of smoke that ascended with the ease of thought from a Japanese incense-stick', and as the effects became more powerful they fell silent and closed their eyes. Jünger 'enjoyed the colourful phantasmagoria of oriental images; I was on a trip among Berber tribes in north Africa, saw coloured caravans and lush oases'.[68] But the dose that was sufficient for Hofmann was far too cautious for Jünger, who concluded that 'compared with the tiger mescaline, your LSD is, after all, only a pussycat'.[69]

Jünger reported on his experience to Frederking, who sourced some LSD from Hofmann and introduced it into his psychiatric practice. As one of the few clinicians who had been using mescaline for years, he was able to make a closer comparison than most of the early researchers. Putting aside the huge difference in potency, he concluded that mescaline was the more 'overpowering' of the two, with a deeper psychic reach, and should be preferred to LSD 'in cases where the strongest possible emotional upheaval is desired'.[70] LSD, by contrast, was easier to dose with precision and more 'circumscribed' in its effects, concerned mostly with 'pleasurable and unpleasant sensations'. In this respect its effect was comparable to manic-depressive mood disorders, whereas mescaline's was often 'interspersed with tensions almost schizophrenic in nature'.[71] As his practice continued Frederking found himself using LSD more frequently than mescaline, since its interventions could be more precisely targeted and it could be 'used more often without the risk of harmful effects'.[72]

🌸　　🌸　　🌸

The discovery of LSD came at a transformative moment for psychiatry. Its first International Congress, held in Paris in September 1950, demonstrated that biological and chemical approaches had attained a critical mass. Delegates were presented with new research on metabolic systems in the brain, findings from chromosome studies, conclusions drawn from EEG data and thyroid activity measured by radioactive isotopes, much of it developed over the previous decade with support from the Rockefeller Foundation and similar funding bodies. Drawn by these advances in brain science, more medical graduates were choosing psychiatry than ever before: in 1951 the American Psychiatric Association had 8,500 members, up from 3,000 in 1940. Their ambitions fuelled a trend away from practice in mental hospitals and towards research programmes that were being driven and shaped by pharmaceutical companies such as Sandoz as much as by the universities. Psychiatry was developing a hard scientific core, with psychopharmacy at its centre.

The first major pharmaceutical breakthrough of the new era was every bit as unexpected as Albert Hofmann's discovery of LSD. The French neurosurgeon Henri Laborit was searching for a compound to potentiate anaesthesia and minimise surgical shock when in 1950 he synthesised an antihistamine derivative, chlorpromazine, that had unusual sedative qualities. In informal trials with patients suffering from psychotic disorders at the Sainte-Anne Hospital in Paris, he found they became not groggy but calm and indifferent to their mental disturbances. In some cases the chronically withdrawn and catatonic were miraculously restored to full consciousness. Chlorpromazine was licensed in the USA in 1954 under the brand name Thorazine by Smith, Kline & French, who were expanding rapidly thanks to their successful antidepressant Dexamyl, a combination barbiturate and amphetamine. Thorazine was orginally marketed as an anti-emetic but as news of its remarkable calming effects on schizophrenic patients spread it was prescribed by psychiatrists and became a mainstay of mental hospital regimes. The optimism with which it was adopted was such that it was given to around 50 million people before it became clear that its side effects included tardive dyskinesia, an incurable neurological condition.

The near-simultaneous arrival of chlorpromazine and LSD transformed research into psychotic disorders, in particular schizophrenia. If mescaline and LSD could instigate a model psychosis, chlorpromazine could now switch it off. The classification of mental disorders proposed by Emil Kraepelin fifty years previously had always lacked an essential component: it was a list of diseases without a corresponding list of cures. Now the combination of 'psychotomimetics', as mescaline and LSD were known in the new psychiatry, and 'antipsychotics' – chlorpromazine and its successors such as haloperidol – promised to unlock the mysteries of mental illness. If psychoses responded to chemical stimuli, they must have a biochemical basis and potentially a pharmaceutical cure.

Mescaline's new role as psychotomimetic brought it into the mainstream of psychiatric research for the first time, but it pushed its subjective effects to the margins. The experience it produced was not under investigation; researchers rarely took it themselves, administering it instead to lab rats or day-old chicks. Dozens of studies attempted to establish whether its effects were associated with changes in metabolism, such as endocrine activity; whether its metabolites could be detected in urine; whether it produced electrical or biochemical changes in the brain; how soon after birth its functions were detectable. Some psychiatrists, such as Herbert Denber at the Manhattan State Hospital in New York, experimented with administering mescaline in combination with chlorpromazine to mental patients with diagnoses of schizophrenia. Denber recorded some of his patients' responses, which included 'like an emotional brain wash' and 'a horror, a torture chamber'.[73] He noted that 'aggressivity and hostility' was often directed at figures of authority, 'usually the physician'.[74]

In psychotomimetic terms, LSD's extraordinary potency made it a precision tool. Mescaline, in common with other psychoactive drugs such as cannabis and opium, had been regarded by early psychiatrists such as Emil Kraepelin and Karl Jaspers as a poison that achieved its mind-altering effects by flooding or overwhelming normal brain functions. The effect of LSD at tiny microgram doses, by contrast, suggested that it was acting on a very specific chemical trigger mechanism, and it quickly rose to become the research chemical of choice. But mescaline had one quality that LSD lacked, and which generated the boldest of the early biological hypotheses. It was the brainchild of two British psychiatrists, Humphry Osmond, a senior psychiatric resident at St George's Hospital in London, and John Smythies, a young researcher with multi-disciplinary interests that spanned neuroanatomy, philosophy and psychical research, who began a residency at St George's in 1951.

Within two weeks of his arrival Smythies, who had been drawn to the mind sciences after a spontaneous mystical experience while studying medicine at Cambridge, began researching mescaline and its hallucinations. During his survey of the literature he came across the illustration in Alexandre Rouhier's *Le peyotl* of its molecular structure, which Rouhier presented alongside those of peyote's other alkaloids.[75] Smythies was struck by its simplicity and at the same time by its resemblance to adrenaline, the hormone produced in the adrenal glands that was known to modulate the activity of the sympathetic nervous system. Adrenaline was also a phenethylamine, and had been synthesised in the laboratory as far back as 1904. Along with Osmond, who shared his interest in the mental phenomena of schizophrenia, Smythies ordered a sample of mescaline from the London medical suppliers Lights Chemical.

Osmond was the guinea pig for an experience that he would within a few years christen 'psychedelic' but at this point conceived as psychotomimetic. He took 400mg of mescaline in Smythies' apartment just off Wimpole Street, in the centre of London's medical district, accompanied by Smythies, his wife Vanna, who was a nurse, and another friend with a tape recorder. The drug announced itself to Osmond with a building sense of unease and tension, summoning vivid memories of 'dangerous times in the past',[76] particularly London during the Blitz, which Osmond had endured while at Guy's Hospital medical school. The tape recorder glowed with menacing purples and reds, and the room shivered: 'I knew that behind those perilously unsolid walls something was waiting to burst through.'[77] Osmond's companions took him outside for some fresh air but the city's streets seemed even more threatening, with passers-by covered in warts and a child with a pig-like face staring through a window. They quickly returned. The apparently imagined fears of schizophrenics, Osmond realised, were acutely real. 'We should listen seriously to mad people,' he wrote afterwards; they experience 'voyages of the human soul that make the wanderings of Odysseus seem no more than a Sunday's outing'.[78]

Osmond's experience, combined with Smythies' observations about the mescaline molecule, prompted them to a hypothesis that they rushed into print in the *British Journal of Psychiatry*. The 'adrenosympathetic system', they argued, was 'one of the most constant features' of schizophrenia's signature symptoms of mental excitement and disturbances. Might it therefore be a 'synthetic illness', produced by a toxic substance in the brain?[79] This line of reasoning was supported by the similarity between mescaline's effects and the symptoms of schizophrenia, and also by 'the striking implications of the relationship between the bizarre Mexican cactus drug and the common hormone' adrenaline, which had 'so far as we know, never been recorded before'.[80] They summarised the similarities between mescaline and psychosis in a tabulated checklist that included sensory disorders, motor disorders, thought disorders, delusions and depersonalisation.[81]

The list was similar to the one that Wilhelm Mayer-Gross had compiled back in the 1920s; but Mayer-Gross, now at Crichton Royal Hospital in Scotland, had recently published a new paper on the subject in the *British Medical Journal* that highlighted some significant differences. Subjectively, it appeared, the two were quite easy to distinguish. 'If mescaline was given to a chronic schizophrenic,' Mayer-Gross had found, 'the patient distinguished the new phenomena and remarked on their appearance, usually laying blame for them on the same persecutors who had molested him before.'[82] Osmond and Smythies responded that 'the remarkable thing is that these these acute reactions have so much in common', and that 'mescaline reproduces every single major symptom of schizophrenia, although not always to the same degree'. The difference, in their view, was between a brief, acute intoxication with the drug as a known cause and a 'psychosis of indefinite duration in an unprepared subject'.[83] The symptoms of schizophrenia were capacious enough to find support for their hypothesis even in Mayer-Gross's report that Christian missionaries among the Native Americans 'insist that its regular intake leads to increasing laziness and impairment of will power'.[84] 'Surely,' they argued, 'a lay person might describe a chronic schizophrenic in such a phrase?'[85]

On this evidence Osmond and Smythies proposed their biological theory. It had recently been suggested that adrenaline was produced in the brain from noradrenalin by transmethylation, a breakdown process whereby a methyl group is transferred from one compound to another. Similar processes had been well studied in plants. Could transmethylation of adrenaline in the brain produce a substance similar to mescaline? The pathological process might be triggered by stress overworking the adrenal glands; there might also be a hereditary disposition to it. The presence of this substance in the brain would create distortion of perception and thoughts: in other words, the symptoms of schizophrenia. 'We therefore suggest,' they concluded, 'that schizophrenia is due to a specific disorder of the adrenals in which a failure of metabolism occurs and a mescaline-like compound or compounds are produced, which for convenience we shall refer to as "M-substance".'[86] Once triggered, the physical symptoms of schizophrenia would be compounded by social factors. Faced with an unfamiliar and threatening world of distorted perceptions, as Osmond had been in his mescaline experiment, the subject's 'painfully learned patterns of behaviour suddenly become useless and he is left isolated and enmeshed in his own fantasies and the phantasmagoria produced by M-substance'.[87]

Osmond was unable to find funding in Britain to pursue their research; he recalled that one of the directors of the Maudsley Hospital 'literally laughed at him'.[88] Smythies suspected that the consultants at St George's, committed to Freudian orthodoxies, considered newfangled biochemical theories of the mind to be 'rather bad form'.[89] Instead, Osmond answered an advertisement in the *Lancet* for a deputy director of Saskatchewan Mental Hospital, a remote institution deep in the Canadian prairie but one administered by a social democratic government committed to progressive mental health approaches, where research could be conducted with minimal bureaucratic interference.

On arrival at the hospital, a cluster of four-storey blocks among flat grasslands that receded to the horizon, Osmond teamed up with Abram Hoffer, the director of psychiatric services and a former colleague of Heinrich Klüver, who lent his distinguished support to the prospect of further mescaline research. Hoffer had begun his career as a biochemist studying vitamins and nutrition and was a skilled administrator who succeeded in attracting funding from the Canadian federal government and the Rockefeller Foundation. Smythies joined the pair in 1952 to continue the search for M-substance, working systematically through the compounds intermediate between mescaline and adrenaline. They narrowed their search to substances that 'produce psychological disturbances similar to mescaline', for which they coined a new term, 'hallucinogens'. 'As Klüver has observed,' they explained, 'when we take these remarkable compounds we enter a world beyond language', which must be expanded to accommodate them. The new category at this point included mescaline, LSD, harmine, ibogaine and hashish.[90]

As their investigations proceeded they made the curious discovery that asthmatic patients who injected themselves with adrenaline occasionally reported odd, short-lived hallucinatory effects, particularly with old pharmacy stock that had taken on a pink colour. This turned out to indicate the presence of adrenochrome, an unstable oxidisation product of adrenalin first identified in 1937 and suspected to be present in trace amounts in the human body. Its molecular structure was based around an indole nucleus, a characteristic shape combining two rings that was shared by all the recently designated hallucinogens. Hoffer, Osmond and their wives self-experimented with small amounts of the substance, which turned out to be painful to inject unless mixed with blood from the subject's vein. After a larger dose Osmond noted swarming dots across his visual field: they 'were not as brilliant as those which I have seen under mescal, but were of the same type'. He felt that he was 'in an aquarium among a shoal of brilliant fishes. At one moment I concluded that I was a sea anemone in this pool.'[91] When he left the laboratory, the world seemed 'sinister and unfriendly'; he was disconnected from his colleagues and 'felt no special interest in our experiment and had no satisfaction at our success, though I told myself it was very important'.

Hoffer, on a large dose of 5mg, had a similar sense of alienation – 'I didn't have a flicker of feeling' – and 'began to wonder whether [he] was a person anymore'.[92] They concluded that they had both experienced the depersonalisation associated with psychosis and consequently that 'adrenochrome is the first substance thought to occur in the body which has been shown to be a hallucinogen'.[93] This demonstrated, at the very least, that 'M-substance could exist' and that it might produce 'a wide variety of clinical pictures'.[94] It could be the cause of schizophrenia; it could also lead to its cure.

Based on notes that Smythies had brought with him from London, he and Osmond worked up a paper that set the potential consequences of their researches in a broader frame. Psychological medicine, they wrote, currently stood where physical medicine had in the eighteenth century; the task facing it was 'the replacement of a huge amount of inspired guesswork . . . by an ever increasing amount of surer knowledge based on the careful disciplines of science'.[95] At the same time, it was crucial to recognise that the mental phenomena with which they were dealing were not mere pathologies and their patients were more than 'skinfuls of psychochemical automata'.[96] The new biological psychiatry needed to accommodate subjective experience, bringing brain and mind into a new synthesis. The horizons of human potential were expanding, illuminated by a range of fields from electronic computing to extra-sensory perception, captured in Carl Jung's notion of the unconscious mind as 'a vast, strange and beautiful inner world more akin to the Eastern view of man'. Such vistas could readily be experienced by anyone prepared to submit themselves to a dose of mescaline, and the authors 'would have thought that anyone, concerned in devising systems of psychology based on the unconscious mind, would have utilized such a prolific source as mescaline offers, but none has yet done so'.[97]

Osmond and Smythies' paper was accepted by the *Hibbert Journal*, a British quarterly which since 1902 had published scholarly essays on religion, theology and philosophy. One of its long-time readers responded with an enthusiastic letter to the paper's authors. If Osmond or Smythies were ever passing through Los Angeles, Aldous Huxley would be most interested in trying mescaline.

CHAPTER NINE

THE DOORS BLOWN OPEN

1953–59

CALIFORNIA, WISCONSIN, MEXICO, PARIS,
ATLANTIC CITY, OXFORD

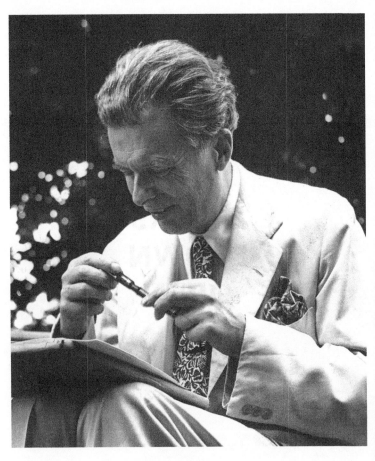

Aldous Huxley, 1952.

Osmond and Smythies' paper found Aldous Huxley at a moment of physical, mental and spiritual fragility. The process of writing his most recent book, *The Devils of Loudun*, a narrative of demonic possession in seventeenth-century France, had drained and depressed him, and he was not cheered by the book's reception, which focused on its distasteful and grotesque details of mass possessions, exorcisms and tortures. It was received more in sorrow than in anger by critics who had admired Huxley's early novels but lamented, in Osmond's paraphrase, his 'unfortunate mystical trends in his later years'.[1] He was in great pain from an eye infection and, his wife Maria wrote, 'he feels in an off mood and that he never has anything to say'.[2] He retreated into psychological and spiritual explorations – Dianetics, 'E therapy', hypnosis, extra-sensory perception – and attempts to reach his 'deeper self'. 'As one goes down through the subliminal,' he wrote, 'one passes through . . . a layer of Original Sin, if one likes to call it so – into a layer of "Original Virtue", which is one of peace, illumination and insight, which seems to be on the fringes of Pure Ego or Atman.'[3] What he sought was, in the summary on the dust jacket of his mystical anthology *The Perennial Philosophy* (1946), the 'Highest Common Factor of all theologies', which he was increasingly convinced could be accessed by neuroscientific as well as spiritual means.

His views on the role of drugs in this quest were evolving rapidly. In his early novels they had been treated, as they commonly were during the Progressive Era, as agents of dehumanisation. Most famously in *Brave New World* (1932), they were tools in the service of mental and social pacification: 'there is always *soma*, delicious *soma*, half a gramme for a half-holiday, a gramme for a week-end, two grammes for a trip to the gorgeous East . . .' *Soma* was the drug of choice for a blank post-Christian hedonism in which its devotees toasted 'I drink to my annihilation.'[4] As recently as 1952 Huxley was still writing of intoxicants as 'toxic short cuts', their 'moment of spiritual awareness' bought at a price of 'subhuman stupor, frenzy or hallucination, followed by dismal hangovers and, in the long run, by a permanent and fatal impairment of bodily health and mental power'.[5] In the epilogue to *The Devils of Loudun*, however, he had speculated that drugs might have a positive function as paths to self-transcendence. 'From poppy to curare, from Andean coca to Indian hemp and Siberian agaric', countless cultures had used them to 'go beyond the limits of the insulated ego'. Osmond and Smythies' claims for mescaline, with their bracing mix of biochemistry, parapsychology, Jung and eastern philosophy, were the perfect stimulus for his new-found curiosity.

Huxley's initial letter to Osmond shared some of his recent thinking. The self, he suggested, might be transcended by all sorts of physical and mental means: 'disease, mescaline, emotional shock, aesthetic experience and mystical enlightenment'.[6] He hoped that Osmond or Smythies might be visiting Los Angeles for the Psychiatric Congress in May, and wondered if they could bring some mescaline. Maria was worried that they might regret the invitation: 'he may have a beard and we may not like him'. But once Osmond arrived all quickly relaxed in each other's company. Both men were diffident in proposing the experiment, and Maria helped them over their British reserve by suggesting a mescaline session for the following day. Despite some residual anxiety about becoming infamous as 'the man who drove Aldous Huxley mad', Osmond returned the next morning and administered him a dose of 400mg.[7]

The effect was not at all what Huxley had anticipated. Having immersed himself thoroughly in the literature on mescaline, he envisaged that he would 'lie with my eyes shut, looking at visions of many-coloured geometries, or animated architectures, rich with gems and fabulously lovely, of landscapes with heroic figures, of symbolic dramas trembling perpetually on the edge of intimate revelation'.[8] But, as well as being partially sighted, Huxley was by his own account a poor visualiser, and his trip was far less ocularcentric than most of his predecessors'. Instead, he experienced something more remarkable: the real world, through open eyes, subtly but profoundly transformed.

Curiously for the trip that would wrest mescaline away from the psychiatrists and transform it into a tool for spiritual enlightenment,

Huxley's description reads in many respects like the 'aura' or onset of a psychotic episode. Every detail was suddenly pregnant with meaning, every thought an insight into the essence of being; the objects on which he focused were, as he put it, 'all but quivering under the pressure of the significance with which they were charged'.[9] In the psychiatrist Louis Sass's description of the phenomenology of the psychotic break, 'this sense of an uncertain yet definite shift in experience can fascinate the individual, causing him to stare intently at the world'.[10] Mescaline did not drive Huxley mad, as Osmond had feared, but it triggered what Sass called 'the truth-taking stare'. His account has the urgent, supercharged quality of what psychotherapists might describe as a 'spiritual emergency' or 'breakdown/breakthrough'. It brought a long period of accumulated mental and psychic stress to an explosive moment of truth, from which he emerged with a new narrative and direction.

Though mescaline turned out to be quite different from what he had anticipated, much of *The Doors of Perception* consists of ideas he had formulated in advance. The epiphany for which the book is best remembered is that the brain is a 'cerebral reducing valve',[11] filtering out the higher consciousness of the 'Mind at Large' that would otherwise overwhelm our ability to make sense of mundane reality. Huxley attributed this idea to the philosopher Henri Bergson, and he conceived it as an explanation for the effects of mescaline some time before he took it: he had outlined it in his first letter to Osmond a month previously.[12] Repeating the challenge that concluded Osmond and Smythies' paper, he insisted that mescaline had unaccountably been ignored by philosophers, psychologists and other explorers of the subconscious, yet he echoed many of the previous descriptions of its effects. Besides Havelock Ellis, the influence of William James is perhaps the most conspicuous, presiding over Huxley's conclusion that 'the various "other worlds" with which human beings erratically make contact' merit the scrutiny of science as 'so many elements in the totality of awareness belonging to the Mind at Large'.[13]

Huxley wrote *The Doors of Perception* fast and fluently, in a month either side of his fiftieth birthday. It was a breakthrough on every level: personal, professional and spiritual. The persona that emerged was a hybrid of old-fashioned scholar–mystic and prophet of a new age of scientific and spiritual possibility. The most striking and best remembered moment of self-description is the moment when he gazes down at his legs: 'Those folds in the trousers – what a labyrinth of endlessly significant complexity! And the texture of the grey flannel – how rich, how deeply, mysteriously sumptuous!'[14] As he stared at them he pronounced, 'This is how one ought to see.'[15] He had apparently been wearing blue jeans during the experiment, but Maria suggested he change them in the text: 'she thought I ought to be better dressed for my readers'.[16] It was an inspired suggestion. The image of Huxley on a psychedelic voyage in his grey flannels captured precisely the book's winning sense of intellectual gravitas surprised by joy.

The Doors of Perception's insights can be traced back through the decades, but its sensational reception showed how eloquently it spoke to its moment. Previous decades had lacked the germ of a mass culture of spiritual transcendence or the belief that drugs might be a route to it. Huxley's erudite synthesis wove into a multicoloured tapestry the many faces that mescaline had shown at different points throughout the twentieth century: the marvel of science, the native spirit medicine, the sublime stimulus to art, the miracle drug of psychiatry, the revealer of hidden dimensions of mind. It reigned over the short years of mescaline's ascendancy, during which it became both a talisman for an emerging generation of seekers and a source of fascination for a mainstream readership who were being informed daily of a revolution in the chemical understanding of the mind. Huxley was emblematic of both constituencies: an adept of spiritual self-discovery, but also a stand-in for a sober general public to whom, until the arrival of mescaline, all mind-altering drugs had been 'dope', of interest only to bohemians, foreigners and criminals.

In the months before Huxley published *The Doors of Perception*, the psychiatric claims for mescaline had already become a topic of general interest. In July 1953 *Time* magazine presented Hoffer, Smythies and Osmond's theories in a feature entitled 'Mescaline and the Mad Hatter', with Smythies describing visions of 'the utmost poetical integrity' and urging further studies of their transmethylation hypothesis, after which it 'will either join countless others on the scrap heap of psychiatry or the cause of schizophrenia will be known'.[17] *Newsweek* followed with a piece on 'Mescal Madness' that quoted G. Tayleur Stockings' obscure paper from 1940, with its claim that the drug was 'of the greatest importance as a method of approach to the understanding of mental disorder'.[18] The buzz of scientific currency breathed fresh life into Huxley's perennial philosophy: what the literary critics had dismissed as dreary metaphysics and crank theories was now grounded in the neurochemistry that was transforming the understanding of the brain.

The book's fusion of science and spirituality was perfectly captured in John Woodcock's design for the jacket of the British edition, perhaps the first that could be classed, slightly *avant la lettre*, as psychedelic. Three brightly coloured diagrammatic eyes – along with Heinrich Klüver's spirals, the defining visual motif of the psychedelic era to come – are stacked upon one another, their pupils filled with atomic particles, strange geometrical structures and abstract red flashes of energy: the visual language of science warped and stretched into mysterious cosmic dimensions. Huxley had struggled, as William James had before him, to explain how a chemical compound could extend the reach of the mind beyond normal consciousness to unveil the mysteries of the cosmos. The image captured this paradox and gestured at its resolution in a radically expanded conception of science and human possibility, in which the galactic realms of space and the infinitesimal world of subatomic particles are ultimately motes in the mind's eye.

✴   ✴   ✴

Mescaline captured the spirit of the age, but behind the headlines LSD was already replacing it. By 1956 Alfred Hubbard – a former huckster and alleged spy turned president of the Uranium Corporation of Vancouver – had become the 'Johnny Appleseed of LSD', ordering forty-three cases of liquid vials of Delysid from Sandoz with which he would later turn on Timothy Leary. The same year, the Beverley Hills psychiatrist Oscar Janiger began using Delysid in trials that developed into a lucrative therapy practice in which he treated Hollywood stars such as Cary Grant. Huxley took LSD for the first time in December 1955 with Hubbard, together with his old friend and mystic fellow-traveller Gerald Heard. He found it more potent physically, producing a sensation of intense cold, but 'the psychological effects, in my case, were identical with those of mescaline'. It produced for him the same transfiguration of the external world and the recognition, as on mescaline, that 'Love is the One, and that this is why Atman is identical with Brahman, and why, in spite of everything, the universe is all right'.[19] Huxley never took mescaline again, continuing with LSD all the way to his famous final experiment on his death bed in 1963.

Back in Saskatchewan, Osmond also switched to LSD after his first experiment with it. 'That stuff,' he pronounced, 'carries a punch like a mule kick.'[20] His reasons were the same ones that prompted most clinical researchers to make the switch. LSD was similar to mescaline but much stronger, with fewer physical side effects at high doses, cheaper to produce and just as easily available, in Osmond's case from the Sandoz branch in Quebec.

LSD had a freshly minted novelty, perfectly suited to the rhetoric of scientific revolution: a new drug for a new era of the mind. Mescaline, conversely, had a history and a hinterland that LSD lacked, and its new public profile drew attention to older strands of its story. In *The Doors of Perception* Huxley praised the Native American Church, which he presented as an example of the 'direct and illuminating' religious experience mescaline could generate and the group identity it forged: 'peyote-eating and the religion based upon it have become important symbols of the Red Man's right to spiritual independence'.[21] His description of the NAC was based on a study by the anthropologist

James Sydney Slotkin, who spent the summers of 1949–51 living with the peyotists of the Menominee people, an Algonquian tribe in Wisconsin. They had invited Slotkin and his wife to make a written record of their history, rituals and beliefs. Although a small and remote group they became, thanks to Huxley as much as Slotkin, among the best-known and studied representatives of the religion.

Slotkin's report and subsequent book included lengthy interview transcripts that brought authentic Indian voices to a mainstream white readership for the first time. Their language was often conventionally Christian, avoiding exoticising terms such as 'ceremony' and often any direct mention of peyote, speaking simply of meetings where worshippers would sit together and pray. Most were reluctant to discuss their visions, and many replied that they saw nothing special. Slotkin noted that they tended to consider visions 'at best, as a means of learning from Peyote; at worst, as distractions resulting from not concentrating on proper subjects'.[22]

The NAC by this time had spread beyond the Southern Plains into almost every corner of the USA, and the original structure was under strain. The Menominees were a chapter of the Wisconsin state NAC that had only been incorporated in 1939; charters had by now been granted in most Midwestern states up to the Canadian border. In 1944 an umbrella organisation, the Native American Church of the United States, was formed under the dynamic leadership of Frank Takes Gun, a Crow leader from Montana who had worked with John Collier in 1937 to oppose the federal ban, together with members from the mother church in Oklahoma, including the founding signatory Mack Haag. At the NAC's 1954 convention James Sydney Slotkin was invited to become a trustee, the first non-Indian representative of the church. He used his position to undertake research into the membership and publish a quarterly bulletin. In 1955 the charter was amended to rename it the Native American Church of North America (NACNA), allowing it to include Canadian chapters. The confident, organised and accessible face it now presented to white society embodied John

Collier's vision of a culture that had 'turned from anticipated death to anticipated life, from fatalism to action, from inferiority to healthful pride'.[23]

In October 1956 Humphry Osmond and Abram Hoffer were invited by the NACNA to the peyote meeting of a Cree chapter of the church in Saskatchewan. The Canadian government had been investigating allegations of assault and rape among the Cree Nation in Alberta, and the superintendent of their agency had pointed his finger at the peyote 'cult' and its 'demoralising effect'.[24] The director of the Indian Health Services added his concerns about 'disgusting orgies' and 'peyote sprees'.[25] A night in the tipi, during which Osmond participated and Hoffer observed, presented them with a quite different picture. 'I found the ceremony extremely beautiful,' Osmond wrote to Frank Takes Gun, 'and felt that I had a much greater understanding of the Indian's way of life . . . and the part that peyote may play in giving him back the confidence and self-respect that he had almost lost.'[26] Far from being a debauch, he and Hoffer were struck by the great success of the NAC in combatting alcoholism, and they became excited by the idea of trialling mescaline or LSD in its clinical treatment. They advised the government that peyote should not be classified as a narcotic and lent their authority to the campaign to maintain its legal use for religious purposes.

Non-Indian perceptions of peyote were reshaped by positive media portrayals that challenged the old language of cults and degenerate orgies. In September 1954 the *New Yorker* published a narrative by the Oklahoma historian Alice Marriott that she felt would be of interest to readers of *The Doors of Perception*, a description of a peyote healing ceremony that had taken place a few years previously while she was an ethnography student working with a tribe in South Dakota. She was many months into her fieldwork before she learned about peyote, since her interpreter Mary, an ardent Christian, refused to translate conversations about it: 'It is heathen. It pretends to be Christian but it's not. It calls itself the Native American Church, and that's blasphemous.'[27]

Over the scorching summer Marriott lost her appetite and became weak and ill, and Mary's elderly and blind uncle decided to convene a peyote meeting for her. A Cheyenne roadman was invited, along with a dozen or so other participants. Before the meeting Marriott was given a sweat-lodge treatment that left her even weaker than before. She was then taken to the tipi where the fire was lit, tobacco was smoked and she was given a tufted dry peyote with an 'indescribable, rank, green cactus taste'.[28] At midnight the eagle-bone whistle blew, and she took another button with the prescribed four swallows of water. After that point the fire and the singing took hold, and 'light and colour and beauty had embraced us'. By daybreak she felt 'full of life and health once more'; she slept deeply, and woke with a huge appetite. 'The tremendous first exhilaration lasted for several days, and there was no sudden drop following it.' The effect was, as best she could describe it, 'like seeing the door to life swing open'.[29]

In 1957 the journalist Karl Eskelund travelled to Mexico on an assignment for a Danish weekly magazine to investigate a cactus that, he persuaded his editor, would make him 'filled with love toward all your fellow beings'.[30] The resulting travel book, *Cactus of Love*, included Eskelund's journeys in Huichol country, where his enquiries about peyote were politely rebuffed: 'They ate it only at religious ceremonies and had not brought any with them.'[31] He eventually acquired a specimen from a Belgian cactologist, chewed it down with difficulty and after a few hours 'it was as if I had suddenly discovered the third dimension'. He was indeed filled with love: 'for four hours I went around loving . . . I felt the same deep love for everyone.' It was, Eskelund concluded, 'far better than marijuana'.[32]

Peyote was by now making appearances in underground literature and the emerging drug culture. William Burroughs, on the lookout as always for the next kick, noted that it was not controlled under the Harrison Narcotics Act and could be had by mail order from the right supplier. In Mexico in 1952 he sourced some from a local herb dealer, ground the buttons down and swallowed them with tea. Ten minutes later he felt sick: 'Everyone shouted, "Keep it down, man"' but despite his best efforts 'the peyote came up solid like a ball of hair'. Eventually he felt 'something like a benzedrine high. You can't sleep and your pupils are dilated. Everything looks like a peyote plant.' When he finally slept he was assailed by nightmares in which he had a chlorophyll habit. 'Me and about five other chlorophyll addicts are waiting to score on the landing of a cheap Mexican hotel. We turn green and no-one can kick a chlorophyll habit. One shot and you're hung for life. We are turning into plants.'[33]

Burroughs' collaborator Allen Ginsberg also encountered peyote in 1952 via the bohemian harpsichord-maker Bill Keck, one of the 'subterraneans' of the San Remo café, the beat epicentre in the Greenwich Village neighbourhood where Mabel Dodge's coterie had made their ill-starred experiment several decades earlier. Ginsberg took the dried buttons in his bedroom at the family home, choking them down with difficulty. He was roused from the resultant nausea by the beauty of a cherry tree in blossom outside his window; wandering outside, he fixated on a rock 'serried and worn by years, so old'. He was struck by how much longer it would last than any human alive: as he wrote later that night, 'we're flowers to rock'. He went back indoors, put some Tito Puente on the record player, and went round 'grinning idiotically at people'. 'Peyote is certainly one of the world's great drugs,' he thought; and 'I have to find, among other things, a new word for the universe, I'm tired of the old ones.' Where Ellis and Huxley had reached across time for Wordsworth, Ginsberg felt sure that the poet William Carlos Williams was the only other person in New York who would fully appreciate it.[34] Peyote, he decided, was rather like a combination of marijuana and Benzedrine, with the mind-stretching qualities of the former and the stimulant kick of the latter. With devotees such as Burroughs and Ginsberg, mescaline was beginning the next phase of its cultural life in which it would become one mind-altering drug among many, not merely for a few outsiders such as Crowley, Witkiewicz or Jünger, but for a generation.[35]

Ginsberg continued to take peyote on occasion over the next three years as he developed the open poetic form based around breath-length that culminated in *Howl*. It was 'like telepathy, like electricity', he recalled; it 'could turn your eyes into X-rays so that you could see the insides of things'.[36] He oscillated between New York and San Francisco, the twin poles of beat culture. His West Coast haunts bore traces of the old peyote mystique that had passed from Tony Luhan via Jaime de Angulo and Frank Waters to Gary Snyder, whom he pegged as a 'peyoteist [*sic*] . . . hung up on Indians'.[37] During one cactus trip in San Francisco in 1954 Ginsberg looked out of the window of the Nob Hill apartment where he was staying into a city of mist and fog, through which the lights of the buildings down the hill glimmered. Their hulking shapes were transformed into 'the robot skullface of Moloch', the bloodthirsty Canaanite god 'whose eyes are a thousand blind windows'.[38] Afterwards he found himself muttering 'Moloch, Moloch', and around this vision coalesced the central image of Part II of *Howl*: the idol of money and technocracy to which his generation were being sacrificed.

※　　※　　※

Howl was published in 1956, the same year as Henri Michaux's *Misérable Miracle*, the first instalment in what would become the twentieth century's most sustained creative engagement with mescaline. Over the following years Michaux subjected the drug to the closest possible phenomenological scrutiny, producing five essays, a film and dozens of drawings under its influence. His project was rooted in the experimental modernism of pre-war Paris, where he had begun his career as an iconoclastic poet, author of esoteric travelogues, composer of imaginary alphabets and associate of Max Ernst and Paul Klee. He had written about his experiences with hashish, opium and ether in the 1920s but didn't encounter mescaline until he was fifty-five, when he was supplied with it in medical ampoules by a Spanish neurologist of his acquaintance. Secreting himself in a darkened room with the curtains drawn, pen and paper before him, 'in a state of great uneasiness, of anxiety, of inner solemnity . . . in a state of expectancy, an expectancy that becomes with each minute more pregnant', he submitted himself to the bitter solution.[39]

Across both his writing and his drawing, Michaux experimented with techniques for trapping mescaline's elusive spirit through what he called *chevauchements*: 'encroachings', 'vaultings' or 'overlappings' that aimed to probe behind its ever-changing visions to their underlying mechanism. He developed a style of parallel texts, one commenting on the other, sometimes pushing beyond the limits of language into recursive trails of sounds, homonyms, repetitions and oscillations. In his drawing he surrendered control to his nervous system, depriving his hand of conscious guidance and hoping to catch the movements of the loom behind the tapestry it was weaving. 'Mescaline makes everything tremble with constant little tremblings,' he wrote, and 'undulate with an almost imperceptible microscopic swell.'[40] Sometimes his attempts to shadow it produced a palimpsest of vibrations like sound waves or EEG tracings, at other times delicate lattices resembling cell walls, or illegible cursive script dissolving in and out of abstraction.

The process was exhausting. Michaux often felt as if the drug was playing hide and seek, deliberately frustrating and subverting his attentions. 'I haven't seen any colours yet, no really brilliant colours. Perhaps I am not going to see any,' he would sulk; then 'I am submerged in thousands of little coloured dots. A tidal wave!' Then they would vanish: 'No longer any colours at all. Yet they are not really absent either. Or are they vanishing too quickly now to be really perceptible?' The constant flux infected his will: 'I should like to get up. No, I'd like to lie down, no, I'd like to get up immediately, no, I'd like to lie down at once.'[41] Mescaline, he concluded, was the enemy of poetry, of art, of any attempt to achieve 'fixation of the idea . . . one cannot "settle" anywhere'.[42] Like Sartre, he felt pressed close up against the fabric of reality, but in his case the response was not nausea as much as enervation. 'Ludicrous!' he found it; 'Intolerable!' When it eventually began to wear off, he gasped with relief. 'Cessation! at last!'[43]

He persevered, finding the process more unpleasant every time. 'Mescaline and I were more often at odds with each other than together,' he wrote later. Once he had its measure, he found its displays 'tawdry', a 'stupid phantasmagoria'. In the end it was 'really like a robot. It only knew how to do certain things.' As per the title of his first book on the drug, it was a 'miserable miracle'. His attempts to track it to its source led him only into the hall of mirrors of his own mind. 'Should I speak of pleasure? It was unpleasant.' It was an assault in which 'my cells were brayed, buffeted, sabotaged, sent into convulsions'.[44] Ultimately 'mescaline is an experiment in madness', but even on this subject 'it told me more about the madness of others than about my own, and more about symptoms than fundamentals'.[45] It dictated to him relentlessly, but its clumsy attempts to manipulate a consciousness beyond its comprehension shared the limits of the science that had synthesised it.

On his fourth experiment Michaux, 'through an error of calculation', took 600mg, 'six times what is for me a sufficient dose'. As 'the waves of the mescalinian ocean' began to break over him, he realised that 'the torture [was] going to last for hours'.[46] It was pure agony: 'with mad speed, hundreds of lines of force combed my being which could never reintegrate itself quickly enough for, before it could come together again, another line of rakes began raking it, and then again, and then again'. Eventually he was reduced simply to a line, 'a line that breaks up into a thousand aberrations', 'the metaphysical taken over by the mechanical'.[47] Four nights later, attempting sleep, he found himself 'in intimate relations with horror', trapped in a subterranean vault reminiscent of the nightmare architectures of Piranesi or De Quincey.[48] It took more than three months before he began to feel that 'though not fully recuperated, I am getting farther from this drug which is not the drug for me'. His conclusion was that 'My drug is myself, which mescaline banishes.'[49]

Misérable Miracle, together with Michaux's subsequent mescaline writings *L'infini turbulent* (1957) and *Paix dans les brisements* (1959), his drawings and sketches and his film *Images du monde visionnaire* (1963), can hardly be faulted for stamina and determination, yet their author considered them a failure. The limits against which he repeatedly flung himself were of his own making; his determination to dissect it leached the experience of meaning. Lying alone in a shuttered room, suffering the torments of nausea and cold extremities, he turned himself into an invalid and the drug into an illness. He never seems to have considered changing the form of his experiments, or exploring the natural history behind the synthetic drug. He had no interest in the experience of peyote users in traditional cultures, who, 'probably but little accustomed to dreaming, have no visions, or at least not visions strong enough to be interesting'.[50] He sought escape from the self but gave mescaline nothing else to work on, and it reflected back at him his own nausea, passivity and *anomie*.

The arch-experimenter William Burroughs observed drily of Michaux's method, 'I had my most interesting experiences with mescaline when I got outdoors and walked around – colors, sunsets, gardens.'[51] By the end of the 1950s Allen Ginsberg was occasionally mailing mescaline pills to Burroughs in Tangier, and Michaux worked his way into one of their private routines. 'A friend of mine [who] calls himself Micheaux [*sic*] sometimes,' Burroughs wrote to Ginsberg, 'had just taken a mescaline pill when Mr. B [Burroughs] saw him in a Tangier café. Mr. B proposed a drink but he replied, "No! No! I must go home and see my visions", and he rushed home and closed the door and bolted it and drew the curtains and turned out the light and got into bed and closed his eyes and there was Mr. B and Mr. M said, "What are you doing here in my vision?" and Mr. B replied: "Oh, I live here." '[52]

❦   ❦   ❦

In May 1955 the American Psychiatric Association held a symposium in Atlantic City on 'Lysergic Acid Diethylamide and Mescaline in Experimental Psychiatry', at which Aldous Huxley was invited to speak to the profession he described in a letter to Humphry Osmond as 'the

Electric Shock Boys, the Chlorpromaziners, and the 57 Varieties of Psychotherapists'. He observed that the other speakers' accounts had all treated the effects of these drugs as pathological, 'coloured by fear and anxiety', yet 'the classic mescaline experience', as he presented it, was quite different: a transport far beyond the concerns of the individual self to a strange Antipodes of the mind, a metaphor he had recently developed in *Heaven and Hell*, his follow-up essay to *The Doors of Perception*. 'The mental climate of our age is not favourable to visionaries,' he observed; their tales of distant lands, radiant light and cosmic revelations were likely these days to get them locked up.[53] He proposed that mescaline and LSD should not be connected to mental disease but rather to the abode of gods in classical civilisation, the animal–human hybrids that populated archaic religions, or the numinous otherworlds of Celtic and Teutonic folklore.

Huxley's was the only lecture to concentrate on mescaline. Some of the other presentations included it but the majority focused exclusively on LSD, and the symposium was sponsored by Sandoz, LSD's sole US distributor. The most congenial of the speakers to Huxley's outlook was the British psychiatrist Ronald Sandison, an early adopter of LSD therapy at Powick Hospital in Worcestershire. 'Just as dreams have come to be regarded as a source of material for Freudian and Jungian analysts,' Sandison predicted, 'so the experiences of patients under LSD might be similarly used.' A 'new era in treatment' beckoned, made possible by 'drugs which compel the unconscious, willy-nilly, to unlock its secrets'.[54] This possibility naturally also interested the CIA, who had launched their covert MK-ULTRA research programme into brainwashing and psychological warfare agents in 1953. They too experimented with mescaline but moved quickly on to LSD, the extraordinary potency of which meant that a small suitcase could hold enough to dose the entire population of the USA. As one agent later recalled, 'we thought about the possibility of putting some in a city water supply and having the citizens wander around in a more or less happy state, not terribly interested in defending themselves'.[55]

Abram Hoffer was also invited to the Atlantic City symposium, presenting research that aimed to show that niacin suppressed the effects of LSD; but by this time the search for an adrenaline-like M-substance was attracting less interest. Financed by a series of grants from the Canadian government and the Rockefeller Foundation and drawing on his previous biochemical work, Hoffer was pursuing the theory that Vitamin B3, in the form of niacin, might help the body flush out excess adrenaline. In a small initial trial on schizophrenic subjects, massive doses of niacin apparently resulted in remarkable therapeutic effects – suspiciously so, for some of his colleagues. A second study was more ambiguous, as were the urine and serum tests for the metabolites that would demonstrate niacin's action. The profession's attention was already waning by 1956 when Hoffer's announcement that he had found adrenochrome in human blood was rejected by the National Institute of Mental Health, which concluded the positive result was an artefact of the presence of ascorbic acid. Hoffer never retracted his claims but the wider profession fell in behind Seymour Kety, the head of NIMH's clinical laboratory, who pronounced that the 'evidence supporting them was hardly compelling'.[56]

M-substance theory and niacin therapy were never entirely discredited, but it came to seem implausible that they would yield up the psychiatric revolution that had been advertised. Chlorpromazine, in the estimation of most clinicians, was far more effective than niacin in the treatment of schizophrenia. Despite Osmond and Hoffer's self-experiments, the established view remained that adrenochrome was not significantly psychoactive; even Smythies came to believe that his associates' accounts 'may well have been due to placebo effects, the extraordinary range of which was not fully realized at the time'.[57] There was much new evidence to suggest that brain activity was controlled not by washes of hormones but by neurochemicals such as dopamine and the recently discovered serotonin interacting with specific receptors in the brain.[58] After the Swedish researcher Arvid Carlsson established in 1956 that chlorpromazine worked by blocking dopamine receptors, schizophrenia research came to cluster round the dopamine hypothesis.

The new paradigm called into question the assumption, central to Hoffer, Osmond and Smythies' work, that mescaline produced a 'model schizophrenia'. During the early 1950s emergency hospital wards saw a large increase in patients presenting with psychotic symptoms such as voice-hearing and delusions of persecutions who turned out to have taken large doses of amphetamines. In 1958 the term 'amphetamine psychosis' was coined, and the drug's powerful action on the dopamine system added to the growing body of evidence that drew schizophrenia research in this direction.[59] By the early 1960s the notion that mescaline and LSD were 'psychotomimetics' was in retreat. Rather than compiling lists of the resemblances between their effects and the symptoms of schizophrenia, a new generation of medical pharmacologists such as Leo Hollister addressed their fundamental differences. Hollister administered mescaline, LSD and psilocybin to 'normal' volunteer subjects, including Ken Kesey, at Menlo Park Mental Hospital in California and found their responses had little in common with psychotic disorders. The broad clinical category of 'hallucination', he argued, was unhelpful and misleading. In most subjects on LSD or mescaline, typical psychotic symptoms such as 'disorientation, paranoid ideation, disturbed thinking, and auditory, gustatory, olfactory or tactile hallucinations were uncommon'.[60] In particular, the core feature of psychosis – the subject's lack of insight into their condition and its causes – was by definition absent in subjects who had knowingly just taken a drug.

At the beginning of the 1950s, Osmond and Smythies' mescaline hypotheses had been dismissed as biologically reductive by the Freudian establishment. By the decade's end, they were rejected as unscientific by a new generation of biological researchers. Mescaline's long association with psychiatry, which had run through the twentieth century in an erratic but unbroken line from the founding era of Emil Kraepelin, was coming to an end.

✻   ✻   ✻

Within the nascent world of psychedelic studies, Huxley's advocacy for mescaline was divisive. Albert Hofmann read *The Doors of Perception* and *Heaven and Hell* as soon as they appeared and was initially enthralled. His own commitment to a mystical pietist Christianity was never far beneath the surface and he rejoiced that 'the gift of spontaneous visionary perception (which belongs to mystics, saints and great artists)' was now being offered to all.[61] His mentor Ernst Jünger, however, wrote to Hofmann, saying 'I cannot agree with Huxley's idea, that hereby the masses can be given possibilities for transcendence.'[62] Jünger, an instinctive aristocrat of the spirit, recoiled from promoting mescaline to the general public as 'a kind of substitute for religion'.[63] 'One must take into account that mescaline reinforces the initial state of the person who takes it, which might be weak or confused': the effect could just as easily be delusion, psychopathy or sheer banality.[64] As the 1960s progressed Hofmann became ever more convinced that Jünger was right and Huxley wrong. 'Psychotic breaks, accidents and criminal activity, consequent on states of confusion, multiplied in a frightening way,'[65] he wrote in his 1979 memoir. LSD remained, in the phrase of Hofmann's title, his problem child.

Many of Huxley's literary and intellectual readers baulked, as the author himself had until recently, at the paradoxical concept of a mystical drug. The novelist Thomas Mann, sent *The Doors of Perception* by an enthusiastic friend just before his death at the age of eighty, judged it 'the most audacious form of Huxley's escapism, which I could never appreciate in this author. Mysticism as a means to that escapism was, nonetheless, reasonably honourable. But now that he has arrived at drugs I find it rather scandalous.' It would be 'repulsive to me', Mann felt, to be in 'a position in which everything human becomes indifferent to me and I should succumb to unscrupulous aesthetic self-indulgence . . . This, however, is what he recommends to the whole world.'[66]

Carl Jung had been interested enough in Osmond and Smythies' mescaline reports to invite them to tea at his home in Küsnacht, Switzerland, in 1952, and Smythies had visited just before leaving for Saskatchewan. 'The point of interest for both of us,' Smythies recalled, was that mescaline's 'mind pictures of such transcendental beauty' seemed independent of the subject's personality; they concurred that 'the collective unconscious must indeed be a strange and marvellous place'.[67] But Jung, too, was diffident about Huxley's claims. He wrote to a friend in 1955:

The LSD-drug, mescaline: it has indeed very curious effects – *vide* Aldous Huxley! – of which I know far too little. I don't know what its psychotherapeutic value with neurotic or psychotic patients is. I only know there is no point wishing to know more of the collective unconscious than one gets through dreams and intuition . . . I am profoundly mistrustful of the "pure gifts of the Gods". You pay very dearly for them.

Here Jung conflates LSD and mescaline, yet at other times he seemed to regard them as opposites or shadows of one another. 'It is quite awful that the alienists have caught hold of a new poison to play with, without the faintest knowledge or sense of responsibility,' he wrote of LSD, before continuing: 'I can only hope that the doctors will feed themselves thoroughly with mescaline, *the alkaloid of divine grace*, so that they learn for themselves its marvellous effect.'[68]

One formidable reader was sufficiently scandalised by Huxley's claims to undertake his own experiment. R.C. Zaehner, professor of eastern religions and ethics at Oxford University, was appalled by the implication that the mescaline experience could be equivalent both to a schizophrenic breakdown and to the communion of the saints. He had entered the Roman Catholic church after experiencing a 'Beatific Vision, namely, the direct experience of God in His unutterable holiness', and refused to take Huxley's word that his drug-induced 'mystical experience has any connection with that Vision'.[69] (He shared, at least, Huxley's fondness for capitalising abstract nouns.) On 3 December 1955 he invited John Smythies to his rooms in All Soul's College to administer him with 400mg of mescaline, and half a Dramamine tablet for nausea.

After several hours of feeling little more than light-headed, Zaehner was accompanied by Smythies to Oxford Cathedral where finally 'things began to happen'.[70] The stained-glass rose windows expanded and contracted in ways that Zaehner found irritating and less beautiful than their normal state. Back in his rooms, when he was asked to contemplate a reproduction of Gentile da Fabriano's altarpiece painting *Adoration of the Magi*, it struck him as uproariously funny. One of the magi seemed to be trying to remove his crown; the eldest was approaching the Christ Child's feet and 'was trying to bite them and the child would not let him'. Zaehner 'could only laugh until I cried'.[71] Smythies gave him further objects to examine but he insisted, through paroxysms of laughter, 'This is the silliest test I have ever had to go through. You take it all so seriously.'[72] Smythies recalled the day's events as hilarious: Zaehner became 'quite manic – bubbling over with unrestrained wit and licence'.[73] As the paroxysms wore off he listened to a piece of music of great religious significance to him, Berlioz's *Te Deum*, but found the drug once more an irritating distraction. He wrote up the experiment in withering terms: 'I would not presume to draw any conclusions from so trivial an experience' (a conclusion in itself). 'In Huxley's terms "self-transcendence" of a sort did take place, but transcendence into a world of farcical meaninglessness.'[74]

Another author who took mescaline in a spirit of challenge to Huxley was the English philosopher, novelist and critic Colin Wilson, who had been urged by Huxley to try it when they met in the Athenaeum Club in London in 1959. Three years later Wilson was writing about Sartre's experiences on mescaline and decided he should sample it for himself. A psychologist friend wrote him a prescription, and he paid £5 for a gram from a medical supplier that arrived in the post in a sealed vial a week later. He reread *The Doors of Perception* that evening and 'had a strong intuition that taking mescaline would be pointless for me'. His was a strenuous world view in which 'the basic answer to the problem of existence lies in will and determination', and he was suspicious of Huxley's blithe promises of gratuitous grace.[75]

And so it proved. Wilson took roughly 250mg, noticed nothing, and took the same again. He felt some nausea (he had been drinking heavily in advance) and made himself sick. He fell asleep – 'all I wanted now was for the filthy stuff to wear off' – and woke to feel 'a wonderful sweetness flowing through my body'. But his strenuous habits of mind rebelled at this unwarranted pleasure: 'I couldn't simply relax into the mescaline experience.' His responsibilities as a husband and father nagged at him, and as it went on 'this feeling of being lapped in a sea of universal love was debilitating, rather like an orgasm that trickled on indefinitely'. He asked his wife to cook him a lamb chop but 'it was underdone, and I was too aware that it had been a lamb'. This ushered in 'a bad phase of the experience', in which he felt 'as if I was in a telephone exchange with messages coming from all around me'. As with Sartre, reality had become intimate in a most unpleasant way: it was 'like waking up on a train and finding a stranger with his face within an inch of your own'. It came down, he decided, to a question of outlook. 'If, like Sartre, you basically mistrust the universe, your response is to scream. If, like Huxley, you trust the universe, then your response is one of wonder and delight.'[76]

⁂ ⁂ ⁂

The day before John Smythies administered mescaline to R.C. Zaehner in Oxford, Humphry Osmond had done the same, in a BBC television studio in London, to Christopher Mayhew MP. Mayhew was an excellent televisual surrogate for Huxley: an old schoolfriend of Osmond, a former president of the Oxford Union, a distinguished veteran of the Second World War, a documentary filmmaker in his own right and genuinely wearing grey flannel trousers. The experiment took place in the drawing room of his Surrey home, where despite the initial nausea he quickly formed a comfortable relationship with both the drug and the camera. An hour after swallowing his 400mg in water he was 'in the full flood of the extraordinary visual phenomena described in *The Doors of Perception*'.[77]

As the experiment progressed, however, the visual effects were over-whelmed by another of mescaline's signature phenomena: the derange-ment of time. Between the hours established by Osmond and the film crew as 12.30 and 4 p.m., Mayhew was convinced that 'I existed *outside* time.' First, the usual sequence was scrambled: 'I was experiencing the events of 3.30 before the events of 3.00; the events of 2.00 after the events of 2.45, and so on': in the film he frequently refers to present events having occurred previously. Second, and even stranger, he was convinced that he had made lengthy 'excursions' in which clock time stood still but he experienced another life. At one point, while obeying Osmond's instruction to count backwards from one hundred in sevens, he announced in clipped and genial tones, 'I'm off again for a long period. But you won't notice that I've gone away at all.' Later he wrote that during these excursions 'I enjoyed an existence, fully conscious of myself, for what seemed like several years.'[78]

The film had been intended for the *Panorama* documentary strand, but the BBC decided against showing it on the grounds that Mayhew's effusive positivity might encourage the wider use of mescaline.[79] The experiment made its way into the public domain through an article by Mayhew published in the *Observer* the following year titled 'An Excursion out of Time'. It was sensationally popular and the *Observer* was 'overwhelmed with letters' in response.[80] It drew admiring comment from figures such as Mircea Eliade, the Romanian anthropologist whose work on shamanism had defined the subject in western scholar-ship. Although Eliade was notoriously reluctant to allow that drugs were an important or time-honoured element of shamanic practice, he 'trembled with joy' at Mayhew's account, which 'helps us to understand ecstatic situations . . . in which time is left behind'. It demonstrated that 'these are not aberrant or peripheral experiences without interest for everyday man. On the contrary, I would say there exists in the soul of each one of us a secret longing for this sort of ecstasy.'[81]

The exceptionally large postbag that Mayhew received in response to the article reflects the fusion of science, mysticism and intoxicating future possibility captured in *The Doors of Perception*. Many of the correspondents proposed that mescaline was a form of mystical technology that potentialised latent psychic powers, a short-cut to the mental self-conditioning mastered by over many years by mystics and yogis. Others argued that the states produced by telepathy or yogic practices were superior to 'borrowed and forced experiences, via drugs'.[82] Some explained Mayhew's excursion out of time in neuroscientific terms: brainwaves, disturbances of the memory centres or the nervous system. Some dismissed it as pathological, the same 'fantasy of superior knowledge' that manifested in schizophrenia.[83] One reader announced that he had achieved the same results by a 'long spell of abstracted thinking' about mathematic equations.[84] Two had had similar experiences under gas at the dentist. Several referred Mayhew to J.W. Dunne's popular book about precognitive dreaming, *An Experiment with Time* (1927), and others to ESP, astral bodies, the third eye, the fourth dimension and the atomic nature of light.

Notably absent were any readers who confessed to having tried mescaline themselves or who expressed an interest in seeking it out, apart from one who asked if she might be a guinea pig in any future experiments. The handful of early adopters among the general public who have left their traces in writing, urban legend or (in my case) family history seem at this point to have been exceptional. Over the following decade, things would change.

CHAPTER TEN

TRIPPING WITH MESCALITO

1960–2014

NEW YORK, CALIFORNIA, TEXAS,

ARIZONA, LAS VEGAS

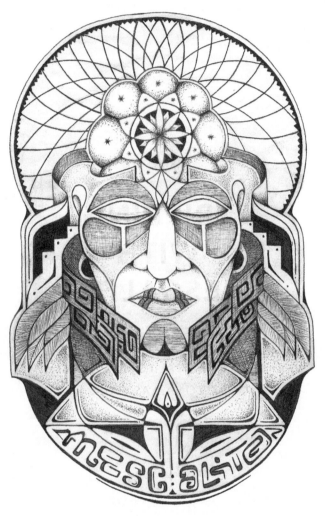

'Mescalito', tattoo art.

In 1960 Weston La Barre, whose 1938 monograph *The Peyote Cult* had been long established as the standard scholarly work on the subject, undertook another ethnographic field trip from his academic base at Duke University. This time his destination was not Oklahoma but New York, where he had heard reports of a new peyote cult centred round the Dollar Sign coffee house at 306 East 9th Street on the Lower East Side. There was no name above the door, merely a dollar sign, and the window was dominated by a cage containing eight monkeys. La Barre discovered that the 'bearded and barefoot proprietor', a twenty-eight-year-old Harvard graduate named Barron Bruchlos, was selling gelatine caps filled with powdered peyote for 50 to 75 cents apiece.[1]

La Barre was scornful of Aldous Huxley's claims that peyote – 'which Huxley persisted in calling by the long-discarded and quite incorrect name "mescal"' – was 'a chemical key to the mystical state, a sort of instant Zen'.[2] Generally, he was of the opinion that most white peyotists from Havelock Ellis onwards had been 'ethnologically spurious, meretricious and foolish poseurs'.[3] He was shocked, however, to learn that two undercover federal officers had recently visited the Dollar Sign, bought some peyote capsules and then raided the premises, confiscating 145 capsules and over 300 pounds of dried buttons. Bruchlos had been buying his peyote from registered wholesalers around Laredo, Texas, and even had stock that he had bought directly from federal government auctions, stamped with Department of Agriculture seals certifying that they were pest-free. There was, as La Barre observed, 'no federal law against the transportation, sale and use of peyote' and charges were eventually dropped.[4]

La Barre's interview with Bruchlos revealed a trade with a healthy profit margin. He was buying his peyote from Laredo at $8 per hundred buttons and selling them processed for around five times that amount. Had he sold all his stock, he would have cleared between $2,000 and $5,000. Bruchlos closed the Dollar Sign and opened another store nearby, which was by now one of several in lower Manhattan selling dried or powdered buttons. At the San Remo, Allen Ginsberg's Greenwich

Village haunt, the writer Terry Southern recalled that 'people started chopping them up and eating them like figs'.[5]

'Peyote and mescaline,' according to La Barre, 'were now becoming well known to every practising bohemian and beatnik.'[6] They were equally familiar on the west coast, especially in North Beach boho circles where they were consumed and traded alongside marijuana, Benzedrine and heroin. In 1958 the underground filmmaker Lawrence Jordan produced a short piece, *Triptych in Four Parts*, that spliced images of the bearded and barefoot North Beach artist John Reed with dazzling colour footage of *peyoteros* harvesting, cutting and drying hundreds of buttons under azure skies in the Laredo cactus gardens. Further south in the jazz clubs and burlesque joints of Hollywood, peyote buttons from Exotic Gardens in El Paso circulated as the hipster comedian Lord Buckley entertained the likes of Lenny Bruce, Ken Kesey and Henry Miller with his routine about the Church of the Living Swing, where the Sacrament was mescaline.[7]

In marked contrast to the bohemians of the 1920s, who had regarded Indian peyote use as inauthentic and degenerate, for those of the 1960s it was a powerful attractor towards Native American culture and spirituality. At the solar eclipse in February 1962 a group of North Beach and Big Sur bohemians including Stewart Brand and Peter Coyote convened at Mount Tamalpais in Marin County for what was perhaps the first non-Indian peyote ceremony in the US since Mabel Dodge's catastrophic salon in 1916. Brand, who later founded the *Whole Earth Catalog*, was among the first of the new generation to seek out Native American Church groups and participate in peyote meetings. By 1965 going 'up the cactus trail' was an established route for spiritual seekers.[8] In Colorado, the activist Linda Pedro recalled first hearing about peyote from fellow beatniks on the University of Colorado's Denver campus in 1963, and almost immediately being given three buttons by a stranger as he walked past her. Struck by the synchronicity, she set up a peyote altar in her room and was promptly presented by another friend with a copy of Frank Waters' *The Man*

Who Killed the Deer. Peyote 'seemed to be coming from everywhere at once'. She seized the moment and moved to Santa Fe, where she attended her first peyote ceremony in an apartment on East Alameda Street in 1965.[9]

In Texas, the home state of the peyote gardens, the connection with the local beatnik culture was made as early as 1960. In the Ghetto club in Austin, where marijuana circulated discreetly, peyote was introduced by University of Texas anthropology students to a crowd who were taught to consume it seriously in improvised NAC-style rituals. They were overseen by sober 'babysitters' and the bitter cactus was powdered and packed in gel caps to reduce nausea. Tommy Hall, soon to become a core member of the 13th Floor Elevators, made trips to Hudson's cactus farm outside Laredo to procure supplies, and used his chemistry background to perform rough extractions of mescaline. These home-made preparations, along with the morning glory milkshakes he also experimented with, were abandoned in 1965 when the first vials of blue liquid LSD arrived in town.

Around the same time the anthropology student John Kimmey, who had encountered peyote while travelling in Mexico and developed his own spiritual ceremony around it, took peyote with a group of friends in a cave at Pyramid Lake, Nevada. During the ceremony he heard the word 'Taos' spoken clearly inside his head. Kimmey and his fellow travellers moved to the environs of Taos in 1965 and established a commune they called New Buffalo, which aimed to live in harmony with the land as the continent's original inhabitants had.[10] Few of the residents of Taos pueblo were prepared to cooperate with them, but one, Little Joe Gomez, visited and taught them how to build tradition-ally in adobe. Gomez was from a peyotist family and his father had once had a vision that the peyote religion would pass from Indians to whites in generations to come. He presided over ceremonies at New Buffalo, initiating the participants into the ritual uses of fire, staff, drum, rattle and feathers and holding the circle together despite the nausea and vomiting of his novice congregation.

New Buffalo achieved immortality through its inclusion in *Easy Rider* (1969), and is among the few communes from that era that survives today as a self-sufficient agricultural community. By the early 1970s most had collapsed in the face of the harsh high desert conditions and increasing tensions with the Taos pueblo, which were mirrored across the pueblos and reservations of the Southwest. The new arrivals often assumed incorrectly that all Indians were peyotists, which made them insensitive to the delicate issues it raised between tribes, families, generations and the Indian and Hispanic communities. They also tended to assume that peyotists approved of marijuana and alcohol; in fact most NAC members were firmly opposed to them. They failed to respect Indian land, or to appreciate many Native Americans' patriotic support of army veterans and the Vietnam War. The huge popularity of Frank Waters' *Book of the Hopi* led to an invasion of the Hopi reservation by free spirits who found a strict and ascetic caste of elders appalled at the prospect of their younger generation becoming hippies.

After the release of *Easy Rider*, its director and star Dennis Hopper bought Mabel Dodge Luhan's now-crumbling adobe house and filled it with fine contemporary art just as its architect had. He nicknamed it 'the Mud Palace' and famously rode his Harley across its roof. An apocryphal tale circulated among his visitors that D.H. Lawrence had once taken peyote there, thrown off all his clothes and had to be chained up in the courtyard, howling like a coyote.

The 1960s were a period of rapid growth for the Native American Church, which by some estimates doubled its membership during the decade. The Indian activist Vine Deloria Jr recalled growing up on the Oglala Lakota reservation of Pine Ridge, South Dakota, close by Wounded Knee, where during the post-war years the NAC was no more than a distant and notorious rumour. By the late sixties he estimated that around 40 per cent of his people had become members of the church. 'It appears to be the religion of the future among the Indian people,' he wrote at the end of the decade.[11] The white Christianity of the missionaries was dying; it failed to satisfy the Indian appetite for religion or to make sense of Indian society, and allied itself too uncritically with the dominant culture's money-worship and racial discrimination. The circumscribed Christian notion of 'giving' was much less generous than true Indian 'sharing', the spirit of mutualism nurtured by the NAC.

🌿   🌿   🌿

By 1970, however, the American counterculture's understanding of peyote was being shaped by a quite different narrative. Ten years previously, in 1960 (so the story went), Carlos Castaneda, a young UCLA anthropology student, was waiting for a Greyhound bus in the Sonoran Desert on the Arizona–Mexico border when his local guide directed his attention to 'a white-haired old Indian' who was 'very knowledgeable about plants, especially peyote'.[12] Castaneda introduced himself to the old man, Don Juan, and asked if he would teach him. In August of the following year he visited Don Juan in his house on the Arizona side of the border. In the presence of five other Indian men, but without any ceremony, Castaneda was given seven dried buttons, or *mescalitos*, from a coffee jar. He chewed them down, washing the bitterness away with tequila, and soon noticed that 'my vision had diminished to a circular area in front of my eyes'. In this circle a black dog appeared and came to drink from a pan of water; as Castaneda watched, the dog became a being of radiant light. He knelt to share the water and as he drank 'I saw the fluid running through my veins setting up hues of red and yellow and green . . . I was all aglow. I drank until the fluid went out of my body through each pore and projected out like fibers of silk, and I too acquired a long, lustrous, iridescent mane. I looked at the dog and his mane was like mine.' Castaneda and the dog wrestled and played together for hours, and by the time he returned to consciousness 'I had forgotten I was a man!'[13]

When Castaneda asked Don Juan the next morning whether all this had really happened, the old man replied sternly, 'Goddammit! It was not a dog!'[14] Nor would he permit Castaneda to use the word peyote:

he insisted on referring to the cactus as Mescalito, a person, and rebuffed his student's attempts to talk about him directly. In his book Castaneda described how, over a sequence of four encounters, he learned to use peyote to enter the world of the *nagual*, or shaman, in which the rules of everyday reality no longer applied. On a night-time excursion to the desert he encountered Mescalito face to face for the first time, as a human figure with green, warty skin like a peyote and a hole in his hand through which scenes from Castaneda's future life flashed. Mescalito turned away and 'hopped like a cricket for perhaps fifty yards. He hopped again and again, and was gone.'[15]

The Teachings of Don Juan: A Yaqui Way of Knowledge was the block-buster opening to a series of adventures that went on to sell over 25 million copies. Their success was not notably impacted by the procession of anthropologists who pointed out the absence of a peyote tradition among the Yaqui people, who lived to the west of its natural habitat;[16] that much of the plant lore related by Castaneda, such as the smoking of dried hallucinogenic mushrooms, was unknown in any indigenous tradition;[17] and that many of the stories he attributed to Don Juan had clear sources in the work of anthropologists such as Michael Harner, Peter Furst and Barabara Myerhoff. In 1976 the investigative journalist Richard de Mille published *Castaneda's Journey*, a forensic analysis of the uncredited borrowings in the Don Juan stories, which concluded that Castaneda's fieldwork and reportage was 'a swindle, a sham, a masquerade, a spoof, a hoax, or what you will'.[18]

In his books, Castaneda sidestepped the question of where his teacher's knowledge came from: 'He never mentioned the place where he had acquired his knowledge, nor did he identify his teacher. In fact, Don Juan disclosed very little about his personal life.'[19] He had travelled extensively, so Castaneda's story went, and lived for extended periods in the centre and south of Mexico. His shamanism was eclectic and unique; or, as de Mille and other scholars concluded, he was a fictional repository for an assemblage of ethnographic accounts that spanned Mesoamerica, the Andes and the Amazon.

One of the major sources was the anthropological studies of the Huichol. De Mille documented thirty-seven passages in Castaneda's books that appeared to be plagiarised from the work of Barbara Myerhoff and Peter Furst. It turned out that Castaneda had visited Myerhoff when she was staying with the Huichol, and she had introduced him to Ramón Maria Silva, who was, it seemed, a real-life model for Castaneda's mysterious teacher. Nonetheless, Castaneda's experiences with peyote had little connection to Huichol traditions. The anthropologist Jay Fikes, who spent several seasons living with the Huichol, learning their language and observing healing sessions and rituals, concluded that the main source for Castaneda's Mescalito was 'Jiminy Cricket, Walt Disney's cartoon character'.[20]

Fikes tracked the tangled lines of influence back to UCLA's anthropology department, where Castaneda had studied and won a doctoral degree on the basis of what subsequently became his first book. This was where Myerhoff and Furst were based, along with other scholars and champions of shamanism such as Carlo Ginzburg and Marija Gimbutas. Fikes and Furst traded accusations of academic fraud and persecution that escalated to a series of lawsuits.[21] In Mexico, meanwhile, the effect of Castaneda's books was to turn the Huichol into poster children for the psychedelic counterculture. Fikes was distressed by the young tourists who were now descending on them from the United States and beyond, demanding peyote and showing little respect for their traditions. Castaneda's first wife Margaret claimed, perhaps with some exaggeration, that her husband's books had 'led millions of young people' to seek shamanic powers 'with the aid of mescaline and peyote'.[22]

After his academic exposure, Castaneda's writings gradually disappeared from the footnotes and bibliographies of his UCLA teachers, though some continued to defend him against the debunkers. When Richard de Mille asked Myerhoff whether 'the fact that the Don Juan books were a transparent fraud [didn't] invalidate the model', she replied, 'No, it doesn't . . . the message is needed.'[23] In appropriating aspects of Don Juan's peyote shamanism from Ramón and the Huichol, Castaneda was popularising a new sensibility that took indigenous beliefs seriously. Douglas Sharon, the first anthropologist to immerse himself in Peru's San Pedro healing traditions and a UCLA acquaintance of Castaneda's, concurred: 'In spite of the fact that his work may be fiction, the approach he was taking – validating the native point of view – was badly needed in anthropology.'[24] Whether fact or fantasy, his books articulated an indigenous perspective in which 'power plants' were not simply intoxicants but spiritual allies with which skilled users could develop a deep and reciprocal relationship.

The popularity of Castaneda's work did not depend on the imprimatur of the academy; in many ways, quite the opposite. Like Huxley's, his sensational success owed as much to timing as to content. He wrote for a generation that was discovering psychedelics for itself, and offered them a charter stitched from a variety of indigenous traditions that, precisely because it had no actual real-life referent, could be freely appropriated. He plagiarised but also showcased for non-academic readers the work of a new generation of anthropologists who were immersing themselves in practices that their seniors had typically dismissed as inebriation, self-poisoning or cultural decadence.

Castaneda also provided a corrective to the dominant rhetoric of the psychedelic sixties, which prophets of LSD such as Timothy Leary had presented as a radical form of modernity, even a new stage in human evolution. He told an alternative story in which psychedelics had long been part of cultures from which the modern west had much to learn. His peyote visions bore little resemblance to any described before or since, but they worked perfectly as narrative devices for shifting the protagonist and the reader into the world of the *nagual*. He presides in spirit over today's mass-cultural phenomenon of the ayahuasca journey, which has for better or worse transformed both tourism and shamanism in the Amazon. Far more than peyote, the DMT-rich ayahuasca potion reliably generates the kind of hallucinatory spirit encounters that Castaneda attributed to Mescalito.

✳   ✳   ✳

During the sixties mescaline made a parallel journey into the emerging counterculture, not from the Mexican desert but from the laboratory. In the early years of the decade it was largely replaced in clinical research by LSD and psilocybin, which Albert Hofmann had isolated from Mexican mushrooms in 1958 and synthesised in 1959, and which Sandoz subsequently marketed under the name Indocybin. Mescaline still had some research uses, particularly in trials that aimed to compare the effects of a range of psychoactive drugs. These included CIA-funded trials under the MK-ULTRA programme, such as those begun in 1957 by Dr Paul Hoch of the US Army Chemical Corps to test his theory that mescaline and LSD were essentially 'anxiety-producing drugs' that might be used to instil fear in a target population. Hoch used mescaline to induce paranoia and recorded that 'the mental picture was that of a typical schizophrenic psychosis while the drug influence lasted'. He proceeded to combine mescaline with electroshock treatment, and found that 'it did not influence the clinical symptoms at all'.[25]

Hoch's studies were funded by the Josiah Macy Foundation, a medical research body with close links at that time to the CIA. In 1959 it organised a conference on LSD research that was attended by the clinical pharmacologist Leo Hollister, a sceptic of the psychotomimetic model that viewed the effects of psychedelics as model psychoses. Hollister argued that double-blind controls were needed in which these drugs were administered to 'normal' subjects alongside schizophrenic patients, and he received funds indirectly from the CIA to conduct trials at his place of work, the Veterans Affairs Hospital at Menlo Park near the university campus in Stanford, California. He acquired a battery of psychoactive drugs including LSD, mescaline, psilocybin and deliriants such as Ditran derived from chemical warfare agents, and advertised for volunteers with good physical and mental health. He offered compensation of $25 for the first session and up to $75 for subjects prepared to stay the course. The trials took place in the hospital, in small sanitised rooms with wired-glass windows, during which the volunteers were put through tests for motor skills, cognition and memory. Among them was an aspiring writer named Ken Kesey.

Kesey's first session, with a little blue pill that turned out to be Sandoz LSD, was a revelation. He was already familiar with marijuana and Benzedrine, but this was of a different order: it seemed 'to give you more observation and insight, and it [made] you question things you [didn't] ordinarily question'.[26] He continued with the trial and, having established where the research chemicals were kept, took a job as janitor in the hospital, giving him illicit but easy access to them. He worked night shifts, during one of which he took a huge dose of mescaline and 'managed the night by mopping fervently whenever the nurse arrived so she couldn't see my twelve-gauge pupils'.[27] He spent long hours with the psychiatric patients, during which he conceived the notion that the hospital was a microcosm of the systems of power and control that operated in society at large, and he began to sketch out what would become *One Flew Over the Cuckoo's Nest*. He also discovered that peyote buttons could be ordered from Smith's Cactus Ranch in Laredo, the same wholesaler that was supplying Barron Bruchlos in New York. During one hospital stint on eight buttons, the character of Chief Bromden, the huge, docile Native American patient, 'just appeared' in his mind: a narrator who stood outside the drama of sanity and madness in which all the other characters were enmeshed.[28]

'We need a messiah to tell the people,' Kesey announced, and he was one of several charismatic figures who over the next few years made it their mission to introduce psychedelics to the culture at large.[29] None of these figures, however, made mescaline their drug of choice. For Kesey and his anarchic cohort the Merry Pranksters, LSD became the sacrament; when their scene expanded to a scale that demanded its own supply, the underground savant Augustus Owsley Stanley III taught himself how to synthesise it in his kitchen, working backwards from a little blue Sandoz pill. Timothy Leary and Richard Alpert began their psychedelic experiments with the Mexican mushroom and switched to its Sandoz-supplied active ingredient for their Harvard Psilocybin Project of 1961–63, before turning their researches and proselytising energies to LSD. Alan Watts listed mescaline along with psilocybin, LSD and DMT as a stimulus to the expanded consciousness he described in *The Joyous Cosmology* (1962), but he never described his experiences with it.[30] Tom Wolfe's *The Electric Kool-Aid Acid Test* (1965) unfolds with no mention of mescaline at all.

By the early sixties chemical suppliers were subjecting orders of all psychedelics to closer scrutiny, and permission for psychedelic research studies became harder to obtain. In 1962 the Kefauver–Harris Amendment to the codes of the Food and Drug Administration (FDA), passed in the wake of the Thalidomide tragedy, tightened the rules further by mandating that new drugs had to be medically approved for their intended use, and a subsequent editorial in the *Journal of the American Medical Association* informed its members that any drug which altered 'mental and emotional equilibrium' should be available only 'under medical control'.[31] In the new climate, the high potency of LSD made it the most obvious choice among the psychedelics for clinical research, with the fewest 'side effects' – meaning, in this context, anything not related to cognitive function. Mescaline's physicality, large dosage and long duration all counted against it. Among the psychedelic vanguard, mescaline's physical effects ('body load') also made it second-favourite to LSD, for which there were a growing number of non-medical sources.

Those who specifically sought out mescaline after 1960 did so largely as a result of reading *The Doors of Perception*. The physician Andrew Weil, as a Harvard freshman in 1961, was inspired by reading Huxley to approach the psychology lecturer Timothy Leary, who told Weil he wasn't permitted to recruit undergraduate volunteers for his psilocybin research but recommended to him that mescaline might be the easiest psychedelic agent to get hold of. 'It took only two months and moderate ingenuity,' Weil recalled, to obtain a supply from a US chemical research company, after which he formed a group with seven other undergraduates to investigate and report carefully on its effects.[32] Although 'insights were gained that have had lasting importance' he found mescaline overall to be unreliable. Most sessions produced 'nothing more than intensifications of pre-existing moods with promi-nent periods of euphoria', and many of the effects were undesirable: 'the prolonged wakefulness, for example, and the strong stimulation of the central nervous system with resultant dilated eyes, cold extremities, and stomach butterflies'.[33] In 1964 he had a much more powerful experience with psilocybin, and later found LSD to be the most rewarding psychedelic for his researches.

Experimenters had always found it impossible to separate out mescaline's peculiar combination of mental, physical, visual, psychic and emotional effects, and by the sixties they no longer needed to: LSD and psilocybin could deliver similar alterations in consciousness with significantly less of what were now conceived as 'side effects' or 'residue'. After 1963, however, legal and commercial controls tight-ened around all three. In the wake of Leary's expulsion from Harvard, Sandoz withdrew LSD and psilocybin from sale in the US except for orders where specific clearance had been given by the FDA. Concerns about the non-medical 'abuse' of psychedelics dovetailed with growing evidence, particularly from trials on US military subjects, that LSD carried both acute and long-term risks of serious mental illness such as psychosis and depression.[34]

In 1965 mescaline and LSD were prohibited by the US Drug Abuse Control Amendments for everything but government-approved research, and from this point on clinical research with mescaline became vanishingly rare. One of the few later examples was at Freiburg medical school in Germany, where in the mid-1980s the remainder of Kurt Beringer's sixty-year-old vials of Merck mescaline were brought to light. They were used in a small-scale trial that aimed to validate Beringer's concept of 'mescal psychosis' by elucidating, once again, the common-alities between its effects and the symptoms of psychotic disorders.[35]

The study proved, if nothing else, that properly stored mescaline can remain viable for a lifetime.

＊　　＊　　＊

Mescaline, alongside LSD and psilocybin, was placed under Schedule 1 of the US Controlled Substances Act (high potential for abuse and no recognised medical application) in 1970, and prohibited internationally under the UN Convention on Psychotropic Substances of 1971. By that time it had largely vanished from the streets just as it had from the laboratory and the clinic. The economics of the illicit market overwhelmingly favoured LSD: the process of synthesising the two compounds was comparable in cost and risk, but the rewards of LSD were thousands of times greater. At a standard dose of around 250 to 400mg, a gram of mescaline amounts to around three doses; a gram of LSD can provide up to thirty thousand.

Mescaline retained a powerful mystique, however, and underground chemists not motivated by financial return produced it occasionally in small batches for the connoisseur market. Various new syntheses had been developed since Ernst Späth's original discovery: the one most commonly deployed was a seven-step process first published by Makepeace Tsao in the *Journal of the American Chemical Society* in 1951 which begins with gallic acid, a relatively accessible precursor used in industrial pharmacy.[36] But in an illicit market it was anyone's guess what was actually in the pills or powders: anything could command a high price from those who believed it to be mescaline. It was sometimes sold to the unwary in the microdot or blotter formats used for microgram doses of LSD, which are incapable of holding anything like a full dose of mescaline. Even when the size of pill or quantity of powder was plausible, 'mescaline' might be anything from LSD to methamphetamine, PCP ('angel dust') or the synthetic phenethylamine known as DOM or STP. *Microgram Journal*, the bulletin of street drugs and laboratory analysis circulated by the US

Bureau of Narcotic and Dangerous Drugs in the 1960s, lists mescaline in its expanding inventory of target drugs and makes reference to the 1951 Tsao synthesis, but includes no reports of verified street purchases or seizures.[37]

A handful of rock legends from the era invoke mescaline: in his memoir Arthur Lee recalls taking it along with his band, Love, and Jimi Hendrix during an all-night session at Olympic Studios in London in 1970, and the Grateful Dead's 'mescaline show' at Springfield, Massachusetts, in 1978 is still fondly recalled.[38] But the trip from this era that redefined mescaline for the rest of the twentieth century and beyond was Hunter S. Thompson's white-knuckle ride in *Fear and Loathing in Las Vegas* (1971). Thompson arrives at his Vegas hotel already badly twisted on cocaine and LSD, together with his companion, a 'Samoan attorney', who is gibbering 'I *must* have some drugs! What have you done with the mescaline?'[39] The pair dig some 'pellets' (pills? rolled-up peyote buttons?) out of their medical bag and are driving down Main Street when 'the fiendish cactus juice took over, plunging me into a sub-human funk'.[40]

The mescaline is temporarily subsumed in the polydrug frenzy; they arrive at a bikers' gun club and the madness spools on. Some while later, in the Circus-Circus casino, Thompson feels the gears cranking up – 'good mescaline comes on slow' – to a pitch of 'that fearful intensity that comes at the peak of a mescaline seizure'.[41] There is no further mention of the drug through the chaos that follows, which concludes many hours later with the show-stopping scene of his attorney, now with 'a head full of acid and the sharpest knife I've ever seen',[42] demanding that Thompson throw the hotel radio into his bath at the moment when Jefferson Airplane's 'White Rabbit' peaks.

The roots of *Fear and Loathing*'s mescaline trip are exposed in Thompson's 1969 article 'First Visit with Mescalito',[43] a more single-minded account of his first mescaline experience and, with hindsight, a dry run for his masterpiece. Its title was a riposte to Castaneda's recently published first book, which he had just read: 'Very weird; that old man really fucked the kid around, eh? . . . a Yaqui way of publicity. Fuck it; I'm tired of all that bullshit.'[44] Thompson's experiment took place before dawn in a hotel on Sunset Strip, after several days and nights awake on Dexedrine, when he found himself with a flight to catch to Denver and nothing in his drugs bottle but 'a big spansule [time-release capsule] of mescaline and "speed"'. Even for this street pharmacologist *par excellence*, the pill was something of a mystery – 'I don't know the ratio of the mixture, or what kind of speed is in there with the mescaline'[45] – and it seems odd that a substance as rare and expensive as mescaline should have been mixed with a cheap and unspecified amphetamine. But, whatever its chemistry, the psychedelic overdrive is captured in persuasive and excruciating detail. Thompson's typewriter clatters at top speed as 'the keys sparkle, glitter with high-lights' and the typist finds himself 'buzzing all over . . . the little red indicator that moves along with the ball on this typewriter now appears to be made of arterial blood. It throbs and jumps along like a living thing.'

As dawn breaks and harsh reality intrudes, elements of the *Fear and Loathing* scenario snap into place. Oscar Acosta, the prototype for the book's 'Samoan' attorney,[46] is summoned on a rescue mission to supply beer and human cover as Thompson attempts to pack, check out of the hotel and make it to the airport. 'White Rabbit' even makes a cameo appearance as the stream of consciousness rushes on: 'I seem to have leveled out, like after the first rush of acid. If this is as deep as it's going to bore, I think we can make it to the plane, but I dread it. Getting in a steel tube and shot across the sky, strapped down . . .' After a flight relayed in paranoid fragments – 'warn the pilot – this plane feels very wormy at this altitude' – Thompson comes down, still jangling and disconnected, on the prosaic but solid tarmac of Denver airport.[47]

Fear and Loathing situated mescaline within an exotic pharmaco-poeia, and by extension a streetwise drug culture that was leaving the utopian dreams of the sixties in its dust. The hippies were not going to save the world with their transcendental medication; mescaline was no longer the portal to Huxley's transcendent 'Mind at Large' or Castaneda's world of the *nagual*. It had become one among a 'whole galaxy of multi-colored uppers, downers, screamers, laughers' that included everything from cocaine to ether and amyl nitrate, sheets of blotter acid to rum and tequila.[48] In the process it scrambled the image of mescaline once more, in some respects returning it to the nineteenth century and the Wild West, where 'mescal' labelled a confused territory in which peyote, strong spirits and poison berries overlapped. 'Fiendish cactus juice' might be either mescaline or a mezcal spirit such as tequila: the two sat next to each other in the trunk of Thompson's car (which 'looked like a mobile police narcotics lab').[49]

Fear and Loathing was also the source of the urban legends around adrenochrome, Osmond, Smythies and Hoffer's candidate for 'M-substance', a compound that would have passed from popular memory had it not been for the unforgettable narrative Thompson constructed around it in the chapter entitled 'A Terrible Experience with Extremely Dangerous Drugs'. Thompson's attorney horrifies him by announcing that 'one of those Satanism freaks' has gifted him a bottle of adrenochrome, a legendary substance that can only be obtained from 'the adrenal glands from a *living* human body'. Thompson delicately dips a match head into the bottle. 'That's about right,' his attorney nods, 'that stuff makes pure mescaline seem like ginger beer.' It comes on 'like a combination of mescaline and methedrine': the spansule in the Sunset Strip hotel.[50] When Osmond and Hoffer announced that adrenochrome was the first psychoactive substance to be identified in the human body, they can hardly have imagined that this was how their discovery would be best remembered.

🌺　　🌺　　🌺

In the drug culture of the twenty-first century, mescaline has two faces: the sacred and the profane. The first is identified with peyote and the magical tales of Carlos Castaneda, the second with a legendary white crystal and the twisted exploits of Hunter S. Thompson. The two might be seen as the culminating points of two strands of western engagement that ran in parallel throughout the twentieth century: Castaneda as heir to the spiritual explorations of William James, Aleister Crowley, Frederick Smith and Aldous Huxley, and Thompson to the creative derangement of the senses pursued by Havelock Ellis, Stanisław Ignacy Witkiewicz, Henri Michaux and William Burroughs. Both of their narratives are tangled webs of fact and fiction, and both have been further mythologised through an echo-chamber of references that extends across the mainstream of pop culture from *The Matrix* to *The Simpsons*.[51]

Mescaline itself has almost entirely vanished from the modern drug scene – or perhaps, one could argue, it has metamorphosed to become the beating heart of it. The most consequential mescaline trip of the sixties was, with hindsight, the one taken in April 1960 by Alexander Shulgin, a biochemist at Dow Chemical Company in California who had recently completed his postdoctoral studies in pharmacology at Berkeley. He had read Huxley and followed his footsteps back to Beringer and Rouhier, and was surprised by how little pharmacological work had been done on mescaline's wider chemical family. When a psychologist offered him the chance to try it, he accepted eagerly, and the experience 'unquestionably confirmed the entire direction of my life'. He was awoken to colour and visual detail as never before, and continually struck with novel insights, but 'more than anything else, the world amazed me, in that I saw it as I had when I was a child'. He found himself immersed in 'a space wherein I had once roamed as an immortal explorer, and I was recalling everything that had been known authentically to me then, and which I had abandoned, then forgotten, with the coming of age'.[52] He decided on the spot that if there were similar compounds as yet unknown, he would discover them.

Shulgin quickly established that there were only two known chemicals with a phenethylamine structure and effects that resembled those of mescaline, trimethoxyamphetamine (TMA) and methylenedioxyamphetamine (MDA). During the early sixties he synthesised and sampled

TMA, and experienced severe nausea and some slight changes in perception and mood. Bitten by the bug of discovery he turned his attention to the essential oils of nutmeg, which included the psychoactive compound myristicin and looked as if they could be tweaked to produce TMA- or MDA-like drugs. His first attempt yielded the previously unknown 3-methoxy-4,5-methylenedioxyamphetamine, or MMDA, which turned out to be 'a truly fascinating compound. It did not have the bells and whistles, the drama of mescaline, but it was considerably more benign.' Its effects lasted only a couple of hours as opposed to a gruelling ten or twelve, and the visuals it produced were 'just on the verge of mescaline or psilocybin'.[53] Another substituted phenethylamine, DOM (2,5-dimethoxy-4-methylamphetamine), turned out to be active at a much smaller dose than mescaline, around 4mg. (In 1967 Owsley manufactured a batch that was sold through his Bay Area networks under the name STP, supposedly an acronym for 'Serenity, Tranquillity and Peace'. Its effects were anything but: a decimal point error, most unusual for the fastidious Owsley, had produced wildly over-strength tablets of 20mg that led to a wave of emergency hospital admissions.)

In 1961 Shulgin developed one of the first biodegradable pesticides, marketed by Dow as Zectran. It was hugely profitable and he was thereafter allowed great latitude in directing his own laboratory work, which he used to further his psychopharmacy research. In 1965 he synthesised an N-methylated version of MDA, 3,4-methylenedioxymethamphetamine or MDMA, which had originally been patented by Merck in 1912 but never made available for research. When Shulgin tried it two years later he found it 'unlike anything I had taken before. It was not a psychedelic in the visual or interpretative sense, but the lightness and warmth of the psychedelic was present and quite remarkable.'[54] He began taking it regularly, carrying a vial around with him and dosing himself at parties, where he referred to it as his 'low-calorie martini'.[55] He shared it with friends, who found it euphoric and emotionally therapeutic, and he introduced it to a psychotherapist who discreetly used LSD and MDA with some of his clients. The therapist reported that it had unique potential for drug-assisted therapy, and MDMA spread rapidly through California's psychotherapeutic community. It was, one psychiatrist pronounced, 'penicillin for the soul'.[56]

By the early 1980s MDMA had made the transit, like LSD before it, from the clinic to the street. At this point still a legal substance, it circulated initially in the dance clubs of Texas, Chicago and New York. Its original marketeers named it 'empathy' to stress its open-hearted and euphoric effects, but the street name that took hold was 'ecstasy'. It was, in many respects, mescaline tamed for the new chemical generation. Its physical effects still included a tendency to nausea at onset but the warm, tingling euphoria of mescaline's spectrum predominated, and its duration was reduced to a manageable three or four hours. Its psychedelic effects were less disorientating and challenging than a large dose of mescaline, but not dissimilar to those produced by the lower doses of peyote and San Pedro used in their traditional contexts. It didn't yield the brilliant visions prized by mescaline's early experimenters, but rather what Shulgin called 'a special magic' that made the world sparkle and glow.[57]

By nudging its physical symptoms in a milder and more pleasurable direction, MDMA turned what scientists and psychonauts alike had considered to be mescaline's undesirable side effects into a delicious 'body high' of rushes, waves and tingles. It was a trip for the senses as well as the mind, and it reconfigured drug culture to its needs: expansive dance spaces in warehouses or open-air festivals, extended hypnotic beats and vibrant dayglo visuals. It evolved a ceremony that accommodated its sacrament in many of the ways that native peyote traditions had, using rhythmic movement to banish chills and nausea and intense group bonding to lift the spirits.

✳ ✳ ✳

The 1990s were designated the 'Decade of the Brain' by President George H.W. Bush, a former director of Prozac manufacturers Eli Lilly, and the same discoveries in neurochemistry that flooded the pharmaceutical market with antidepressants also stimulated underground chemists to develop a galaxy of new stimulants and euphoriants. Shulgin, now working from his DEA-licensed laboratory in a shed behind his house, led the field. He synthesised, assayed and reported on some two hundred new psychedelic phenethylamines, many of which had properties that overlapped with one or another part of mescaline's spectrum. MDMA was joined in the illicit marketplace by compounds such as 2C-B and 2C-T-7[58] that combined the tingling euphoria of ecstasy with the swirling visual patterning of mescaline. Before Shulgin's death in 2014 he began exploring new 'fly' and 'dragonfly' structures, wing-like extensions on such molecules that created new and more potent variations on his already vast repertoire. Mescaline itself may have disappeared from both the laboratory and the street, but its progeny are everywhere and their future permutations potentially infinite.

UNDER A COMANCHE MOON

7–8 OCTOBER 2017
OKLAHOMA

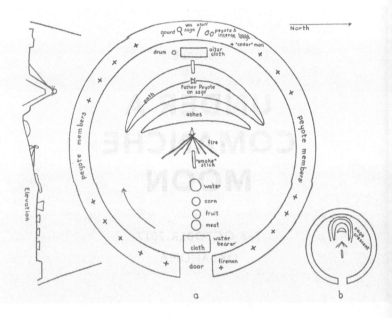

A peyote meeting.

When Quanah Parker, first and last chief of the Comanches, died in 1911 his 'grandfather peyote', a large and perfect dried specimen, was sitting on the table by his bedside in its dark wooden glass-lidded box. On 7 October 2017, the ninety-ninth anniversary of the signing of the charter that incorporated the Native American Church (NAC) in the state of Oklahoma, this peyote was taken from its climate-controlled conservation room and set on the horseshoe-shaped mound of rich red earth inside a tipi, to preside over a ceremony for the first time since Quanah's passing.

The meeting was one of many convened that night by NAC chapters across the state to mark the occasion. This one took place on a 160-acre plot on the northeast fringes of the former reservation, originally allocated to the Comanche woman Louise Looking Glass. The tipi was erected on rolling farmland, the Wichita Mountains visible as a smudge against the flat western horizon. As dusk fell four golden eagles, guests from a world-renowned Comanche breeding programme that makes available sacred feathers from federally protected species, were tethered on perches around the tipi for the all-night vigil, facing out in the cardinal directions.[1]

Night fell, and a full moon rose in a clear sky: a sight the other inhabitants of the Southwest used to call a Comanche moon, as they battened the hatches of their forts and homesteads against night-raiding warbands. The roadman led the celebrants into the tipi where the fire was already burning. Tobacco and corn shucks were passed round the circle, were rolled and lit; clouds of smoke merged with the flames and spiralled up through the tipi's open apex to the circle of stars above. A mutter of prayers in Comanche, Kiowa and English rose with the smoke, echoed and multiplied by the enclosing canvas. The roadman and his assistant unwrapped the drum and gourd rattle, wreathed them in cedar incense and passed them to the drum chief. They were followed around the circle by a large jar of dried and powdered peyote, fibrous and feather-light, heaped into palms and swallowed down with a demijohn of cold tea.

The drum and rattle made their way round the circle, each singer accompanied on the drum by his neighbour. The songs, sung from deep in the throat over the insistent, driving rhythm, were amplified inside the tipi into the sound of a galloping warband. The fire leapt with electric flashes as the fireman fed the long sticks into its heart, raking the mounting pile of coals into a glowing sculpture of two eagle wings that fanned out in display to the grandfather peyote and to the circle of night above. At intervals between the songs, when a celebrant was moved, they rolled tobacco and, with the smoke carrying their prayers upwards, opened their heart to the Creator. The prayers began humbly and often tearfully, confessing the celebrants' weak and pitiful state, gradually gaining force and rising to soaring flights of oratory. As song and prayer alternated and built on one another, fed by fire, incense, tobacco and peyote, the tipi became a world outside time.

In the twenty-first century mescaline in its crystal form has almost vanished. It can occasionally be found for sale on the markets of the dark web, along with every other designer psychedelic imaginable, but even here it is rarely listed and has no discernible subculture of connoisseurs. Its salts, usually the hydrochloride, are still offered by some pharmaceutical companies, still including Merck and my uncle Peter's old suppliers, now Sigma-Aldrich. It is listed as a certified reference material for use in drug testing, forensic analysis and criminal toxicology and its sale is, naturally, highly controlled. Its role in biomedical research is currently limited to the perennially well-supported fields of illicit drug detection and addiction studies.[2]

By contrast, the ceremonial use of the peyote and San Pedro cacti is thriving. In 1959 the United Nations Narcotics Division described the NAC as 'an ethnographical curiosity rather than an important movement', its peyote use an anomaly in the international drug control system that was not expected to endure.[3] Today it has well over a quarter of a million members. The most spectacular growth has been among the Navajo (Diné) people, of whom over 100,000 are now estimated to be NAC members, including the current president of the NAC of North America, Andrew Tso. A generation ago it was unusual for a Navajo family to be peyotists, but today it appears the most popular form of worship. The huge weekend flea market in Gallup, New Mexico, the largest in Navajo country, is dominated by stalls selling ceremonial accessories and CDs of peyote songs from Comanche, Kiowa and Cheyenne ceremonies as well as their own. In Gallup's dedicated NAC trading stores their eclectic creativity is on full display, with drums, wands, feathers and water buckets in a profusion of styles and decorations, drawing on traditions from across indigenous America: historical motifs from the Wild West, Huichol yarn designs, modern ayahuasca art from the Amazon with its inflections of western psychedelia.

Unlike the art of the Huichol, this is work produced essentially for its creators' own people rather than the wider marketplace. The NAC remains generally discreet about its sacrament and disengaged from psychedelic culture in the wider world. It keeps its distance from the current interest in psychedelics as western medicines, the global vogue for shamanic healing with ayahuasca and San Pedro, and the movements for the legal regulation of marijuana. History has taught it that there is nothing to gain from presenting its religious practice as an aspect of drug culture.[4] As Quanah Parker and James Mooney recognised at the start, it was important to embed peyote in Indian culture as a whole and to resist the western tendency to reduce it to its psychedelic properties. These days NAC elders advise younger members to use language with particular care on social media: 'peyote ceremony' will attract sensational interest, but 'prayer meeting' passes beneath the radar. Peyote remains alien to the white culture that surrounds it and constantly vulnerable to the persecution that has been a consistent feature over five centuries from the Spanish conquistadors to the US Drug Enforcement Agency (DEA).

Since 1994 the NAC has in theory full protection under US law, yet its future is precarious in two crucial respects. In legal terms the supply of peyote from the gardens of south Texas, on which the church has always depended, hangs by a thread. Under US law peyote is illegal except when collected by registered traders and supplied to legitimate branches of the NAC. The handful of legal suppliers – today's *peyoteros*, in some cases family businesses dating back to the early days – were until recently administered by the state of Texas but are now controlled directly by the DEA. The legitimacy of the hundreds of NAC branches and chapters rests essentially on tradition and bureaucratic precedent, and remains vulnerable to aggressive legal moves by the federal government.

Cultivation of peyote is strictly illegal under US law, whether in the peyote gardens or anywhere else, and in consequence the cactus, slow growing and with only a tiny corner of its natural range in US territory, is also threatened by over-demand. Even when properly managed, harvests are stretched by the legitimate supplies to the NAC, and illicit gathering stretches them further. The licensed harvesters supply around 1.4 million buttons a year, and country where old-time ranchers recall 'walking on mattresses of peyote' has since been cleared for pasture and agriculture.[5] The combination of decreasing supply and increased demand makes it impossible to hand-pick peyote with the care and experience of previous generations. When peyote roots are damaged, inevitable with hurried or inexperienced pickers or any form of mechanical harvesting, the cacti are unable to recover.

On the Mexican side of the border, peyote's more extensive habitat is under pressure from the unregulated market in peyote-based patent medicines: bottles and tubs of herbal *aciete* or *pomada*, liquids and pastes advertised with pictures of Huichol shamans and promising relief from rheumatic pain or bronchitis.[6] Around the Huichol pilgrimage grounds of Wirikuta, peyote has been the driver for an influx of New Age tourism and a boom in neo-shamanic rituals: organised therapy sessions, drumming circles, temazcal sweat-lodges and spas, spiritual retreats and alternative cancer cures. Peyote tours are organised to Huichol villages; where cacti used to be found on their nearby slopes, it now requires a two-day trek to see them. Harvesting for medical preparations is commonly by mechanical digger, taking up roots and all.

The Huichol themselves are more conspicuous than ever in the twenty-first century, as artists and ambassadors for the indigenous cultures of Mexico at home and abroad. On high days and holidays their celebrations in and around Real de Catorce are a magnet for young western and Latin American travellers in their hundreds. They are far more visible than the NAC on the global scene, travelling to conduct ceremonies at international festivals and prehistoric sacred sites across Europe and a regular presence on the psychedelic conference circuit. Their travels are motivated by a millennial project they describe as the 'renovation of the world': the offerings of their ancestors that kept the world's spiritual forces in alignment are running low, and rituals are required to restore their balance. Like the global network of travelling *ayahuasceros* from Brazil, Colombia, Peru and Ecuador, their extended pilgrimage is a source of income for their community, allowing them to buy land that maintains their independence by staving off the encroachment of mining and agriculture. Taking their message to the wider world entails change, compromise and a level of commercialism that risks corrupting their traditions, but is part of a longstanding process of negotiation between their traditional lifeways and modernity.

San Pedro, even more than peyote, is conspicuously thriving in the twenty-first century. Abundant, fast growing, legal in most countries and readily available through online suppliers, the *curandero* healing potion that was until recently confined to the coast of Peru and Ecuador is being carried on the same currents that have turned ayahuasca from an obscure Amazonian plant brew to a global phenomenon. In California, where sophisticated San Pedro preparation techniques have circulated since the 1990s, a cosmopolitan network of neo-shamans, often with roots in urban Peru and apprenticeships with traditional *curanderos* on the coast, have set up healing circles and retreats. Their ceremonies are usually based around the traditional *mesa* ritual but often replace the cheap synthetic *agua florida* perfumes with natural essences more to western taste. Many centres in the Peruvian, Colombian and Brazilian Amazon that host ayahuasca retreats now also have resident San Pedro shamans, and like ayahuasca the ceremony has spread through long-established nodes of spiritual exchange – Goa, Ibiza, Thailand – to the global marketplace. In 2013 a movie starring Michael Cera, *Crystal Fairy and the Magical Cactus*, introduced a mainstream youth audience to a pair of American back-packers on a pilgrimage through South America in search of San Pedro's illumination.

*   *   *

At midnight in the tipi, the thunder of voice and drum paused and the roadman gave a series of sharp blasts on his eagle-bone whistle. A silver pail of drinking water was passed round the circle, which thinned out temporarily as some took the opportunity to leave the tent and stretch their legs, massage away cramps, relieve themselves or find an extra blanket. The long 'dark hours' of the ceremony are an ordeal, and intended as such. Suffering, as the roadman observed in encourage-ment, raises prayer more urgently up to heaven. After midnight the tempo of the ceremony picked up. Any queasiness or discomfort from the peyote was subsiding; the jar circulated once more, lifting up the participants with a brisk current of physical and psychic energy. In the pounding of rattle and drum, whispered words formed and dissolved like a radio tuned to a distant station. The column of sparks spiralled up from the fire to the sky; as the pile of glowing coals heaped, it was spread with practised sweeps into jewelled feathers.

In response to a request for healing made before the ceremony, the roadman stood and approached the fire, summoning the patient to join him. He scattered cedar incense from his embroidered bag across the coals, and the fragrant smoke enveloped them both as he passed his hands across the celebrant's back, arms, torso and legs: both massage and blessing, medical and spiritual, harnessing the power of the ritual to its purpose. It was medicine in the expansive indigenous sense of the word: a power that resides not simply in a drug but in the ritual and the occasion, the support and witness of the whole community, with the will of the patient as important as the skill of the doctor.

This type of doctoring is hard to encompass within the western clinical paradigm, which is predicated on separating the action of a drug from the 'non-pharmacological variables' of placebo response or faith-healing. For peyote's traditional practitioners, there is no such distinction. It is both a medicinal plant and an omniscient spirit: it is crudely reductive to attempt to separate the peyote from the ritual as a whole, even more so to reduce the power of the cactus to the mescaline it contains. Even the word 'peyote' is used sparingly: the general term for 'medicine' in the native tongue is often used in preference. In English, the terms 'medicine' and 'sacrament' are used more or less interchangeably. It is 'mescaline' or a 'drug' only to outsiders, usually those with hostile intent.

In the century since its laboratory synthesis, western culture has attempted to instrumentalise mescaline in ways as diverse as western culture itself: as a medicine, a brainwashing tool, a creative stimulus, a spiritual catalyst, an instrument of science or of pleasure. For all these purposes its bewildering spectrum of effects has made it fascinating, tantalising and frustrating. In its indigenous worlds, by contrast, the cactus is granted personhood, all its properties accepted as facets of a complex and irreducible character. Rather than attempting to bend it to a preconceived purpose, its traditional users have always taken it on its own terms and shaped their world around it.

　　　🌵　　　🌵　　　🌵

After the healing the cycle of songs and prayers resumes, powering the celebrants through the final stretch of the night. The dark hours are receding; this is the time of reward and illumination, when the spirit is at its height and new songs may be received and composed. Outside, coyotes circle the tipi with their howling, one pack setting off the next. The peyote jar passes round once more, and the celebrants produce their feather fans, bound with leather onto embroidered handles. In Quanah's day the eagle-feather fan was the preserve of the roadman; today they are displayed by all, treasured possessions and badges of lineage. The singer masks his face behind the fan, and the celebrants twist and flutter their feathers before them, whirling the smoke and prayers upwards and making the fire dance, currents of energy almost visible as they spin round the circle and ascend to the stars. Around the eagle wings of the glowing embers and Quanah's altarpiece, the circle is suspended in the rainbow shimmer of the peyote, held weightless by voice, rattle and drum.

ENDNOTES

1. Huxley 2004 [1954], 3.
2. Huxley 1980, 42.
3. Huxley 2004 [1954], 7.
4. Huxley 1980, 107.
5. Huxley 2004 [1954], 2.
6. Ibid., 48.
7. *Life*, 3 June 1957, 16.
8. Heywood 1964, 229–30.
9. Bird 2010, 9.
10. For example, *The Doors of Perception* also draws on his friend William Sheldon's then-fashionable somatotype theory of ectomorphs, endomorphs and mesomorphs; his previous book, *The Devils of Loudun* (1952), was underpinned by William Sargant's Cold War-era theories of brainwashing and mind control.
11. He refers to him incorrectly as 'Ludwig Lewin'.
12. Ellis 1898, 7.
13. Ibid., 13.
14. Huxley 2004 [1954], 14.
15. Nahua refers to speakers of the Nahuatl language, which includes those often referred to in western sources as Aztec. There are still many native speakers of Nahuatl in Mexico today.
16. There is no single satisfactory term for the indigenous inhabitants of America. 'Indian' is of course a post-colonial concept – there was no need of it before the arrival of Europeans – but many native American groups have used and continue to use the word to describe themselves. In the Pueblo cultures of the American Southwest, for example, it is preferred to 'Native American'; however, it is rarely used among the First Nations of Canada. According to the US Census Bureau in 1995, 50 per cent of indigenous respondents chose to identify as 'American Indian' and 37 per cent as 'Native American'. Given the diversity of indigenous American cultures and the breadth of historical contexts, I have not attempted consistency; I use what I hope is the most appropriate term in each case. I make a distinction between the more general 'native American' and the capitalised 'Native American', which has a specific meaning in the USA (and, as we see in chapter 5, was originally adopted in the context of the peyote religion).
17. Arthur Heffter, the chemist who first extracted mescaline from peyote in 1897 along with five other related alkaloid compounds, asserted that it was entirely responsible for the cactus's visionary effects. This claim now requires some qualification. It turns out that mescaline is one of over fifty alkaloids found in different quantities in the cacti; some are closely related to mescaline, while others contribute a different spectrum of effects such as lowering blood pressure, increasing heart rate and boosting dopamine levels. For the alkaloids present in peyote, see Anderson 1996 [1980], 138–44; for their medical properties see Perrine 2001, 7–10.

I CACTUS MYSTERIES

1. Huxley 2004 [1954], 1.
2. The taxonomy of the San Pedro cacti is tangled. The genus *Trichocereus* was subsumed in many classificatory systems into the larger genus *Echinopsis* before recently being restored (see Albesiano and Kiesling 2012). In Albesiano and Kiesling's scheme *pachanoi* is a subspecies of what they regard as the type species in the genus (*Trichocereus macrogonus* subsp. *pachanoi*). The closely related *Trichocereus peruvianus* is sometimes referred to as San Pedro and sometimes by a different common name, Peruvian Torch. Some cactologists and growers have reverted to *Trichocereus* while others still use *Echinopsis*. No nomenclature is universally accepted. See also Trout 2005, 106.
3. See Fung 1972. She doesn't confirm the identity of the cactus or explain why the skins have been separated and rolled; however the mescaline in San Pedro is concentrated in the cortex area under the skin, and the rolls may have been a mode of preparation or storage.
4. Forbes and Clement 2011 claimed to identify mescaline in some species of acacia in south Texas, but their findings have been questioned and remain unconfirmed. They also claim to have found amphetamine, methamphetamine and nicotine in their samples.
5. See Trout 2005, 272 for a list of around eighty cacti which have been reported to contain mescaline, some unconfirmed.
6. Anderson 2001, 136. Early surveys suggested that as many as 90 per cent of the cactus family contained alkaloids, but the pharmacologist and peyote specialist Jan Bruhn's 1971 survey put the figure at around 40 per cent.
7. Mescaline has a lower affinity for serotonin receptors than the tryptamines, which is why it requires a larger dose to achieve its psychoactive effects. It is also less effective at penetrating the blood–brain barrier, which accounts for its longer onset time. There are many subtypes of serotonin receptors; although their relative contributions are unclear, it seems that mescaline's distinctive spectrum of effects is related to the subtypes with which it has a particular affinity and the adrenergic responses that it elicits alongside them. See Kennedy 2014, 100–1.
8. Fogleman and Danielson 2001 and Kopp 2012 describe the emergence of a new species of fruit fly in the Sonoran Desert that evolved to tolerate the alkaloids in a species of columnar cactus that is toxic to flies of related species.
9. The range of perspective techniques deployed in Chavín art makes it possible that the grooved ribs are a two-dimensional schematic representation of a plant with a larger number of sections (see Cordy-Collins 1977, 356, Trout 2005, 17).
10. The main psychoactive compounds in *Anadenanthera* seeds are bufotenine and N,N-dimethyltryptamine.
11. See Torres 2008 for an illustrated overview of the iconography of psychoactive plants at Chavín-era sites. Mulvany de Peñaloza 1984 has argued that all the plant designs on the Tello obelisk, a carved pillar at Chavín decorated in a similar style to the *Lanzón*, may be representations of psychoactive species.
12. For example the Wichí in Bolivia and Argentina.
13. Torres 2018, 247. It is unclear whether and how DMT in *chicha* could be orally active; it has been argued that the metabolites of the ethanol might include beta-carbolines that inhibit the enzymes that break it down, much as the DMT in the ayahuasca brew is potentiated by the beta-carbolines present in the *yagé* vine. In the northwest Amazon, people such as the Yanomami sometimes chew the *yagé* vine while snuffing *vilca*; this may be a historical antecedent of the oral preparation ayahuasca.
14. See Cordy-Collins 1977 and Burger 1992, 157: 'The central role of psychotropic substances at Chavín is amply documented by its graphic representations on the sculptures'. This has been confirmed by the more recent archaeological work of Shady Solís 2007 and Fux (ed.) 2013, though none of them have proposed in more detail how the plants might have been used ceremonially.
15. Burger 1992, 226.

16. See Mulvany de Peñaloza 1994.
17. Sharon 1978, 43.
18. There is wide variation in assays of mescaline content in both peyote and San Pedro; average estimates may be skewed by outlying and inaccurate readings but they probably also reflect a wide range of potencies between different specimens. Broadly, San Pedro is typically around 0.5–1 per cent mescaline by dried weight (though it may reach 2 per cent), while peyote is around 3–4 per cent but may reach 6 per cent. See Erowid Plant Vaults: Psychoactive Cacti, online at https://erowid.org/plants/cacti (accessed 29 October 2018).
19. Sharon 1972, 132.
20. This was probably prompted by the claim that Fischinger was one of the subjects in Kurt Beringer's mescaline experiments in Heidelberg in the 1920s (described in chapter 6), and became obsessed with putting the 'furious succession' of images he experienced onto film. His animation for *Fantasia*, to Bach's 'Toccata and Fugue in D Minor', was allegedly the result of this obsession. Unfortunately this claim seems to have no earlier verifiable source than an unreferenced assertion in Stafford 1992, 113, and is probably an urban legend that emerged after the film was re-released in 1969 with a psychedelic-style promotional campaign.

2 THE DEVIL'S ROOT

1. Šnicer, Bohata and Myšák 2008.
2. Bruhn, De Smet, El-Seedi and Beck 2002 dated the samples to 3700 BCE; Terry et al. 2006, working with the same material, found a slightly older date of 4045–3690 BCE.
3. Stewart 1987, 19.
4. Clendinnen 1991, 221.
5. Burkhart 1992, 91.
6. Stewart 1987, 19.
7. Anderson 1996 [1980], 8.
8. Taylor 1944, 176.
9. Cervantes 1994, 16.
10. Earle 2014, 83–99.
11. See Dawson 2018 and Jenkins 2004, 94–5.
12. United Nations, 'Single Convention on Narcotic Drugs', 1961; online at https://www.unodc.org/pdf/convention_1961_en.pdf (accessed 29 October 2018); preamble: '. . . a serious evil for the individual . . . fraught with social and economic danger to mankind'.
13. Cervantes 1994, 63.
14. Nesvig 2017, 37. >
15. Edict of the Holy Office, ANG-1, Vol 3, exp. 35, 1620, quoted in Leonard 1942, 325–6.
16. Stewart 1987, 25–6.
17. La Barre 1938, 36.
18. Lumholtz 1903, vol. 1, 357.
19. Ibid., 363.
20. Ibid., 365.
21. Ibid., 368.
22. Ibid., 375.
23. Ibid., 377.
24. Ibid., vol. 2., 156.
25. Ibid., 177.
26. Ibid., 268.
27. Ibid., 277.
28. Myerhoff 1974, 73.
29. Ibid., 189.

30. Ibid., 149.
31. Furst, Royal Anthropological Institute, RA55, film, 22 minutes.
32. Ibid., 34 minutes.
33. Myerhoff 1974, 164.
34. Ibid., 226–7. 'A man's life . . .': Among the Huichol both men and women take peyote and participate in the peyote hunt. The pilgrimage Myerhoff joined was 'typical in its wide age range and inclusion of both sexes' (ibid., 118) comprising five men and two women.
35. Ibid., 262.
36. Furst (ed.) 1990 [1972], 137.
37. Fikes 1993, 170.
38. Myerhoff 1974, 190.
39. Kennedy 1978, 148.
40. Zingg 1938, 383–5.
41. Ibid., 259–60.
42. Myerhoff 1974, 74.

3   MAKING MEDICINE

1. Bass 1954, 253.
2. Ibid., 250.
3. Ibid., 917.
4. Moses 2002 [1984], 61.
5. Bass 1954, 254.
6. Mooney recorded its name in Comanche (Numunu) as *wokowi*, in Mescalero as *ho* and Tarahumara as *hikori*.
7. Mooney 1896b, 10.
8. Ibid., 8.
9. Bass 1954, 255.
10. Moses 2002 [1984], 20.
11. Mooney 1896a, 777.
12. Moses 2002 [1984], 68.
13. Mooney 1896a, 657.
14. Ibid., 929.
15. Ibid., 940.
16. Ibid., 942.
17. Mooney 1896b, 8.
18. Subsequent anthropologists have noted that the conditions against which peyote has been regarded as most powerful, such as consumption and alcoholism, are diseases of the white man (see Calabrese 2013, 103).
19. Mooney 1896b, 10.
20. Ibid., 9.
21. Mooney 1910, 237.
22. Mooney 1896b, 11.
23. Morgan 1976, 72.
24. Bender 1968, 160.
25. Bruhn and Holmstedt 1974, 357.
26. Ibid., 356.
27. Bender 1968, 160.
28. Parke, Davis & Co., 1975 [1885].
29. Hoefle 2000, 30.
30. Bruhn and Holmstedt 1974, 358.
31. Mitich 1971, 210.

32. Morgan 1976, 44.
33. Ibid., 66.
34. It was perpetuated by William Safford, botanist at the US Department of Agriculture in Washington, whose 1915 paper 'An Aztec Narcotic' identified peyote with *teonanacatl*, the 'flesh of the gods' recorded by Sahagún and other early Spanish sources. *Teonanacatl* was subsequently identified by Richard Schultes and others as the psychedelic mushroom *Psilocybe mexicana*.
35. Weston La Barre and others have argued that the older 'mescal bean cult' prefigured and prepared the ground for the adoption of peyote by the Plains tribes (La Barre 1969 [1938], 105).
36. *New Orleans Picayune*, 30 September 1856, 1.
37. Bruhn and Holmstedt 1974, 354.
38. Ibid., 360.
39. Ibid., 362.
40. Perrine 2001, 46.
41. Bender 1968, 164.
42. In a feature by Lida Rose McCabe, *Chicaco Inter Ocean*, illustrated supplement 20 August 1893.
43. La Barre 1937, 42.
44. Ibid., 109 ff., Stewart 1987, 45 ff.
45. Mooney 1897, 330.
46. I am indebted to Sia, the Comanche Nation Ethno-Ornithological Initiative and Piah Puha Kahni (Mother Church) of the Numunuh (Comanche) Native American Church, for many details of their people's story. The names of their deceased are traditionally not spoken and I thank them for their permission to record them here.
47. Hagan 1993, 31.
48. Ibid., 60.
49. Ibid., 53.
50. Ibid., 55.
51. University of Oklahoma, Western History Collection, Indian Pioneer Papers 9452, 309.
52. Hagan 1993, 57.
53. For the classic description of the Comanche rite see La Barre 1937, 43–53.
54. Perrine 2001, 23.
55. Cornell University Library, House Resolution 2614, 1918, 71.
56. Perrine 2001, 24.
57. Cornell University Library, House Resolution 2614, 1918, 71.
58. Ibid., 72.
59. Perrine 2001, 21–2.
60. In 1901 the core of the reservation was designated a national park, now the Wichita Mountains Wildlife Refuge. In 1956 Quanah's house was moved a few miles away to Eagle Park, on the edge of the small town of Cache. It was registered as a National Historical Site in 1972 and is still standing, though in a severely dilapidated state.
61. The glass plate negative is held in the Smithsonian's National Anthropological Archives (BAE GN 01778a 06305400, undated, labelled as 'Peyote Ceremony').
62. Cornell University Library, House Resolution 2614, 1918, 72.
63. Mooney 1896b, 10.

4 BRILLIANT VISIONS

1. Prentiss and Morgan 1895, 580.
2. Ibid.
3. Coppin and High 1999, 36.
4. Ewell 1896, 624.

5. Ibid., 626.
6. Prentiss and Morgan 1895, 580.
7. Ibid., 581.
8. Ibid., 582.
9. Prentiss and Morgan 1896, 6.
10. Peyote: Hearings on House Resolution 2614, pt. 1, Feb 21–25 1918, 52–3.
11. Ibid., 62.
12. Mooney 1896b, 11.
13. It now seems likely that it was the species known today as *Lophophora diffusa*, which has a smaller and more southern distribution than *L. williamsii* and little or no mescaline among its alkaloids.
14. Bruhn and Holmstedt 1974, 365.
15. Ibid.
16. Mitchell is perhaps best remembered today for his 'rest cure' for neurasthenia, which has become infamous through Charlotte Perkins Gilman's novella *The Yellow Wallpaper* (1892), a fictionalised narrative of the treatment to which he subjected her.
17. Earnest 1950, 154.
18. Mitchell 1877, 52.
19. Mitchell 1896, 1,625.
20. Ibid., 1,626.
21. All ibid., 1,627.
22. All ibid., 1,628.
23. Ibid., 1,627.
24. Earnest 1950, 154.
25. Ibid.
26. Nicotra 2008, 210.
27. James 1890, 224.
28. Ibid., 620.
29. Nicotra 2008, 210.
30. James 1985 [1902], 388.
31. Ellis 1898, 7.
32. Ellis 1897, 1,541.
33. Ellis 1898, 8.
34. Ibid.
35. All ibid., 9–10.
36. Ong 2002 [1982], chapter 4.
37. Benjamin 2003, 328.
38. Ellis 1898, 11.
39. *Review of Reviews*, January 1898, 55.
40. *British Medical Journal*, 5 February 1898, 390.
41. Ellis 1898, 10.
42. Ibid.
43. 'And yet I am the lord of all, / And this brave world magnifical . . .'; 'Haschisch', December 1896.
44. Beckson 1987, 169.
45. Symons 2014 [1899], 6.
46. Ellis 1898, 12.
47. *Ibid.*
48. Perrine 2001, 11.
49. Ibid., 43.
50. Holmstedt and Liljestrand 1963, 208.
51. Ibid., 209.
52. Lewin 1998 [1924], 3.

53. Ibid., 81.
54. Ibid., 89.
55. Holmstedt and Liljestrand 1963, 209.

5 HIGHER POWERS

1. Holmstedt and Liljestrand 1963, 209
2. *British Medical Journal*, 11 November 1899, 1,357.
3. Dixon 1899, 71.
4. Ibid., 72.
5. Ibid., 79.
6. Ibid., 80.
7. Ibid., 83.
8. Crowley's oeuvre is the context in which Louis Lewin's nomenclature is best remembered today.
9. King 1987 [1977], 63.
10. *Daily Sketch*, 24 August 1910.
11. Archer 1932, 94.
12. Ibid., 101.
13. Ibid., 102.
14. Ibid., 103.
15. Ibid., 105.
16. Ibid., 107.
17. Everitt 2016 offers the most detailed analysis to date and proposes that Crowley's magickal diaries and rites contain many concealed and coded references to peyote and its extracts.
18. *Equinox* 1.2, 1909, 36.
19. *Equinox* 1.3–6, 1910–11.
20. Everitt 2016, 38.
21. Sutin 2002, 229.
22. Ibid., 230.
23. Crowley 1929, 386.
24. Sutin 2002, 253.
25. *Equinox* 3.1, 1919, 16.
26. Sutin 2002, 282.
27. Smith 1918, 111.
28. Ibid., 213.
29. James 1914, 9.
30. Ibid., 16.
31. Smith 1918, 62.
32. Ibid., 42.
33. Ibid., 107.
34. Ibid., 111.
35. Ibid., 112.
36. Ibid., 181.
37. Barnes 1998, 98.
38. Tommasini 1997, 84. I'm very grateful to Alan Piper for the references from his 2016 paper, 'A 1920s Harvard Psychedelic Circle with a Mormon Connection: Peyote Use among the "Harvard Aesthetes" '.
39. Piper 2016.
40. Tommasini 1997, 84.
41. Rudnick 1984, 74.

42. Ibid., 64.
43. Luhan 1936, 266.
44. Ibid.
45. Ibid., 268.
46. Ibid., 270.
47. Ibid., 275.
48. Ibid., 277.
49. Ibid., 278.
50. Rudnick 1984, 129.
51. William James wrote of New Thought as an integral part of the 'mind-cure movement' and believed its growth through the late nineteenth century meant that 'it must now be reckoned with as a genuine religious power' (James 1902, 94).
52. Rudnick 1984, 150.
53. Rudnick 1996, 16.
54. Ibid., 91. 'Red Atlantis' invoked the teachings of Theosophy and the belief of its founder, Madame Helena Blavatsky, that native American rock art and pictographs were the survival of an ancient system of knowledge dating back to Atlantis.
55. Smith and Snake (eds) 1996, 126.
56. Jenkins 2004, 95.
57. It seems that peyote had been known in some Pueblo cultures as a medicine, though not as the focus of an organised religion. Spanish records show that as far back as 1719 a Taos pueblo resident was tried for having drunk a beverage of 'the herb peyote' (Parsons 1996 [1939], 1,095).
58. Ibid., 1,094.
59. Luhan 1937, 176.
60. Ibid., 287.
61. Ibid., 288.
62. Ibid., 289.
63. Ibid., 310.
64. Ibid., 331.
65. Cornell University Archives, House Resolution 2614, 1918, 3.
66. The pattern and timing of peyote's diffusion across the US between 1890 and 1920 is complex and disputed. Mooney's account was revised by Ruth Shonle (1925) and hers has subsequently been challenged and amended by, among others, La Barre 1938 and Stewart 1987.
67. Ibid., 176.
68. Ibid., 20.
69. Ibid., 45.
70. Cornell University Archives, House Resolution 2614, 1918, 21.
71. Ibid., 60.
72. Ibid., 52.
73. Ibid., 53.
74. Ibid., 63.
75. Ibid., 74.
76. Ibid., 82.
77. Ibid., 74.
78. Ibid., 99.
79. Ibid., 144.
80. Ibid., 143.
81. Ibid., 146.
82. Ibid., 79.
83. Kavanagh (ed.) 2008, 6.

84. I am indebted for this and many of the following stories to Charlie Haag, grandson of Mack and current president of the Native American Church of Oklahoma (interview, 10 October 2017).
85. Stewart 1987, 135.
86. Marriott and Rachlin 1971, 86.
87. Stewart 1987, 224.
88. Smith and Snake (eds) 1996, 136.
89. Moses 2002 [1984], 204.
90. Stewart 1987, 222.
91. Moses 2002 [1984], 216–17.

6 DER MESKALINRAUSCH

1. Späth 1919.
2. Anderson 1996 [1980], 147.
3. Bruhn and Holmstedt 1974, 367. Heffter had suggested in 1901 that mescaline was 3,4,5-trimethoxybenzylmethlyamine, but reversed this identification in 1905.
4. Klüver 1929a, 446.
5. Knauer and Maloney 1913, 427.
6. Ibid., 426.
7. Ibid., 425.
8. Ibid., 427.
9. Ibid., 428.
10. Ibid., 426.
11. Prentiss and Morgan 1895, 581.
12. Moreau 1973 [1845], 17.
13. Knauer and Maloney 1913, 429.
14. Ibid., 432.
15. Ibid., 435.
16. Beringer 1969 [1927], 31 (my translation).
17. Klüver 1966 [1928], 51–5.
18. Mayer-Gross 1951, 318.
19. Beringer 1969 [1927], 113–14.
20. Klüver 1966 [1928], 17.
21. Ibid., 19.
22. Ibid., 40.
23. Ibid., 41.
24. Ibid., 30.
25. Klüver's 'form-constants' have been recognised in a wide range of conditions including epilepsy, migraine and out-of-body experiences. They were used by Ernst Gombrich in his studies of the history of decoration in art. Since the sixties they have become a common motif in op-art and other psychedelic styles. They are the basis for the theory popularised by David Lewis-Williams in *The Mind in the Cave* (2002) that patterns and motifs in Palaeolithic and hunter–gatherer cave art are depictions of entoptic or drug-induced visual phenomena.
26. Klüver 1966 [1928], 22.
27. Ibid., 23.
28. Ibid., 31.
29. Ibid., 53.
30. Ibid., 55.
31. Ibid., ix.
32. Ibid., viii.

33. Hofmann 2013 [1980], 39.
34. Klüver 1966 [1928], 54.
35. Fernberger 1932, 375.
36. Rouhier 1989a [1926], 233.
37. Rouhier 1989b [1926], 5.
38. Ibid., 10.
39. Rouhier 1989a [1926], 340.
40. Ibid., 348.
41. The other alkaloids originally isolated by Heffter – pellotine, anhaline (hordenine), anhalonine, anhalonidine and lophophorine – are, as Rouhier argued, quite varied in their pharmacology: for a summary see Perrine 2001, 8–10.
42. Rouhier 1989a [1926], 353.
43. United Nations 1959, 25–6.
44. Klüver 1929b, 421.

7 PROFANE ILLUMINATIONS

1. Kandel 2012, 205.
2. 'Surrealism, noun, masc.', First Surrealist Manifesto, 1924.
3. Balakian 1974, 99.
4. Lotringer 2015 [2003], 179. In response to persistent rumours about his use of mescaline, mushrooms and LSD, Salvador Dalí famously pronounced in 1982: 'I don't do drugs. I *am* drugs!'
5. Gerould 1981, 15.
6. Ibid., 16.
7. A list that included nicotine, alcohol, cocaine, morphine, ether, hashish, Eukodal and harmine.
8. Witkiewicz 1992 [1932], 250.
9. Ibid., 258.
10. Witkiewicz 2018 [1932], 67–8.
11. Witkiewicz 1992 [1932], 247.
12. Ibid., 259.
13. Ibid., 260.
14. Witkiewicz 2018 [1932], 79.
15. Witkiewicz 1992 [1932], 262.
16. Witkiewicz 2018 [1932], 79.
17. For example, Brzecki, Kobel-Buys and Buys, 2002.
18. Witkiewicz 2018 [1932], 92.
19. Witkiewicz 1992 [1932], 261.
20. According to Oisteanu 2010, 356–8 Marinescu experimented with a total of seven artists; apart from Michailescu he has identified two others, Paul Molda and Ludovic Basarab.
21. Marinesco 1933, 1,864 (my translations). Marinescu generally published in French medical journals, where he used the Italianate spelling of his surname.
22. Ibid., 1,865.
23. Ibid., 1,866.
24. ten Berge 1999, 259.
25. Bakewell 2017, 39.
26. Boon 2002, 236.
27. Sartre and Gerassi, 2009, 62–3.
28. Ibid., 194.
29. Merleau-Ponty 2002 [1945], 397.
30. Ibid., 391.

31. Ibid., 393.
32. Ibid., 396.
33. Ibid., 399–400.
34. Benjamin 2006, 1
35. Benjamin's fragmentary writings on hashish and mescaline were published in German in 1971 and translated for *On Hashish* (2006), which includes valuable introductory material and extracts of his writings on drugs from previously published sources.
36. Ibid., 117.
37. Ibid., 123.
38. Ibid., 132–3.
39. Ibid., 87.
40. Ibid., 95.
41. Ibid., 88.
42. Ibid., 97.
43. Ibid., 133.
44. Ibid., 122.
45. Ibid., 132.
46. Ibid., 96.
47. Ibid., 126.
48. Ibid., 95.
49. Ibid., 97.
50. Artaud 1976 [1947], 77.
51. Ibid., 82.
52. Knapp 1980 [1969], 125.
53. Artaud 1976 [1947], 3.
54. Ibid., 20.
55. Ibid., 24.
56. Ibid., 77.
57. Le Clézio 1993, 170.
58. Ibid., 166.
59. Artaud 1976 [1947], 27.
60. Ibid., 28.
61. Ibid., 16.
62. Ibid., 32.
63. Ibid., 35.
64. Ibid., 38.
65. Ibid., 42.
66. Ibid., 48.
67. Ibid., 49.
68. Now more commonly referred to as *The Adoration of the Child*; the attribution to Hieronymus Bosch is disputed.
69. Artaud 1976 [1947], 50.
70. Ibid., 26.
71. Le Clézio 1993, 170 observes that there is no authentic detail in Artaud's description of the peyote dance that could not have been drawn from published accounts. He proposes Carlos Basauri's ethnographies of indigenous Mexico in the 1930s as the most likely source.
72. Artaud 1976 [1947], 52.
73. Ibid., 54.
74. Ibid., 94.
75. Knapp 1980 [1969], 147.
76. Ibid., 48.

8 M-SUBSTANCE

1. Stewart 1987 237
2. Smith and Snake (eds) 1996, 128.
3. La Barre 1969 [1938], 8.
4. Ibid., 43
5. Ibid., 54
6. Ibid., 19–20
7. Ibid., 93
8. Ibid., 113
9. Klüver receives a dedication in *Plants of the Gods* (1979), the classic illustrated survey of plant hallucinogens co-authored by Schultes and Albert Hofmann..
10. Lees 2017 has shown that William Burroughs, who met Schultes in Colombia in 1953 while they were independently researching ayahuasca, wrote to him the following year with the observation that the ayahuasca brew derived its power from the combination of the *yagé* vine (*Banisteriopsis caapi*) with the *chacruna* leaf (*Psychotria viridis*). Schultes acknowledged Burroughs' precedence in 1973 after he had unravelled the biochemistry of the combination.
11. Schultes 1937.
12. Davis 1997, 81.
13. Schelling 2017, 11–12.
14. *Oriflamme*, Journal of the Agape Lodge, vol. 1, issue 1 (21 February 1943).
15. Pendle 2006, 218–19.
16. Waters lived in an adobe building beside Tony Luhan's private house, on the edge of the grounds directly bordering pueblo land. Tony's house is currently empty, and Waters' residence was badly damaged by a later fire but still stands as a ruin.
17. Waters 1962 [1942], 83–4.
18. Ibid., 91.
19. Ibid., 93.
20. Rudnick 1996, 179.
21. Angel, Jones and Neve (eds) 2003, 131.
22. Guttman and Maclay 1936, 197. In this paper they use the spelling 'mescalin', a more direct transposition of the German *Mezkalin*; in subsequent papers they also use the more common English spelling, 'mescaline'.
23. Ibid., 201.
24. Guttman and Maclay 1937, 190.
25. Maclay suspected that these colourful and 'disintegrating' cats were produced by Wain during his psychotic episodes, a supposition that was developed by later researchers who assembled some of his cat paintings into a series that purported to illustrated the artist's progression from sanity into psychosis. The sequence is now familiar from its reproduction in dozens of art and psychiatry textbooks, but recent scholarship has shown it to be without foundation. Wain's 'disintegrating' cat pictures are undated and he painted them sporadically throughout his career: he referred to them as his 'wallpaper patterns' (his mother had designed embroideries and carpets). There is no demonstrable match with the various stages of his illness and he was in any case diagnosed with dementia rather than schizophrenia (see Allderidge 2016).
26. Maclay, Guttman and Mayer-Gross 1938, 51.
27. Guttman and Maclay 1937, 190.
28. Beaumont later changed his professional name to Basil Rákóczi.
29. Trevelyan 1957, 74.
30. Ibid., 75.
31. Ibid., 76.
32. Bethlem M03/3, Beaumont report, October 1936.

33. All ibid.
34. Bethlem M03/3, Stephen to Guttman, 27 October 1936.
35. Bethlem M03/3, Guttman to Stephen, 31 October 1936.
36. All ibid.
37. Bethlem M03/3, Beaumont to Guttman, 29 October 1936.
38. Trevelyan 1957, 76.
39. Stockings 1940, 30.
40. Ibid., 46.
41. Ibid., 47.
42. The phrase was apparently coined in a 1922 report in the *Los Angeles Record*, on a case where scopolamine had been used to induce 'twilight sleep' during childbirth (Streatfeild 2006, 37n).
43. Marks 1991 [1979], 6.
44. Streatfeild 2006, 36.
45. The US Naval Technical Mission published their findings in the 300-page 'Technical Report No. 331–45, German Aviation Research at the Dachau Concentration Camp'.
46. Streatfeild 2006, 39.
47. Ibid., 40.
48. Marks 1991 [1979], 5.
49. Frederking 1955, 262.
50. Ibid., 265.
51. Jünger 2013 [1970], § 298. There is no authorised English translation of *Annaherungen*; rather than pagination I have referenced the numbered sections, which are mostly around a page in length.
52. Ibid., § 59.
53. Ibid., § 167.
54. Ibid., § 300.
55. Ibid., § 16.
56. Ibid., § 36.
57. Ibid., § 103.
58. Hofmann 2013 [1980], 113.
59. Jünger 2013 [1970], § 300.
60. Ibid., § 301.
61. Ibid., § 299.
62. Ibid., § 303.
63. Hofmann 2013 [1980], 110.
64. Ibid., 18.
65. Ibid., 19.
66. Ibid., 38.
67. Ibid., 39.
68. Ibid., 114.
69. Ibid., 115.
70. Frederking 1955, 264.
71. Ibid., 265.
72. Ibid., 264.
73. Denber and Merlis 1955, 466.
74. Ibid., 465.
75. Rouhier 1989a [1926], 194–6.
76. Osmond 1952, 4.
77. Ibid., 6.
78. Ibid., 9.
79. Osmond and Smythies 1952, 311.
80. Ibid., 314.

81. Ibid., 312.
82. Mayer-Gross 1951, 320. Patients would of course have been correct in attributing the derangement of mescaline to the same people who were keeping them locked up.
83. Osmond and Smythies 1952, 311.
84. Mayer-Gross 1951, 317. Osmond and Smythies registered their disagreement with Mayer-Gross in a letter to the *British Medical Journal* (vol. 2, issue 4,731 (1951), 607), in which they also acknowledged that 'It remains to be seen what, if any, relationship exists between schizophrenia and mescal intoxication'.
85. Osmond and Smythies 1952, 313.
86. Ibid., 314.
87. Ibid., 315.
88. Barber 2018, 53.
89. Smythies and Smythies 2005, 30.
90. Hoffer, Osmond and Smythies 1954, 30–1.
91. Ibid., 39.
92. Ibid., 40.
93. Ibid., 42.
94. Ibid., 43.
95. Osmond and Smythies 1953, 133.
96. Ibid., 139.
97. Ibid., 141.

9 THE DOORS BLOWN OPEN

1. Huxley 1980, 36.
2. Bedford 1974, vol. 2, 120.
3. Ibid., 130.
4. Huxley 1980, 13.
5. Ibid., 23–5.
6. Ibid., 29.
7. Ibid., 36.
8. Huxley 2004 [1954], 5.
9. Ibid., 7.
10. Nelson and Sass 2008, 348.
11. Huxley 2004 [1954], 13.
12. The antecedents for this idea reach back further than Bergson. A similar metaphor can be found in the first scientific trials of a consciousness-altering drug, the nitrous oxide experiments undertaken by Thomas Beddoes, Humphry Davy and some thirty volunteers at the Pneumatic Institution in Bristol in 1799. One of the subjects, the physician Peter Mark Roget (of *Roget's Thesaurus* fame), described how under the influence of nitrous oxide 'thoughts rushed like a torrent through my mind . . . as if their velocity had been suddenly accelerated by the bursting of a barrier which had before retained them in their natural and equable course' (see Jay 2009, 179).
13. Huxley 1953, 11.
14. Huxley 2004 [1954], 16.
15. Ibid., 19.
16. Bedford 1974, vol. 2, 163.
17. *Time*, 13 July 1953, 40.
18. Siff 2015, 52.
19. Huxley 1980, 86.
20. Dyck 2008, 37.
21. Huxley 2004 [1954], 44–5.

22. Ebin (ed.) 1965 [1961], 242.
23. Philp 1974, 79.
24. Ibid., 81.
25. Ibid., 84.
26. Ibid., 87.
27. 'The Opened Door', *New Yorker*, 25 September 1954, 80.
28. Ibid., 88.
29. Ibid., 90–1.
30. Eskelund 1957, 12.
31. Ibid., 69.
32. Ibid., 76–7.
33. Burroughs 1977 [1953], 145–7.
34. Ebin (ed.) 1965 [1961], 302–4 (originally published in 1960 in the special drugs issue of Birth, a mimeographed magazine edited by Tuli Kupferberg).
35. Ginsberg's 1961 collection *Kaddish and other poems* would include a short poem entitled 'Mescaline', grouped together with 'Laughing Gas' and 'Lysergic Acid'.
36. Torgoff 2004, 60.
37. Jenkins 2004, 147.
38. B. Morgan 2006, 184.
39. Michaux 2002 [1956], 9.
40. Ibid., 59.
41. Ibid., 14–17.
42. Ibid., 63.
43. Ibid., 28–9.
44. Ibid., 7.
45. Ibid., 80.
46. Ibid., 112.
47. Ibid., 126–7.
48. Ibid., 141.
49. Ibid., 85.
50. Michaux 2002 [1956], 38.
51. Interview with Conrad Knickerbocker, 'The Art of Fiction No. 36', *Paris Review*, issue 35 (Fall 1965).
52. Burroughs 2012, 3–5.
53. Huxley 1980, 61–2.
54. Cholden (ed.) 1956, 27.
55. Marks 1991 [1979], 62.
56. Barber 2018, 188.
57. Mills 2010, 18. The psychoactivity of adrenochrome is still disputed, but Osmond and Hoffer's reports remain extreme outliers in the self-experimental literature. The few experience reports filed at Erowid Chemical Vaults: Adrenochrome (online at https://erowid.org/chemicals/adrenochrome; accessed 29 October 2018) suggest slight perceptual changes and markedly unpleasant side effects. It is possible that adrenochrome has a range of different effects in solutions with different pH values.
58. Pearson and Dewhurst 1955, 143.
59. Garson 2017.
60. Hollister 1962, 88.
61. Hofmann 2013 [1980], 127.
62. Hofmann 2008, 65.
63. Jünger 2013 [1970], § 43.
64. Ibid., § 305.
65. Hofmann 2013 [1980], 49.
66. 21 March 1954, quoted in Watt (ed.) 2013 [1975], 394–5.

67. Smythies and Smythies 2005, 36.
68. Jung 1976, 172–3 (italics in original).
69. Zaehner 1957, xx.
70. Ibid., 219.
71. Ibid., 221.
72. Ibid., 222.
73. Personal communication with author, 12 December 2017.
74. Zaehner 1957, 226.
75. Wilson 2004, 231.
76. Ibid., 232–4.
77. Christopher Mayhew, 'An Excursion out of Time', *Observer*, 28 October 1956.
78. All *ibid.*
79. Sections of the film have subsequently been used in other documentaries and some are available, together with later footage of Mayhew recalling the experiment, on YouTube where they have garnered hundreds of thousands of views.
80. Antonio Melechi private collection: *Observer* assistant editor Charles Davy to Mayhew, 3 November 1956.
81. Eliade 1989, 157 (5 February 1962).
82. Antonio Melechi private collection: A.G. Pape, 28 October 1956.
83. Ibid., Philip Metman, 28 October 1956.
84. Ibid., John D Solomon, 30 October 1956.

10 TRIPPING WITH MESCALITO

1. La Barre 1969 [1938], 230.
2. Ibid., 228. Huxley's use of the term 'mescal' in *The Doors of Perception* is perhaps another example of Havelock Ellis's influence.
3. Ibid., xiii.
4. Ibid., 230.
5. Torgoff 2004, 61.
6. La Barre 1969 [1938], 230.
7. R.J. Smith, 'King of the Cats', *Los Angeles Magazine*, 1 June 2005.
8. Smith 2012, 48.
9. Interview recording presented at *Voices of Counterculture in the Southwest*, New Mexico History Museum, Santa Fe, 2017.
10. Ibid.
11. Deloria Jr 1969, 113.
12. Castaneda 1970, 13.
13. Ibid., 38–44.
14. Ibid., 49.
15. Ibid., 100.
16. de Mille 1978 [1976], 113.
17. Letcher 2006, 215.
18. de Mille 1978 [1976], 77.
19. Castaneda 1970, 132.
20. Fikes 1993, 62. Castaneda's notion of Mescalito as peyote's tutelary spirit was co-opted into the personal mythology of Robert Anton Wilson. In *Cosmic Trigger* (1977) Wilson writes that after reading *The Teachings of Don Juan* he recognised Castaneda's description as the warty green-skinned sprite he had himself encountered in 1963, when he experimented with peyote purchased by mail order.
21. Simon Romero, 'Peyote's Hallucinations Spawn Real-Life Academic Feud', *New York Times*, 16 September 2003.

22. Fikes 1993, 13.
23. Znamenski 2007, 208.
24. Ibid., 208–9.
25. Lee and Shlain 1985, 69–70.
26. Dodgson 2013, 117.
27. Stevens 1989, 312.
28. Dodgson 2013, 139.
29. Ibid., 118.
30. Watts 2013 [1962], 97 itemises his chemical allies, without further comment, as 'LSD-25, mescaline, psilocybin, dimethyl-tryptamine (DMT) and cannabis'.
31. Stevens 1989, 256; Oram 2016 argues that although the FDA regulations are commonly described as a ban on psychedelic research, in reality they simply brought it into line with new pharmaceutical guidelines.
32. Weil 1975 [1972], 33–4.
33. All *ibid.*
34. Ross 2017 gives a full account of US Army studies 1955–67 and the follow-up report in 1980.
35. Hermle et al. 1992.
36. Tsao 1951; this synthesis was given in full in underground chemistry manuals such as 'Synthesis and Extraction of Organic Psychedelics', published anonymously in 1969 by the Buzz Communications Company (samizdat, twenty-two typed and stapled pages).
37. Erowid: *Microgram Journal*, Bureau of Narcotics and Dangerous Drugs, US Department of Justice, vol. 1 (1968–69).
38. The Lee and Hendrix session generated 'The Everlasting First' (which appeared on Love's 1970 album *False Start*), two takes of a cover of 'Ezy Rider' and a jam titled 'Loon', which eventually showed up on an acetate offered on eBay in 2009 (it can now be found on YouTube). The Grateful Dead's 'mescaline show' was at Springfield Civic Centre on 11 May 1978 and is archived online at https://archive.org/details/gd78-05-11.moore. minches.18658.sbeok.shnf/gd1978-05-11d3t005.shn (accessed 29 October 2018).
39. Thompson 1972 [1971], 31.
40. Ibid., 33.
41. Ibid., 49–50.
42. Ibid., 58.
43. Published in Thompson 1990.
44. Thompson 2000, 155.
45. Thompson 1990, 101–6.
46. Acosta, an attorney and Chicano activist who had worked with Thompson on some of his investigative assignments, was not pleased at being transposed into a '300-pound Samoan'.
47. Ibid.
48. Thompson 1972 [1971], 12.
49. Ibid. The popular confusion of mescaline and mezcal persists to this day in the urban legend that the worm in mezcal bottles is hallucinogenic. Putting a worm (in fact a cater-pillar) in some commercial mezcal bottles is a relatively recent practice, dating from the 1940s. Its purpose is disputed: some say it's added to show that the spirit is distilled from genuine maguey (agave), others that it demonstrates the alcohol content is high enough to preserve it. Added at the end of the process, just before bottling, the worm contains no mescaline and has no hallucinogenic effects, but it gives customers a sense of authenticity and an opportunity to display machismo by eating it.
50. Thompson 1972 [1971], 122–5.
51. In an early scene in *The Matrix* (1999), the protagonist Neo asks, 'You ever have that feeling where you're not sure if you're awake or still dreaming?' The answer is: 'It's called mescaline. It's the only way to fly.' In *The Simpsons* episode 'D'oh-in' in the Wind' (1998), Homer unwittingly markets a vegetable juice containing peyote that makes his customers

hallucinate; in 'The Mysterious Voyage of Homer' (1997) he eats a super-strength chilli that sends him on a Castaneda-style desert trip where he meets a talking coyote.
52. Shulgin and Shulgin 1991, 16.
53. Ibid., 34–7.
54. Ibid., 69.
55. Ibid., 72.
56. Ibid., 74.
57. Ibid.
58. Full chemical nomenclatures: 4-bromo-2,5-dimethoxyphenethylamine and 2-[2,5-dimethoxy-4-(propylsulfanyl)phenyl]ethan-1-amine.

EPILOGUE   UNDER A COMANCHE MOON

1. Sia, the Comanche Nation Ethno-Ornithological Initiative, have bred, raised and released into the wild several hundred endangered hawks and eagles. Moulted feathers are preserved, microchipped and distributed among Native American tribes for ceremonial use.
2. See Tófoli and Araujo 2016, Dasgupta 2017. In late 2020, the steward-owned pharmaceutical company Journey Colab (www.journeycolab.com) announced their intention to use mescaline in the treatment of alcohol use disorder. They are seeking US Food and Drug Administration (FDA) approval, and plan to begin a preclinical program in 2021.
3. United Nations 1959, 18.
4. Nonetheless, the legal victories of the NAC, particularly the 1994 peyote amendment to the American Indian Religious Freedom Act, established valuable precedents for more recent rulings in favour of ayahuasca worship by the UDV (União do Vegetal) and the Santo Daime Church (see Patchen 2017).
5. Terry and Trout 2016, 2.
6. Terry and Trout 2017, 152–4.

BIBLIOGRAPHY

ARCHIVES

Antonio Melechi private collection
Correspondence of Christopher, Lord Mayhew following his article 'An Excursion out of Time', *Observer*, 28 October 1956.

Bethlem Royal Hospital Archives
Art Collection LDBTH: 43–5, 79, 188–9 [Basil Beaumont], 18–23 [Julian Trevelyan], 81–2 [Herbrand Williams], 191 [Anonymous].
M03/3: Mescaline experiments, Eric Guttman and Walter Maclay.

Cornell University Library
'Peyote: Hearings before a Subcommittee of the Committee of Indian Affairs', House Resolution 2614, US Government Printing Office, 1918.

Erowid (online at https://erowid.org; accessed 28 October 2018)
Chemical Vaults: Mescaline.
Experience Vaults: Mescaline; Peyote; San Pedro.
Microgram Journal, Bureau of Narcotics and Dangerous Drugs, US Department of Justice, vols 1–2 (1968–69).
Plant Vaults: Peyote.

National Anthropological Archives, Smithsonian Institution
Manuscript 1887: James Mooney, miscellaneous notes.
Manuscript 1953: James Mooney, notebook marked 'Trip, 1894–5'.
Manuscript 2537: C.S. Simmons, 'The Peyote Road' (memoir, n.d.).
Manuscript 2537: James Mooney, miscellaneous material regarding peyote.

Royal Anthropological Institute
RA55, film: *To Find Our Life: The Peyote Hunt of the Huichols of Mexico* (1969, dir. Peter Furst).

University of Oklahoma, Western History Collections
Doris Duke Collection, tape transcripts: T-27 (Cecil Horse, Kiowa); T-159, T-235, 248 (Jess Rowlodge, Arapaho); T-245, T-637 (Guy Quetone, Kiowa); T-184, T-223 (Ray Blackbear, Kiowa-Apache); T-344-1 (Leonard Maker, Osage).
Indian Pioneer Papers: Peyote Worship, Methvin J.J., 9452.

Wellcome Library
GC/155: files of Walter E. Dixon and G. Norman Myers, 1865–1949.
PP/CPB/D3 Box 14: 'Subjective Experiences Caused by Mescaline', 1936.
PP/SAN/B/2: 'Mescaline, Psilocybin and other Hallucinogens'.
SADRS DrugScope archive 1920s–2002.

PRINTED SOURCES

Aberle, David F. *The Peyote Religion among the Navajo*, University of Oklahoma Press, 1966.
Albesiano, Sofía and Roberto Kiesling. 'Identity and Neotypification of *Cereus magronus*, the Type Species of the Genus *Trichocereus (Cactaceae)*', *Haseltonia*, vol. 17 (2012), 24–34.
Allderidge, Patricia. *Louis Wain and the Myth of the Disintegrating Cat*, Bethlem Museum of the Mind, 2016.
Anderson, Edward F. *Peyote: The Divine Cactus*, University of Arizona Press, 1996 [1980].
— *The Cactus Family*, Timber Press, 2001.
Angel, Katherine, Edgar Jones and Michael Neve (eds). *European Psychiatry on the Eve of War: Aubrey Lewis, the Mausdley Hospital and the Rockefeller Foundation in the 1930s*, Wellcome Trust Centre for the History of Medicine at UCL, 2003.
Anonymous. 'Why not Try Mescal?', *Contemporary Review*, issue 55 (January 1898).
Archer, Ethel. *The Hieroglyph*, Denis Archer, 1932.
Artaud, Antonin. *The Peyote Dance*, trans. Helen Weaver, Farrar, Strauss and Giroux, 1976 [1947].
Baird, David W. and Danney Goble. *Oklahoma: A History*, University of Oklahoma Press, 2008.
Bakewell, Sarah. *At the Existentialist Café*, Chatto & Windus, 2017.
Balakian, Anna. 'Breton and Drugs', *Yale French Studies*, issue 50, 'Intoxication and Literature' (1974), 95–107.
Barber, P.W. *Psychedelic Revolutionaries*, Zed Books, 2018.
Barnes, Shelby. 'The Higher Powers: Fred M. Smith and the Peyote Ceremonies', *Restoration Studies*, vol. 7 (1998), 86–99.
Barzun, Jacques. *A Stroll with William James*, University of Chicago Press, 1983.
Bass, Althea. 'James Mooney in Oklahoma', *Chronicles of Oklahoma*, vol. 32 (1954), 246–62.
Basset, Vincent. 'New Age Tourism in Wirikuta: Conflicts and Rituals', in Beatriz Labate and Clancy Cavnar (eds), *Peyote: History, Traditon, Politics and Conservation*, Praeger, 2016, 191–210.
Beckson, Karl. *Arthur Symons: A Life*, Clarendon Press, 1987.
Bedford, Sybille. *Aldous Huxley: A Biography*, 2 vols, Chatto & Windus, 1974.
Bender, George A. 'Rough and Ready Research – 1887 Style', *Journal of the History of Medicine*, vol. 23 (1968), 159–66.
Bénitez, Fernando. *In the Magic Land of Peyote*, University of Texas Press, 1975.
Benjamin, Walter. 'On Some Motifs in Baudelaire', *Selected Writings, 4: 1938–40*, Harvard University Press, 2003.
— *On Hashish*, Belknap Press, 2006.
Benzenhöfer, Udo and Torsten Passie. 'Rediscovering MDMA (Ecstasy): The Role of the American Chemist Alexander T. Shulgin', *Addiction*, vol. 105, issue 8 (August 2010), 1,355–61.
Beringer, Kurt. *Der Meskalinrausch*, Springer-Verlag, 1969 [1927].
Berridge, Virginia. 'The Origins of the English Drug Scene', *Medical History*, vol. 32 (1988), 51–64.

Bird, Michael. *Bryan Wynter,* Lund Humphries, 2010.

Boissonnas, Edith, Henri Michaux and Jean Paulhan. *Mescaline 55*, Editions Claire Paulhan, 2014.

Boon, Marcus. *The Road of Excess: A History of Writers on Drugs*, Harvard University Press, 2002.

Booth, Martin. *A Magick Life: A Biography of Aleister Crowley*, Weidenfeld & Nicholson, 1977.

Brant, Charles S. 'Peyotism among the Kiowa-Apache and Neighboring Tribes', *Southwestern Journal of Anthropology*, vol. 6, issue 2 (summer 1950), 212–22.

Bruhn, Jan G. 'Three Men and a Drug: Peyote Research in the 1890s', *The Cactus and Succulent Journal of Great Britain*, vol. 30, issue 2 (1977), 27–30.

Bruhn, Jan G. and Bo Holmstedt. 'Early Peyote Research: An Interdisciplinary Study', *Economic Botany*, vol. 28, issue 4 (October–December 1974), 353–90.

Bruhn, Jan G., P.A. De Smet, H.R. El-Seedi and O. Beck. 'Mescaline Use for 5700 Years', *Lancet*, vol. 359, issue 9,320 (2002), 1,866.

Brzecki, Andrej, Krystyna Kobel-Buys and Guido Buys. 'Hallucinations, Illusions and other Visual Disturbances in Neurology', *New Medicine*, vol. 5, issue 2 (January 2002), 83–8.

Burger, Richard L. *Chavín and the Origins of Andean Civilisation*, Thames & Hudson, 1992.

Burkhart, Louise M. 'The Aesthetic of Paradise in Nahuatl Devotional Literature', *RES: Anthropology and Aesthetics*, issue 21 (spring 1992), 88–109.

Burroughs, William. *Junky*, Penguin, 1977 [1953].

— *Rub Out the Words: Letters 1959–74*, Penguin, 2012.

Calabrese, Joseph D. *A Different Medicine: Postcolonial Healing in the Native American Church,* Oxford University Press, 2013.

Calder-Marshall, Arthur. *Havelock Ellis: A Biography*, R. Hart-Davis, 1959.

Carhart-Harris, Robin L. et al. 'Neural Correlates of the Psychedelic State as Determined by fMRI Studies with Psilocybin', *Proceedings of the National Academy of Sciences of the United States of America*, vol. 109, issue 6 (2012), 2,138–43.

Carroll, Dillon. *Silas Weir Mitchell*, National Museum of Civil War Medicine, http://www.civilwarmed.org/mitchell/ (posted 29 January 2017).

Castaneda, Carlos. *The Teachings of Don Juan*, Penguin, 1970.

— *A Separate Reality*, Penguin, 1973.

Castaño, Victoria Rios. *Translation as Conquest: Sahagún and the Universal History of New Spain*, Iberoamericano/Vervuert, 2014.

Cervantes, Fernando. *The Devil in the New World*, Yale University Press, 1994.

Cholden, Louis (ed.). *Proceedings of the Round Table on Lysergic Acid Diethylamide and Mescaline in Experimental Psychiatry, Held at the Annual Meeting of the American Psychiatric Association, Atlantic City, New Jersey, May 12, 1955*, Grune & Stratton, 1956.

Clendinnen, Inga. *Aztecs: An Interpretation*, Cambridge University Press, 1991.

Collins, John James. 'A Descriptive Introduction to the Taos Peyote Ceremony', *Ethnology*, vol. 7, issue 4 (October 1968), 427–49.

Coppin, Clayton A. and Jack High. *The Politics of Purity: Harvey Washington Wiley and the Origins of Federal Food Policy*, University of Michigan Press, 1999.

Cordy-Collins, Alana. 'Chavín Art: Its Shamanic/Hallucinogenic Origins', in Alana Cordy-Collins and Jean Stern (eds), *Pre-Columbian Art History: Selected Readings*, Peek Publications, 1977, 353–62.

Critchley, Macdonald. 'Mescalism', *British Journal of Inebriety*, vol. 28 (January 1931), 100–8.

Crosby, Alfred W. *The Columbian Exchange: Biological and Cultural Consequences of 1492*, Greenwood Press, 1972.

Crowley, Aleister, *The Spirit of Solitude: An Autohagiography*, 2 vols, Mandrake Press, 1929.

Dally, David W. *Battle for the BIA: G.E.E. Lindquist and the Missionary Crusade against John Collier*, University of Arizona Press, 2004.

Dasgupta, A. 'Challenges in Laboratory Detection of Unusual Substance Abuse', *Advances in Clinical Chemistry*, vol. 78 (2017), 163–86.

Davis, Wade. *One River*, Simon & Schuster, 1997.

Dawson, Alexander S. 'Peyote in the Colonial Imagination', in Beatriz Labate and Clancy Cavnar (eds), *Peyote: History, Tradition, Politics and Conservation*, Praeger, 2016, 43–62.

— *The Peyote Effect*, University of California Press, 2018.

DeGrandpre, Richard. *The Cult of Pharmacology*, Duke University Press, 2006.

Deloria Jr, Vine. *Custer Died for your Sins*, Macmillan, 1969.

de Mille, Richard. *Castaneda's Journey*, Sphere Books, 1978 [1976].

de Mille, Richard (ed.). *The Don Juan Papers: Further Castaneda Controversies*, Ross-Erikson Publishers, 1980.

Denber, Herman and Sidney Merlis. 'Studies on Mescaline VI: Therapeutic Aspects of the Mescaline–Chlorpromazine Combination', *Journal of Nervous and Mental Disease*, vol. 122, issue 5 (November 1955), 463–9.

— 'Studies on Mescaline VII: The Role of Anxiety in the Mescaline-Induced State', *Journal of Nervous and Mental Disease*, vol. 124, issue 1 (July 1956), 74–7.

Desoille, Robert. 'Contribution à l'étude des effets psychologiques du Peyotl', *Revue Métaphysique* (January–February 1928).

Diederichsen, Diedrich. 'Divided Ecstasy: The Politics of Hallucinogens', in Paul Schimmel (ed.), *Ecstasy: In and Out of Altered States*, MIT Press, 2006, 186–95.

Dixon, Walter E. 'The Physiological Action of the Alkaloids Derived from *Anhalonium lewinii*', *Journal of Psychology*, vol. 25, issue 1 (September 1899), 69–86.

Dodgson, Rick. *It's All a Kind of Magic: The Young Ken Kesey*, University of Wisconsin Press, 2013.

Drummond, Paul. *Eye Mind: The Saga of Roky Erickson and the 13th Floor Elevators*, Process Media, 2007.

Dyck, Erika. *Psychedelic Psychiatry: LSD from Clinic to Campus*, Johns Hopkins University Press, 2008.

Earle, Rebecca. 'Indians and Drunkenness in Spanish America', in Phil Withington and Angela McShane (eds), *Cultures of Intoxication*, Oxford University Press, 2014, 81–99.

Earnest, Ernest. *S. Weir Mitchell: Novelist and Physician*, University of Pennsylvania Press, 1950.

Ebin, David (ed.). *The Drug Experience*, Grove Press, 1965 [1961].

Eliade, Mircea. *Journal II: 1957–1969*, University of Chicago Press, 1989.

Ellis, Havelock. 'A Note on the Phenomena of Mescal Intoxication', *Lancet*, vol. 149, issue 3,849 (June 1897), 1,540–2.

— 'Mescal: A New Artificial Paradise', *Contemporary Review*, issue 73 (January 1898), 130–41.

Escohotado, Antonio. *Historia general de las drogas* (3 vols), Alianza Editorial, 1989.

Eskelund, Karl. *The Cactus of Love*, Alvin Redman Ltd, 1957.

Everitt, Patrick. 'The Cactus and the Beast: Investigating the Role of Peyote in the Magick of Aleister Crowley', MA thesis, University of Amsterdam, 2016.

Ewell, Ervin E. 'The Chemistry of the Cactaceae', *Journal of the American Chemical Society*, vol. 18, issue 7 (1896), 624–43.

Fehrenbach, T.R. *Comanches: The Story of a People*, Random House, 1974.

Fernberger, S.W. 'Further Observations on Peyote Intoxication', *Journal of Abnormal and Social Psychology*, vol. 26, issue 4 (January 1932), 367–78.

ffytche, Dominic. 'Visual Hallucinatory Syndromes: Past, Present and Future', *Dialogues in Clinical Neuroscience*, vol. 9, issue 2 (June 2007), 173–89.

ffytche, Dominic and Robert J. Howard. 'The Perceptual Consequences of Visual Loss: "Positive" Pathologies of Vision', *Brain*, vol. 122, issue 7 (1999), 1,247–60.

Fikes, Jay Courtney. *Carlos Castaneda, Academic Opportunism and the Psychedelic Sixties*, Millenia Press, 1993.

Fitzpatrick, Scott M. and Mark D. Merlin. 'Drugs from a Deep Time Perspective', in Scott Fitzgerald (ed.), *Ancient Psychoactive Substances*, University Press of Florida, 2018, 1–19.

Fogleman, James C. and Phillip B. Danielson. 'Chemical Interactions in the Cactus-Microorganism-*Drosophila* Model System of the Sonoran Desert', *American Zoology*, vol. 41, issue 4 (2001), 877–89.

Forbes, T.D.A. and B.A. Clement, 'Chemistry of Acacias from South Texas', *Texas A&M Agricultural Research and Extension Center at Uvalde*, bulletin 15 (May 2011).

Frederking, Walter. 'Intoxicant Drugs (Mescaline and Lysergic Acid Diethylamide) in Psychotherapy', *Journal of Nervous and Mental Disease*, vol. 121, issue 3 (March 1955), 262–6.

Fuller, Robert C. *Stairways to Heaven: Drugs in American Religious History*, Westview Press, 2000.

Fung, Rosa. 'Las Aldas: su ubicación dentro del proceso histórico del Perú antiguo', *Dédalo*, vol. 5, issue 9–10 (1972), 1–208.

Furst, Peter T. (ed.). *Flesh of the Gods: The Ritual Use of Hallucinogens*, Waveland Press, 1990 [1972].

Fux, Peter (ed.). *Chavín: Peru's Enigmatic Temple in the Andes*, Scheidegger & Spies, 2013.

Garson, Justin. 'A "Model Schizophrenia": Amphetamine Psychosis and the Transformation of American Psychiatry', in Stephen T. Casper and Delia Gavrus (eds), *The History of the Brain and Mind Sciences*, University of Rochester Press, 2017, 201–28.

Gerould, Daniel. *Witkacy: Slanisław Ignacy Witkiewicz as an Imaginative Writer*, University of Washington Press, 1981.

Grant, Richard. *Ghost Riders: Travels with American Nomads,* Little, Brown, 2003.

— *God's Middle Finger: Into the Lawless Heart of the Sierra Madre*, Free Press, 2008.

Greenblatt, Stephen. *Marvelous Possessions: The Wonder of the New World*, University of Chicago Press, 1991.

Guttman, E. and W.S. Maclay. 'Mescalin and Depersonalisation: Therapeutic Experiments', *Journal of Neurology and Psychopathy*, vol. 16, issue 63 (January 1936), 193–212.

— 'Clinical Observations on Schizophrenic Drawings', *British Journal of Medical Psychology*, vol. 16, issue 3–4 (1937), 184–205.

— 'Mescaline Hallucinations in Artists', *Archives of Neurology and Psychiatry*, vol. 45, issue 1 (1941), 130–7.

Gwynne, Fred C. *Empire of the Summer Moon: Quanah Parker and the Rise and Fall of the Comanche Tribe*, Scribner, 2010.

Hagan, William T. *Quanah Parker, Comanche Chief*, University of Oklahoma Press, 1993.

Hagenbach, Dieter and Lucius Werthmüller. *Mystic Chemist: The Life of Albert Hofmann and His Discovery of LSD*, Synergetic Press, 2011.

Healy, David. *The Psychopharmacologists*, vol. 1, Chapman & Hall, 1996.

— *The Psychopharmacologists*, vol. 3, Chapman & Hall, 2000.

— *The Creation of Psychopharmacology*, Harvard University Press, 2002.

Hermle, Leo et al. 'Mescaline-Induced Psychopathological, Neuropsychological, and Neurometabolic Effects in Normal Subjects: Experimental Subjects as a Tool for Psychiatric Research', *Biological Psychiatry*, vol. 32, issue 11 (December 1992), 976–91.

Heywood, Rosalind. *The Infinite Hive*, Chatto & Windus, 1964.

Hoefle, Milton L. 'The Early History of Parke, Davis and Co.', *Bulletin for the History of Chemistry*, vol. 25, issue 1 (2000), 28–34.

Hoffer, Abram, Humphry Osmond and John Smythies. 'Schizophrenia: A New Approach – II: Results of a Year's Research', *Journal of Mental Science*, vol. 100, issue 418 (January 1954), 29–45.

Hofmann, Albert. 'The Frontier-Walker: Drugs and Inebriation in the Life and Work of Ernst Jünger', in Amanda Feilding (ed.), *Hofmann's Elixir*, The Beckley Foundation, 2008, 63–71.

— *LSD: My Problem Child*, Oxford University Press, 2013 [1980].

Hogan, Susan. *Healing Arts: The History of Art Therapy*, Jessica Kingsley, 2000.

Hollister, Leo E. 'Drug-Induced Psychoses and Schizophrenic Reactions: A Critical Comparison', *Annals of the New York Academy of Sciences*, vol. 96 (January 1962), 80–92.

Holmstedt, B. and G. Liljestrand. *Readings in Pharmacology*, Pergamon Press, 1963.

Huxley, Aldous. *Moksha: Writings on Psychedelics and the Visionary Experience 1931–1963*, ed. Michael Horowitz and Cynthia Palmer, Chatto & Windus, 1980.

— *The Doors of Perception* and *Heaven And Hell*, Vintage Classics, 2004 [1954/1956].

James, William. *The Principles of Psychology*, vol. 1, Henry Holt & Co., 1890.

— *The Energies of Men*, Moffat, Yard & Co., 1914.

— *The Varieties of Religious Experience*, Penguin, 1985 [1902].

Jarnow, Jesse. *Heads: A Biography of Psychedelic America*, Da Capo Press, 2016.

Jay, Mike. *The Atmosphere of Heaven*, Yale University Press, 2009.

— *High Society: Mind-Altering Drugs in History and Culture*, Thames & Hudson, 2010.

— *Emperors of Dreams: Drugs in the Nineteenth Century*, Dedalus Press, 2011.

— 'Enter the Jaguar', in John A. Rush (ed.), *Entheogens and the Development of Culture: The Anthropology and Neurobiology of Ecstatic Experience*, North Atlantic Books, 2013, 319–32.

— 'A Train of Delightful Visions: Early Scientific Encounters with Psychedelics', in David Luke and Dave King (eds), *Breaking Convention: Essays on Psychedelic Consciousness*, Strange Attractor Press, 2013, 55–68.

— 'The Green Jam of Dr. X: Science and Literature at the Club des Haschischins', in Eugene Brennan and Russell Williams (eds), *Literature and Intoxication: Writing, Politics and the Experience of Excess*, Palgrave Macmillan, 2015, 52–66.

Jenkins, Philip. *Dream Catchers: How Mainstream America Discovered Native Spirituality*, Oxford University Press, 2004.

Jung, Carl. *Memories, Dreams, Reflections*, Pantheon Books, 1963.

— *Letters: Volume 2, 1951–1961*, ed. Gerhard Adler, Princeton University Press, 1976.

Jünger, Ernst. 'Drugs and Ecstasy', in *Myths and Symbols: Studies in Honour of Mircea Eliade*, University of Chicago Press, 1969, 327–45.

— *Annaherungen: Drogen und Rausch*, Klett-Cotta, 2013 [1970].

Kandel, Eric R. *The Age of Insight*, Random House, 2012.

Kaplan, Robert M. 'Humphry Fortescue Osmond (1917–2004), a Radical and Conventional Psychiatrist: The Transcendent Years', *Journal of Medical Biography*, vol. 24, issue 1 (2016), 115–24.

Kavanagh, Thomas W. (ed.). *Comanche Ethnography: Field Notes of E. Adamson Hoebel, Waldo W. Wedel, Gustav G. Carlson, and Robert H. Lowie*, University of Nebraska Press, 2008.

Kennedy, David O. *Plants and the Human Brain*, Oxford University Press, 2014.

Kennedy, John G. *Tarahumara of the Sierra Madre: Survivors on the Canyon's Edge*, Asilomar Press, 1978.

King, Francis, *The Magical World of Aleister Crowley*, Arrow Books, 1987 [1977].

Klor de Alva, J. Jorge, H.B. Nicholson and Eloise Quiñones Keber (eds). *The Work of Bernardino de Sahagún*, Institute for Mesoamerican Studies, State University of New York, 1988.

Klüver, Heinrich. 'Contemporary German Psychology as a "Cultural Science"', supplement to Gardner Murphy, *An Historical Introduction to Modern Psychology*, Harcourt, Brace & Co., 1929a, 443–55.

— 'Contemporary German Psychology as a "Natural Science"', supplement to Gardner Murphy, *An Historical Introduction to Modern Psychology*, Harcourt, Brace & Co., 1929b, 417–42.

— *Mescal* and *Mechanisms of Hallucination*, University of Chicago Press, 1966 [1928/1942].

Knauer, Alwyn and William Maloney. 'A Preliminary Note on the Psychic Action of Mescalin', *Journal of Nervous and Mental Disease*, vol. 40, issue 7 (July 1913), 425–36.

Kopp, Artyom. 'Evolutionary Genetics: No Coming Back from Neverland', *Current Biology*, vol. 22, issue 23 (December 2012), 1,004–6.

Knapp, Bettina. *Antonin Artaud: Man of Vision*, Swallow Press, 1980 [1969].

La Barre, Weston. 'Note on Richard Schultes' "The Appeal of Peyote"', *American Anthropologist*, vol. 41, issue 2 (April–June 1939), 340–2.

— *The Peyote Cult*, Schocken Books, 1969 [1938].

— '*To Find Our Life: The Peyote Hunt of the Huichols of Mexico*', film review, *American Anthropologist*, vol. 72, issue 5 (1970), 1,201.

Langlitz, Nicolas. '*Ceci n'est pas un psychose*: Towards a Historical Epistemology of Model Psychoses', *BioSocieties*, vol. 1, issue 2 (2006), 159–80.

— *Neuropsychedelia*, University of California Press, 2013.

Le Clézio, J.M.G. *The Mexican Dream, or the Interrupted Thought of Amerindian Civilizations*, University of Chicago Press, 1993.

Lee, Martin A. and Bruce Shlain. *Acid Dreams: The CIA, LSD and the Sixties Rebellion*, Grove Press, 1985.

Lees, Andrew. 'William Burroughs: Sailor of the Soul', *Journal of Psychoactive Drugs*, vol. 49, issue 5 (2017), 385–92.

Leonard, Irving A. 'Peyote and the Mexican Inquisition, 1620', *American Anthropologist*, vol. 44, issue 2 (1942), 324–26.

Letcher, Andy. *Shroom: A Cultural History of the Magic Mushroom*, Faber & Faber, 2006.

Lewin, Louis. '*Anhalonium lewinii*', *Therapeutic Gazette*, vol. 4, issue 4 (1888), 231–7.

— *Phantastica*, Park Street Press, 1998 [1924, English trans. 1931].

Lotringer, Sylvère. *Mad Like Artaud*, Univocal Publishing, 2015 [2003].

Luhan, Mabel Dodge. *Intimate Memories*, vol. 3, *Movers and Shakers*, Harcourt, Brace & Co., 1936.

— *Intimate Memories*, vol. 4, *Edge of Taos Desert*, Harcourt, Brace & Co., 1937.

Luke, David. *Otherworlds: Psychedelics and Exceptional Human Experience*, Muswell Hill Press, 2017.

Lumholtz, Carl. *Unknown Mexico: A Record of Five Years' Exploration among the Tribes of the Western Sierra Madre*, 2 vols, Macmillan & Co., 1903.

Lundborg, Patrick. *Psychedelia*, Lysergia Press, 2012.

Macht, David I. 'Louis Lewin', *Annals of Medical History*, vol. 3 (1931), 179–94.

Maclay, W.S., E. Guttman and W. Mayer-Gross. 'Spontaneous Drawings as an Approach in Some Problems of Psychopathology', *Proceedings of the Royal Society of Medicine*, vol. 31, issue 11 (1938), 51–64.

Marinesco, M.G. 'Visions colorées produites par la mescaline', *Presse Médicale*, issue 92 (November 1933), 1,864–6.

Marks, John. *The Search for the 'Manchurian Candidate': The CIA and Mind Control*, W.W. Norton & Co., 1991 [1979].

Marriott, Alice and Carol K. Rachlin. *Peyote*, Thomas Y. Crowell Co., 1971.

Mayer-Gross, Wilhelm. 'Experimental Psychoses and other Mental Abnormalities Produced by Drugs', *British Medical Journal*, vol. 2, issue 4,727 (August 1951), 317–21.

Merleau-Ponty, Maurice. *Phenomenology of Perception*, trans. Colin Smith, Routledge Classics, 2002 [1945, English trans. 1962].

Metzer, W. Stephen. 'The Experimentation of S. Weir Mitchell with Mescal', *Neurology*, vol. 39, issue 2 (February 1989), 303–4.

Michaux, Henri. *Miserable Miracle*, trans. Louise Varèse, New York Review Books 2002 [1956, English trans. 1963].

Miles, Barry. *Ginsberg: A Biography*, Simon & Schuster, 1989.

Mills, David A. 'Hallucinogens as Hard Science: The Adrenochrome Hypothesis for the Biogenesis of Schizophrenia', *History of Psychology*, vol. 13, issue 2 (May 2010), 178–95.

Mitchell, Silas Weir. 'Annual Oration', *Transactions of the Medical and Chirurgical Faculty of Maryland* (1877), 51–68.

— 'Remarks on the Effects of *Anhalonium lewinii* (the Mescal Button)', *British Medical Journal*, vol. 2, issue 1,875 (1896), 1,625–9.

Mitich, L.W. 'Anna B. Nickels: Pioneer Texas Cactophile', *Cactus and Succulent Journal (US)*, vol. 43 (1971), 209–12, 227 and 259–63.

Mitrani, L., S. Sheherdjiiski, A. Gourevitch and S. Yanev. 'Identification of Short Time Intervals under LSD25 and Mescaline', *Activitas nervosa superior*, vol. 19, issue 2 (1977), 102–3.

Mooney, James. *The Ghost-Dance Religion and the Sioux Outbreak of 1890*, Fourteenth Annual Report of the Bureau of Ethnology to the Secretary of the Smithsonian Institution 1892–3, vol. 2, Government Printing Office, 1896a.

— 'The Mescal Plant and Ceremony', *Therapeutic Gazette*, vol. 20 (1896b), 7–11.

— 'The Kiowa Peyote Rite', *Der Urquell*, vol. 1 (1897), 329–33.

— 'Peyote', in Frederick Webb Hodge (ed.), *Handbook of American Indians North of Mexico*, part 2, Bureau of American Ethnology, Smithsonian Institution, 1910, 237.

Moreau, Jacques-Joseph. *Hashish and Mental Illness*, trans. Gordon J. Barnett, Raven Press 1973 [1845].

Moreno, Jonathan. *Undue Risk: Secret State Experiments on Humans*, W.H. Freeman & Co., 2000.

Morgan, Bill. *I Celebrate Myself: The Somewhat Private Life of Allen Ginsberg*, Viking Penguin, 2006.

Morgan, George Robert. 'Man, Plant and Religion: Peyote Trade on the Mustang Plains of Texas', PhD thesis, University of Colorado, 1976.

Morselli, G.E. 'Contribution à la psychopathologie de l'intoxication par la mescaline: le problème d'une schizophrénie expérimentale', *Journal de Psychologie Normale et Pathologique*, vol. 33, issue 5–6 (1936), 368–92.

Moses, L.G. *The Indian Man: A Biography of James Mooney*, University of Nebraska Press, 2002 [1984].

Mulvany de Peñaloza, E. 'Motivos fitomorfos de alucinógenos en Chavín, *Chungara: Revista de Antropología Chilena*, vol. 12 (1984), 57–80.

— 'Posibiles fuentes de alucinógenos in Wari y Tiwanaku: cactus, flores y frutos', *Chungara: Revista de Antropología Chilena*, vol. 26, issue 2 (July–December 1994), 185–209.

Murphy, Gabrielle. 'Mad Art, Bad Art, Sad Art: Surprising Regions of the Mind', *Lancet*, vol. 351, issue 9,100 (February 1998), 455.

Murray, Nicholas. *Aldous Huxley: An English Intellectual*, Little, Brown, 2002.

Myerhoff, Barbara. *Peyote Hunt: The Sacred Journey of the Huichol Indians*, Cornell University Press, 1974.

— 'Peyote and Huichol Worldview: The Structure of a Mystic Vision', in Vera Rubin (ed.), *Cannabis and Culture*, Mouton Publishers, 1975, 417–38.

Nelson, Barnaby and Louis Sass. 'The Phenomenology of the Psychotic Break and Huxley's Trip: Substance Use and the Onset of Psychosis, *Psychopathology*, vol. 41, issue 6 (2008), 346–55.

Nesvig, Martin. 'Sandcastles of the Mind: Hallucinogens and Cultural Memory', in Stacey Schwatzkopf and Kathryn Sampeck (eds), *Substance and Seduction*, University of Texas Press, 2017, 27–54.

Nicotra, Jodie. 'William James in the Borderlands: Psychedelic Science and the "Accidental Fences" of Self', *Configurations*, vol. 16, issue 2 (spring 2008), 199–213.

Norton, Marcy. *Sacred Gifts, Profane Pleasures: A History of Tobacco and Chocolate in the Atlantic World*, Cornell University Press, 2008.

Novak, Steven J. 'LSD before Leary', *Isis*, vol. 88, issue 1 (March 1997), 87–110.

Ó Siadhail, Pádraig. '"The Indian Man" and the Irishman: James Mooney and Irish Folklore', *New Hibernia Review*, vol. 14, issue 2 (summer 2010), 17–42.

Oisteanu, Andrei. *Narcotice în cultura Româna: istorie, religie si literatura*, Pollrom Publishing House, 2010.

Olive, M. Foster. *Peyote and Mescaline (Drugs: The Straight Facts)*, Chelsea House, 2007.

Ong, Walter. *Orality and Literacy: The Technologising of the Word*, Routledge, 2002 [1982].

Oram, Matthew. 'Prohibited or Regulated? LSD Psychotherapy and the United States Food and Drug Administration', *History of Psychiatry*, vol. 27, issue 3 (2016), 290–306.

Osmond, Humphry. 'On Being Mad', *Saskatchewan Psychiatric Services Journal*, vol. 1, issue 2 (September 1952).

Osmond, Humphry and John Smythies. 'Schizophrenia: A New Approach', *British Journal of Psychiatry*, vol. 98, issue 411 (1952), 309–15.

— 'The Present State of Psychological Medicine', *Hibbert Journal*, vol. 51, issue 2 (January 1953), 133–42.

Parke, Davis & Co. *Parke-Davis at 100, 1866–1966*, [Detroit], 1966.

— 'Coca Erythroxylon and Its Derivatives', promotional brochure, reprinted in Robert Byck (ed.), *Cocaine Papers: Sigmund Freud*, Stonehill Publishing, 1975 [1885], 127–50.

Parsons, Elsie Clews. *Pueblo Indian Religion*, vol. 2, Bison Books, 1996 [1939].

Patchen, Jerry. 'Reflections on the Peyote Road with the Native American Church Law, Visions and Cosmology', in Dennis McKenna, Ghillean Prance, Wade Davis and Benjamin De Loenen (eds), *Ethnopharmacologic Search for Psychoactive Drugs: 50 Years of Research*, Synergetic Press, 2017, 257–79.

Pearson, John and Kenneth Dewhurst. 'Mescaline: Apotheosis of "The Devil's Root"', *Irish Journal of Medical Science*, vol. 31, issue 3 (March 1955), 139–43.

Pendle, George. *Strange Angel: The Otherworldly Life of Rocket Scientist John Whiteside Parsons*, Orion Books, 2006.

Perrine, Daniel M. 'Visions of the Night: Western Medicine Meets Peyote, 1887–1899', *Heffter Review of Psychedelic Research*, vol. 2 (2001), 6–52.

Petrullo, Vincenzo. *The Diabolic Root: A Study of Peyotism, the New Indian Religion, among the Delawares*, University of Pennsylvania Press, 1934.

Philp, Kenneth R. 'John Collier and the American Indian', in Leon Borden Blair (ed.), *Essays on Radicalism in Contemporary America*, University of Texas Press, 1974, 63–80.

Pieper, Werner (ed.). *Kurt Beringer und die Heidelberger Drogenforschung der 20er Jahre*, Edition Rauschkunde, 1999.

Piper, Alan. 'Therapeutic Uses of Mescal Buttons (*Anhalonium lewinii*)', *Therapeutic Gazette*, vol. 12 (1896), 4–7.

— 'A 1920s Harvard Psychedelic Circle with a Mormon Connection: Peyote Use among the "Harvard Aesthetes"', *Invisible College Magazine*, vol. 8 (2016).

Pollan, Michael. *The Botany of Desire: A Plant's Eye View of the World*, Bloomsbury, 2001.

— *How to Change Your Mind: Exploring the New Science of Psychedelics*, Allen Lane, 2018.

Powell, Melissa S. and C. Jill Grady (eds). *Huichol Art and Culture: Balancing the World*, Museum of New Mexico Press, 2010.

Prentiss, D.W. and Francis P. Morgan. '*Anhalonium lewinii* (Mescal Buttons): A Study of the Drug, with Especial Reference to Its Physiological Action upon Man, with Reports of Experiments', *Therapeutic Gazette*, vol. 11, no. 9 (1895), 577–85.

Romero, Simon. 'Peyote's Hallucinations Spawn Real-Life Academic Feud', *New York Times*, 16 September 2003.

Roof, Wade Clark. *A Generation of Seekers*, Harper Publishing, 1993.

— *Spiritual Marketplace: Baby Boomers and the Remaking of American Religion*, Princeton University Press, 1999.

Ross, Colin A. 'LSD Experiments by the United States Army', *History of Psychiatry*, vol. 28, issue 4 (2017), 427–42.

Roszak, Theodore. *The Making of a Counterculture*, University of California Press, 1995 [1968].

Rouhier, Alexandre. *Le peyotl: la plante qui fait les yeux émerveillés*, Guy Trédaniel, Éditions de la Maisnie, 1989a [1926].

— 'Les plantes divinatoires', in Alexandre Rouhier *Le peyotl: la plante qui fait les yeux émerveillés*, Guy Tredaniel, Éditions de la Maisnie, 1989b [1926], supp. 5–29.

Rudnick, Lois Palken. *Mabel Dodge Luhan: New Woman, New Worlds*, University of New Mexico Press, 1984.

— *Utopian Vistas: The Mabel Dodge Luhan House and the American Counterculture*, University of New Mexico Press, 1996.

Rusby, Henry H. *Jungle Memories*, McGraw Hill Book Co., 1933.

Sartre, Jean-Paul and John Gerassi. *Talking with Sartre: Conversations and Debates*, Yale University Press, 2009.

Sayre, Matthew P. 'A Synonym for Sacred: *Vilca* Use in the Preconquest Andes', in Scott Fitzgerald (ed.), *Ancient Psychoactive Substances*, University Press of Florida, 2018, 265–85.

Schelling, Andrew. *Tracks along the Left Coast: Jaime de Angulo and Pacific Coast Culture*, Counterpoint Press, 2017.

Schultes, Richard Evans. *Peyote and the Plants Used in the Peyote Ceremony*, Botanical Museum Leaflets, Harvard University, 12 April 1937.

— 'The Appeal of Peyote (*Lophophora williamsii*) as a Medicine', *American Anthropologist*, vol. 40, issue 1 (October–December 1938), 698–715.

Schultes, Richard Evans and Albert Hofmann. *Plants of the Gods*, Healing Arts Press, 1992 [1979].

Schwartzkopf, Stacey and Kathryn E. Sampeck (eds). *Substance and Seduction: Ingested Commodities in Early Modern Mesoamerica*, University of Texas Press, 2017.

Šerko, A. 'Im Meskalinrausch', *Jahrbuch Psychiatrie*, vol. 34 (1913), 355–66.

Sessa, Ben. 'A Brief History of Psychedelics in Medical Practices: Psychedelic Medical History "Before the Hiatus" ', in J. Harold Ellens and Thomas Roberts (eds), *The Psychedelic Policy Quagmire: Health, Law, Freedom, and Society*, Praeger, 2015, 33–60.

— 'The History of Psychedelics in Medicine', in M. von Heydon, H. Jungaberle and T. Majić (eds), *Handbook of Psychoactive Substances*, Springer-Verlag, 2016.

Shady Solís, Ruth. 'America's First City: The Case of Late Archaic Caral', in W.H. Isbell and H. Silverman (eds), *Andean Archaeology III*, Springer, 2006, 28–66.

— *The Social and Cultural Values of Caral-Supe, the Oldest Civilisation of Peru and the Americas*, Biblioteca Nacional de Perú, 2007.

Sharon, Douglas. *Wizard of the Four Winds: A Shaman's Story*, Free Press, 1978.

—'The San Pedro Cactus in Peruvian Folk-Healing', in Furst, Peter T. (ed.). *Flesh of the Gods: The Ritual Use of Hallucinogens*, Waveland Press, 1990 [1972].

Shonle, Ruth. 'Peyote, the Giver of Visions', *American Anthropologist*, vol. X, issue 27 (1925), 53–75.

Shortall, Sarah. 'Psychedelic Drugs and the Problem of Experience', in Phil Withington and Angela McShane (eds), *Cultures of Intoxication*, Oxford University Press, 2014, 187–206.

Shorter, Edward. *A History of Psychiatry*, John Wiley & Sons, 1997.

— *A Historical Dictionary of Psychiatry*, Oxford University Press, 2005.

Shulgin, Ann and Alexander. *PIHKAL*, Transform Press, 1991.

Siff, Stephen. *Acid Hype: American News Media and the Psychedelic Experience*, University of Illinois Press, 2015.

Sjoberg, B.M. and L.E. Hollister. 'The Effects of Psychotomimetic Drugs on Primary Suggestibility', *Psychopharmacologia,* vol. 8, issue 4 (1965), 251–62.

Slotkin, J.S. *The Peyote Religion: A Study in Indian–White Relations*, Free Press, 1956.

Smith, Frederick Madison. *The Higher Powers of Man*, Herald Printing House, 1918.

— 'A Trip among the Omaha Indians', *Saints Herald*, 24 December 1919.

Smith, Huston and Reuben Snake (eds). *One Nation Under God: The Triumph of the Native American Church*, Clear Light Publishers, 1996.

Smith, Roger. *Between Mind and Nature: A History of Psychology*, Reaktion Press, 2013.

Smith, Sherry L. *Hippies, Indians and the Fight for Red Power*, Oxford University Press, 2012.

Smythies, John. 'The Mescaline Phenomena', *British Journal for the Philosophy of Science*, vol. 3, issue 12 (February 1953), 339–47.

— 'The Adrenochrome Hypothesis of Schizophrenia Revisited', *Neurotoxicity Research*, vol. 4, issue 2 (2002), 147–50.

Smythies, John R. and Vanna Smythies. *Two Coins in the Fountain*, BookSurge, 2005.

Šnicer, Jaroslav, Jaroslav Bohata and Vojtěch Myšák. '*Lophophora alberto-vojtechii*, an Exquisite New Miniature from the Genus *Lophophora*', *Cactus & Co.,* vol. 12, issue 2 (June 2008), 105–17.

Späth, Ernst. 'Über die *Anhalonium*-alkaloide', *Monatshefte für Chemie und verwandte Teile anderer Wissenschaften*, vol. 40, issue 2 (1919), 129–54.

Stafford, Peter. *Psychedelics Encyclopaedia*, Ronin Publishing, 1992.

Stevens, Jay. *Storming Heaven: LSD and the American Dream*, Paladin Books, 1989.

Stewart, Omer C. *Peyote Religion: A History*, University of Oklahoma Press, 1987.

Stockings, G. Tayleur. 'A Clinical Study of the Mescaline Psychosis', *Journal of Mental Science*, vol. 86, issue 360 (1940), 29–47.

Streatfeild, Dominic. *Brainwash: The Secret History of Mind Control*, Hodder & Stoughton, 2006.

Stuart, David. *Dangerous Garden*, Frances Lincoln, 2004.

Stuart, R. 'Modern Psychedelic Art's Origins as a Product of Clinical Experimentation', *Entheogen Review*, vol. 13, issue 1 (March 2004), 12–22.

Sutin, Lawrence. *Do What Thou Wilt: A Life of Aleister Crowley*, St Martin's Griffin, 2002.

Swan, Daniel C. *Peyote Religious Art: Symbols of Faith and Belief*, University Press of Mississippi, 1999.

Symons, Arthur. *The Symbolist Movement in Literature*, Carcanet Press, 2014 [1899].

Szummer, Csaba, Lajos Horváth, Attila Szabó, Ede Frecska and Kristóf Orzói. 'The Hyperassociative Mind: The Psychedelic Experience and Merleau-Ponty's "Wild Being"', *Journal of Psychedelic Studies*, vol. 1, issue 2 (July 2017), 1–10.

Taylor, Norman. 'Come and Expel the Green Pain', *Scientific Monthly*, vol. 58, issue 3 (March 1944), 176–84.

ten Berge, Jos. 'Breakdown or Breakthrough? A History of European Research into Drugs and Creativity', *Journal of Creative Behaviour*, vol. 33, issue 4 (1999), 257–76.

Terry, Martin and Keeper Trout. 'Decline of the Genus *Lophophora* in Texas', in Beatriz Labate and Clancy Cavnar (eds), *Peyote: History, Tradition, Politics and Conservation*, Praeger, 2016, 1–20.

— 'Regulation of Peyote (*Lophophora williamsii: Cactaceae*) in the USA: A Historical Victory of Religion and Politics over Science and Medicine', *Journal of the Botanical Research Institute of Texas*, vol. 11, issue 1 (2017), 147–56.

Terry, Martin, Karen L. Steelman, Tom Guilderson, Phil Dering and Marvin W. Rowe. 'Lower Pecos and Coahuila Peyote: New Radiocarbon Dates', *Journal of Archaeological Science*, vol. 33, issue 7 (2006), 1,017–21.

Thompson, Hunter S. *Fear and Loathing in Las Vegas*, Panther Books, 1972 [1971].

— *Songs of the Doomed*, Simon & Schuster, 1990.

— *Fear and Loathing in America*, Bloomsbury, 2000.

Tófoli, L.F. and D.B. de Araujo. 'Treating Addiction: Perspectives from EEG and Imaging Studies on Psychedelics', *International Review of Neurobiology*, vol. 129 (2016), 157–85.

Tommasini, Anthony. *Virgil Thomson: Composer on the Aisle*, W.W. Norton & Co., 1997.

Torgoff, Martin. *Can't Find My Way Home: America in the Great Stoned Age, 1945–2000*, Simon & Schuster, 2004.

Torre, Dan. *Cactus*, Reaktion Press, 2017.

Torres, Constantino Manuel. 'Chavín's Psychoactive Pharmacopeia: The Iconographic Evidence', in William J. Conklin and Jeffrey Quilter (eds), *Chavín: Art, Architecture and Culture*, monograph 61, Cotsen Institute of Archaeology, University of California, 2008, 237–57.

— 'The Origins of the Ayahuasca/Yagé Concept', in Scott Fitzgerald (ed.), *Ancient Psychoactive Substances*, University Press of Florida, 2018, 234–64.

Trevelyan, Julian, *Indigo Days*, Macgibbon & Kee, 1957.

Trout, Keeper. *Trout's Notes on San Pedro*, Better Days Publishing/Moksha Press, 2005.

— 'Mescal, Peyote and the Red Bean: A Peculiar Conceptual Collision in Early Modern Ethnobotany', in Dennis McKenna, Ghillean Prance, Wade Davis and Benjamin De Loenen (eds), *Ethnopharmacologic Search for Psychoactive Drugs: 50 Years of Research*, Synergetic Press, 2017, 234–56.

Tsao, Makepeace U. 'A New Synthesis of Mescaline', *Journal of the American Chemical Society*, vol. 71, issue 11 (1951), 5,495–6.

United Nations. 'Peyotl', *Bulletin on Narcotics*, vol. 11, issue 2 (April–June 1959), 16–29.

Wallace, Anthony F.C. 'Cultural Determinants of Response to Hallucinatory Experience', *Archives of General Psychiatry*, vol. 1, issue 1 (1959), 58–69.

Waters, Frank. *The Man who Killed the Deer*, Neville Spearman, 1962 [1942].

Watt, Donald (ed.). *Aldous Huxley*, Routledge, 2013 [1975].

Watts, Alan. *The Joyous Cosmology*, New World Library, 2013 [1962].

Weatherford, Jack. *Indian Givers*, Crown Publishers, 1988.

Weil, Andrew. *The Natural Mind*, Penguin, 1975 [1972].

Wilson, Colin. *Dreaming to Some Purpose*, Century, 2004.

Witkiewicz, Stanisław Ignacy, *Narcotics: Nicotine, Cocaine, Peyote, Morphine, and Ether* in *The Witkiewicz Reader*, ed. Daniel Gerould, Quartet Books, 1992 [1932], 243–70.

— *Narcotics: Nicotine, Cocaine, Peyote, Morphine, Ether + Appendices*, Twisted Spoon Press, 2018 [1932].

Zaehner, R.C. *Mysticism: Sacred and Profane*, Clarendon Press, 1957.

Zieger, Susan. 'Victorian Hallucinogens', *Romanticism and Victorianism on the Net*, issue 49, 'Interdisciplinarity and the Body' (February 2008).

Zingg, Robert Mowry. *The Huichols: Primitive Artists*, G.E. Stechert & Co., 1938.

Znamenski, Andrei A. *The Beauty of the Primitive: Shamanism and the Western Imagination*, Oxford University Press, 2007.

INDEX

2C-B (phenethylamine), 20, 246
2C-T-7 (phenethylamine), 20, 246
5-HT, *see* serotonin
13th Floor Elevators, 229

achuma, 15; *see also huachuma*; San Pedro
    cactus
Acosta, José de, 40
Acosta, Oscar, 241
Adams, Ansel, 118
Adams, Charles, 71
adrenaline, 193, 196
adrenochrome, 196–7, 216, 242; in *Fear
    and Loathing in Las Vegas* 242; Osmond
    and Hoffer experiments 196–7
Aldrich (pharmaceutical company) 5, 250
Alpert, Richard (Ram Dass), 236–7
American Indian, 257n16; *see also* Apache
    people; Arapaho people; etc.
American Indian Religious Freedom Act
    Amendments (1994), 128
American Philosophical Society, 56
American Psychiatric Association, 191, 214
alkaloids, 18–20, 66, 84–5, 98–100, 144,
    193; in peyote 257n17, 66, 84–5,
    98–100, 144, 193; in San Pedro 18–20
amino acids 18, 19, 131
amphetamines 4, 210, 217, 228, 236, 241,
    242; 'amphetamine psychosis' 217
Anadenanthera spp., *see vilca*
Angulo, Jaime de, 175–6, 211
anhalonidine, 266n41, 98
anhalonine, 266n41, 66, 98, 100
Anhalonium spp., *see* peyote cactus,
    taxonomy
'anhalonium' preparations, *see* peyote
    cactus, pharmaceutical preparations;
    Aleister Crowley; Louis Lewin; Parke,
    Davis & Co.

Apache people, 42, 43, 54, 68, 122, 127;
    see also Lipan; Mescalero
Apekaum, Charlie (Kiowa), 174
Arapaho people, 58, 67, 71, 125, 177
Archer, Ethel, 106–7
Artaud, Antonin, 8, 150, 157, 163–8; in
    Mexico 164–7; peyote experiences 166–7
Augustine, Saint, 37
ayahuasca, 22, 24, 26, 143, 174, 234,
    251, 253
Aztec people, 257n15; *see also* Nahua

Baudelaire, Charles, 92, 143, 150, 161, 187;
    Walter Benjamin on 161; Ernst Jünger on
    186–7
Beaumont, Basil, 180, 181–3; mescaline
    experiment 181–3
Beauvoir, Simone de, 158
Benjamin, Walter, 8, 94, 157, 160–4; on
    Baudelaire 161; mescaline experiment
    162–4
Bennett, Allan, 108
Benzedrine, *see* amphetamines
Bergson, Henri, 203
Beringer, Kurt, 259n20, 135–9, 142, 145–6,
    149, 153, 154, 178, 179, 189, 238, 243;
    Der Meskalinrausch 135–7, 149, 154
Bianco, Ochwiay, (Taos Puebloan), 175–6
Blanc, Albert, 80
Bleuler, Eugen, 133
Board of Indian Commissioners, 123
Boas, Franz, 175
Bonnet, Charles, 140
Bonnin, Gertrude (Yankton Sioux), 123
Bosch, Hieronymus, 166
Botanical Society of Berlin, 66
Brand, Stewart, 228
Breton, André, 150–1, 157; Surrealism and
    drug use 150

288

Briggs, John Raleigh, 62–5, 82, 91
British Journal of Psychiatry, 194
British Medical Journal, 91, 95–6, 194
Bruchlos, Barron, 227–8, 236
Brugmansia (angel's/devil's trumpet flower), 21, 26, 33, 92
Buckley, Lord (Richard Myrle Buckley), 228
Bureau of Ethnology, *see* Smithsonian Institution
Bureau of Indian Affairs (BIA), 53, 59, 119, 122
Bureau of Narcotic and Dangerous Drugs (US), 239
Burroughs Wellcome (pharmaceutical company), 183
Burroughs, William, 4, 5, 209–10, 214, 243; on Henri Michaux 214; and peyote 4, 5, 209–10
Burton, Sir Richard, 65
Bush, President George H.W., 245

cacao (chocolate), 35, 38, 131
cacti, 8–11, 17–19, 80, 209; collectors and enthusiasts 63–4, 80, 209; *see also* peyote cactus; San Pedro cactus
Caddo people, 53, 67, 73, 125; and 'full moon' peyote rite, 73
Camino del Cielo (catechism), 37
cannabis, 4, 82, 103–4, 107, 108, 133–4, 143, 144, 150, 160, 163, 171, 176, 184, 192, 196, 211, 228, 229, 236
Caral (Peru), 16, 27
Cárdenas, Juan de, 36
Carlsson, Arvid, 216–17
Carson, Kit, 118
Castaneda, Carlos, 231–4, 240–1, 242–3; academic controversy 232–4; Huichol influences 233–4; Mescalito 232–4; peyote experiences 231–2; *The Teachings of Don Juan* 232–3
Castaneda, Margaret, 233
chacruna (DMT-containing leaf), 22
Charcot, Jean-Martin, 86, 155
Chatto and Windus (publishers) 3
Chavéz, Dennis, 171, 175
Chavín de Huántar, 15–16, 21–4, 27; ancient use of San Pedro at 15, 21–4
Central Intelligence Agency (CIA), 185, 215, 235; *see also* MK-ULTRA
Cheyenne people, 58, 71, 122, 125–7, 177, 209; and Native American Church charter 125–7
Chicago World's Fair (1893), 53, 64, 79

chicha (maize beer), 22, 42, 47; DMT added to 23; San Pedro added to 23, 24, 25
Chichimeca people, 40, 46
Chief Three Fingers (Cheyenne), 112
Chimú culture, 25
chlorpromazine, 6, 191–2, 216–17; administered with mescaline 192
chocolate, *see* cacao
Chony (Comanche, wife of Quanah Parker), 75
Church of Latter-Day Saints, 110–13, 128
cinchona bark, 25
clairvoyance, 26–7, 143–4, 153
Coahuiltecan culture, 40
Cobo, Bernabé, 25, 143
coca leaf, 21, 131, 143, 202
cocaine, 62, 82, 104, 107, 109, 119, 131, 153, 160, 171, 176, 242
cocoa, *see* cacao
cohoba, *see* vilca
Collier, John, 116, 118–19, 127, 171–2, 207–8; and federal peyote policy 172; as Indian Commissioner 118, 171–2; in New York 116, 172; in Taos 118–19
Comanche people (Numunuh), 54, 67–75, 119, 120, 122, 125–7, 173, 249–50; Fort Sill reservation 68–9, 122; and 'half-moon' peyote rite, 73, 173; Quanah Parker, chief 69–75
Contemporary Review, 92, 95
Controlled Substances Act (US), 239
Cook, Bob, 126
Cook, Philip (Cheyenne), 112
copal (incense), 36, 42, 43
Cortéz, Hernan, 38, 46, 164
Coyote, Peter, 228
Cree Nation, 208
Crichton Royal Hospital (Scotland), 194
Crowley, Aleister, 105–9, 113, 176, 210, 243; use of peyote ('anhalonium') 107–9
Cruz-Sánchez, Guillermo, 15
Cunningham, Carl, 125–6
Cupinisque culture, 25
curanderos, curanderismo, *see* shamans, shamanism
Curtis' Botanical Magazine, 65

Daily Sketch, 105–6
Dasburg, Andrew, 115, 116, 118
Datura sp., *see Brugmansia*
Davis, George S., 62–3; *see also* Parke, Davis & Co.

de Mille, Richard, 232–3
De Quincey, Thomas, 92, 187, 213
Deloria Jr, Vine (Standing Rock Sioux), 230
Denber, Herbert, 192
Department of Agriculture (USA), 80, 123, 227
Desnos, Robert, 150
Dexedrine, see amphetamines
Dixon, Walter, 103–4; mescaline experiments 103–4
DMT (dimethyltryptamine), 19, 237; plants containing 22–4
Dodge, Edwin, 114
Dodge, Mabel, 113–22, 171, 175, 210, 228, 230; anti-peyote campaign 171; house and artist colony in Taos 118–20, 230; and Tony Luhan 118, 120–2; peyote salon in New York 113–16, 121, 175; takes peyote medicine in Taos 121
DOM (phenethylamine), 20, 239, 244
Dow Chemical Company, 243–4
Dreiser, Theodore, 109
Drug Enforcement Agency (USA), 246, 251, 252
Druggists' Bulletin, 62
Dunne, J.W., 223

Eastern Cherokee people, 56
Eastman, Max, 115
Echinopsis pachanoi/peruvianus, 15; see San Pedro cactus
Eli Lilly (pharmaceutical company), 245
Eliade, Mircea, 222–3
Ellis, Henry Havelock, 6–7, 91–8, 103, 107, 114, 138–9 143, 149, 150, 158, 181, 203, 210, 227, 243; gives peyote to Arthur Symons and W.B. Yeats 96–8; 'Mescal: A New Artificial Paradise' 6–7, 92–4; peyote experiments 93–4, 96; progressive politics 92, 114; responses to Mescal 95–6
ephedrine, 131
Equinox, 108, 109
Eschiti (Comanche), 70
Eskelund, Karl, 209
Evans-Wentz, Walter, 177
Ewell, Erwin, 80, 83, 112, 123; enthusiasm for cacti 80; peyote experiment 83
existentialism 8, 146

Federal Bureau of Narcotics (US), 171
Ferdière, Gaston, 150–1

Fernberger, Samuel, 142
Fikes, Jay, 233
Fischinger, Oskar, 29
Florentine Codex, see Bernardino de Sahagún
floripondio, see Brugmansia
Fränkel, Fritz, 160–4
Frederking, Walter, 185–6, 187–8, 190; compares mescaline and LSD 190; friendship with Ernst Jünger 186–8; uses mescaline in therapy 185–6
Food and Drug Administration (FDA), US, 80, 237, 238, 274n2; Kefauver–Harris Amendments (1962) 237
Furst, Peter, 44–6, 233

Ganson, Mabel, see Mabel Dodge
Geneva Opium Convention (1925), 144–5
Gerassi, John, 159
gestalt psychology, 132, 145
Ghost Dance, 53–4, 56–9, 67, 69, 70, 71, 73; James Mooney's reports on 53, 57–8; and Wounded Knee massacre 56–7
Ginsberg, Allen, 4, 210–11, 214, 227; 'Mescaline' poem 271n35; peyote trips 210–11
Glinka, Mikhail, 156
Golden Dawn, Order of, 107, 108
Gombrich, Ernst, 265n25, 149
Gomez, Little Joe (Taos Puebloan), 229
Grant, Cary, 206
Grateful Dead, 240
Graves, Robert, 177
Gray Herbarium, Harvard, 65
Gurdjieff, George, 106, 177
Gutiérrez-Noriega, Carlos 15
Guttman, Eric, 178–83; mescaline experiments on artists 180–3
Guy's Hospital (London), 193

Haag, Mack (Cheyenne), 126–7, 207; signatory of Native American Church charter 127
Hall, G. Stanley, 110
Hall, Tommy, 229
'hallucinogen', term 7, 196
Hapgood, Hutchins, 114
Harrington, Raymond, 114–16, 175
Harrison Narcotics Act (1914), 119, 171, 209
Harvard Botanical Museum, 174; see also universities, Harvard
hashish, see cannabis

Hayden, Carl, 122
Heard, Gerald, 206
Heffter, Arthur, 257n17, 84–5, 98–100, 103, 131, 133, 144; disputes with Louis Lewin 84–5, 100; isolates and names mescaline 99–100
Heidegger, Martin, 187
Hendrix, Jimi, 240
Hennings, Paul Christoph, 32, 66–7; botanical drawing of peyote 32
Hernández de Toledo, Francisco, 35–6
heroin, 4, 165, 228
Hesse, Hermann, 145
Heywood, Rosalind, 5–6
Hibbert Journal, 198
hikuli (Tarahumara), *see* peyote cactus, in Tarahumara culture
Hoch, Paul, 235
Hoffer, Abram, 196–7, 205, 208, 216–17, 242; adrenochrome experiment 197; niacin therapy 216
Hoffman, E.T.A., 143
Hofmann, Albert, 4, 6, 142, 188–90, 191, 218, 235; discovery of LSD 4, 6, 142, 188–9; discovery of psilocybin 4, 235; response to *The Doors of Perception* 218
Hollister, Leo, 217, 235–6; gives mescaline to Ken Kesey 217, 235–6; and psychoto-mimetic model 217
Hopper, Dennis, 230
House of Representatives (US), 122–5, 127, 171
huachuma, 15, 40; *see* San Pedro cactus
Hubbard, Alfred, 205–6
Huichol people, 43–9, 61, 68, 84, 143, 173, 209, 251–3; appropriated by Carlos Castaneda 233–4; art of 47–9, 251–3; international profile 47–9, 233, 252–3; peyote pilgrimage 44–6; 'renovation of the world' 253
Husserl, Edmund, 158; *see also* phenomenology
Huxley, Aldous, 3–4, 5, 6–7, 15, 118, 158, 184, 198, 201–5, 206, 210, 214–15, 218–21, 227, 234, 242, 243; *Brave New World* 201–2; *The Doors of Perception* 3–4, 5, 6–7, 15, 203–5, 206, 208, 218–23, 237; earlier views on drugs 201–2; first mescaline experiment 3, 202–4; *Heaven and Hell* 215, 218; responses to his advocacy of mescaline 218–21; takes LSD 206
Huxley, Maria, 201–2, 204

Ickes, Harold, 171
Idler, 108
'Indian New Deal', 118, 127, 172
Indian Reorganization Act (1934), 127, 172
Indian Rights Association, 123
Inquisition (Mexico), 25, 37, 40–1
International Society for Metaphysical Research, 152

James, Henry, 91
James, William, 89–91, 104, 111, 203, 205, 243; peyote experiment 90–1; and 'second wind' 111; theory of time perception 90, 104
Janiger, Oscar, 206
Jaspers, Karl, 135, 136, 146, 192
Jewish Society, Berlin, 66
Joël, Ernst, 160–1
Johnson, William 'Pussyfoot', 122
Jordan, Lawrence, 228
Josiah Macy Foundation, 235
Journal of the American Chemical Society, 239
Journal of the American Medical Association, 237
Jung, Carl, 118, 145, 175–6, 197, 202, 219; in Taos 118, 175–6; views on mescaline and LSD 219
Jünger, Ernst, 186–90, 210, 218; on Charles Baudelaire 186–7; coins the term 'psychonaut' 187; friendship with Albert Hofmann 188–90; mescaline experiments 187–8; response to *The Doors of Perception* 218
jurema (DMT-containing root), 22

Kennedy, John, 47
Kesey, Ken, 235–6; takes mescaline and peyote 236
Kety, Seymour, 216
Kimmey, John, 229–30; and New Buffalo commune 230
Kiowa people, 53–5, 67, 68, 71, 73, 93, 114–15, 119, 122, 125, 127, 143, 173, 177; and peyote rite 54–5, 60, 73, 114–15, 143, 173, 177; sacred stones ceremony 71
Kiralfy, Imre, 79
Klüver, Heinrich, 132, 138–41, 145, 149, 174, 189, 196, 205; career 138; experiments with mescaline 138; 'form-constants' 140; on German psychology 132, 141, 145; inspiration to Richard Evans Schultes 174

Knauer, Alwyn, 132–5, 128,
Koshiway, Jonathan (Oto), 126
Kraepelin, Emil, 133, 135, 191, 192, 217
Kris, Ernst, 149

La Barre, Weston, 46, 172–5, 227–8;
  fieldwork among the Kiowa 173–5;
  The Peyote Cult 172–3, 227
La Flesche, Francis (Omaha), 124
Laborit, Henri, 191
Lacan, Jacques, 159
Lagache, Daniel, 158
Lakota people, 57
Lambayeque culture, 25
Lancet, 92, 93, 98, 195
Lawrence, D.H., 118, 230
League of Nations, 144–5
Leary, Timothy, 7, 206, 234, 236–8
Lee, Arthur, 240
Lemaire, Charles, 65
Lewin, Louis, 6, 65–7, 80, 84–5, 100; 112,
  disputes with Arthur Heffter 84–5, 100;
  experiments on peyote 66–7, 84;
  Phantastica 100; and self-experimentation
  100
Lewis, Aubrey, 178
LIFE (magazine), 4
Lights Chemicals (pharmaceutical
  suppliers), 193
Lipan (Apache band), 68, 70
Looking Glass, Louise (Comanche), 249
lophophorine, 98
LSD (d-lysergic acid diethylamide), 3, 4, 19,
  33, 142, 187, 188–90, 191, 192, 196,
  205–6, 214–16, 217, 218, 229, 234–40,
  242; comparisons with mescaline 189,
  190, 192, 205–6, 215, 237–8; discovery
  by Albert Hofmann LSD 4, 6, 142,
  188–9; replaces mescaline 7, 205–6, 229,
  235, 236–9; sold by Sandoz as Delysid
  189, 206, 214
Luhan, Mabel Dodge, *see* Mabel Dodge
Luhan, Tony (Taos Puebloan), 118, 120–2,
  176–7, 211; and Frank Waters 176–7;
  peyote use 120–2
Lumholtz, Carl, 42–3, 47, 53, 84, 93, 111;
  peyote experiences 42–3
Lumière brothers, 155

'M-substance', 194–7, 216–17, 242
Mackenzie, Colonel Ranald, 69
Maclay, Walter, 178–83; mescaline
  experiments on artists 180–3

maize beer, *see chicha*
Malinowski, Bronisław, 151
Maloney, William, 132–5, 138,
Manchester Guardian 5
Mangan, Sherry, 113
Manhattan State Hospital, 192
Mann, Thomas, 218
Mansfield, Katherine, 108
mara'akame, *see* Huichol people; shamans
marijuana, *see* cannabis
Marijuana Tax Act (1937), 171
Marinescu, Gheorghe, 155–7
Marriott, Alice, 208–9
Matrix, The, 243
Maudsley Hospital (London), 178–82,
  195
Mayer-Gross, Wilhelm, 136–7, 138, 178,
  194–5; mescaline experiment 136–7
Mayhew, Christopher, 221–3; 'An Excursion
  out of Time' 222–3; mescaline experi-
  ment 222
MDMA (ecstasy), 24, 244–6; synthesised by
  Alexander Shulgin 244
Medical Register, 62
Medicine Lodge, Treaty of (1867), 69
Menlo Park Hospital (California), 217,
  235–6
Menominee people, 207
Merck (pharmaceutical company), 130–2,
  135, 138, 152–3, 238, 244, 250
Merleau-Ponty, Maurice, 159–60
Merry Pranksters, 236
mescal (agave spirit) 64, 242; confusions
  surrounding the term 64–5, 242; *see also*
  peyote cactus
'mescal bean' (*Sophora secundiflora*), 33
Mescalero (Apache band), 65, 68, 74,
  173
mescaline (chemical compound; *see also*
  peyote cactus; San Pedro cactus) 3–11,
  94, 131–46, 149–63, 168, 178–98,
  201–6, 211–23, 229, 235–46, 250, 255;
  art inspired by 5–6, 25, 149–57, 179–83,
  212–14; bad experiences with 158–60,
  181–3, 212–14, 220–1; Basil Beaumont
  experiment 181–3; Walter Benjamin
  experiment 162–4; Kurt Beringer
  experiments 135–7; biochemistry 19–20,
  98–100; as brainwashing tool/truth
  serum 184–5, 215; in clinical research
  178–9, 183–4, 192, 214–15, 217, 235–6,
  238–9, 250; comparisons with LSD 19,
  189, 190, 192, 205–6, 215, 258n7;

cultural prominence in 1950s 4, 204–6; Walter Dixon experiments 103–4; double consciousness (*état mixte*) 8, 29, 104, 133–4, 158, 161; first isolated from peyote 98–100; first laboratory synthesis by Ernst Späth 8, 131–2; Aldous Huxley experiment 3, 202–4; Ernst Jünger experiments 187–8; Ken Kesey trip 236; Gheorghe Marinescu experiments 155–7; Christopher Mayhew experiment 221–3; medical uses 104, 142, 178, 185–6; 'mescal psychosis' 136–7, 141; Henri Michaux experiments 212–14; named by Arthur Heffter 98; Humphry Osmond experiment 193–4; pharmaceutical preparations 5, 131–2, 183, 214, 220, 250; physical symptoms 8, 28, 103–4, 136–7, 181, 237, 245; presence in cacti 8–11, 18–20, 25, 34; prohibition and scheduling 238–9; replaced by LSD 7, 205–6, 229, 235, 236–9; Jean-Paul Sartre experiment 158–60; Alexander Shulgin's trip 243; supplied by Merck 131–2, 152–3; synthetic derivatives 243–6; time distortions 104, 136–7, 182, 222–3; Julian Trevelyan experiment 180–1; Makepeace Tsao synthesis (1951) 239–40; visual hallucinations 8–10, 94, 134–5, 136–42, 145, 153–7, 158–60, 180–4, 185, 222; Andrew Weil experiments 238; Colin Wilson experiment 220–1; Stanisław Witkiewicz experiments 152–5; R.C. Zaehner experiment 220
Methvin, John Jasper, 71
Meyer, Adolf, 178
Microgram Journal (US Bureau of Narcotic and Dangerous Drugs), 239
Michailescu, Corneliu, 155–7
Michaux, Henri, 4, 211–14, 243; William Burroughs on 214; *chevauchements* 212; mescaline experiments 212–14; overdose 213
missionaries, on Indian reservations in USA 59, 60, 71, 72, 119, 195, 230; Spanish in Mexico 35–8
Mitchell, Silas Weir, 6, 86–91, 93, 112, 124, 138, 141, 143, 158; career 86; peyote experiment 87–3
MK-ULTRA, 185, 215, 235
MMDA (phenethylamine), 244
Moche culture, 25
Monardes, Nicolás, 38
Monet, Claude, 7, 93, 95

Mooney, James, 53–61, 65, 67–8, 72–5, 79, 83–4, 93, 94, 111, 114, 123–8, 143, 144, 172, 173, 251; brings peyote to Washington 75, 79; first peyote ceremony 54–5, 60; and Ghost Dance 57–9; and Native American Church 125–8; and Quanah Parker 73–5; testimony to House of Representatives 73–4, 123–5; upbringing 55–6
Moreau, Jacques-Joseph, 133–4, 135–6, 184
Morgan, Francis, 81–3, 85, 86, 90, 93, 98, 103, 112, 133, 138, 142; mescaline experiments 79, 81–3
Mormon church, *see* Church of Latter-Day Saints
morning glory (*Ipomeia purpurea*), 33, 143, 174
morphine, 18, 62, 95, 100, 107, 131, 133, 171, 176
mushrooms, hallucinogenic, 4, 19, 33, 35, 36, 174, 236–7; *see also* psilocybin
Myerhoff, Barbara, 44–7, 49, 233

Nahua culture, 33–8, 46, 95, 119; records of peyote use 8, 35–6
National Institute of Mental Health (NIMH), 216
Native American, 257n16; *see also* Apache people; Arapaho people; etc.
Native American Church (NAC), 6, 11, 28, 126–8, 171, 174, 176, 206–8, 228, 230, 249–51, 254–6; founding charter (1918) 126–7; growth in the 1960s 230–1; recent expansion 250–1; 1994 Supreme Court case 127–8
Native American Church of North America (NACNA), 207–8
Native Christian Church 126
Navajo (Diné) people, 251–2
Neuburg, Victor, 105–6
neurasthenia, 82, 86, 88, 154
New Buffalo commune (Taos), 229–30
New Orleans Picayune, 65
'New Thought' movement, 117
New York Neurological Institute, 133
New York Times, 119
New Yorker (magazine), 4, 208
Newsweek, 4, 205
niacin (Vitamin B3), 216
Nickels, Anna, 63–4, 80
Nietzsche, Elisabeth Förster, 162–3
Nietzsche, Friedrich, 161, 162–3, 187
nitrous oxide, 91, 270n12.

O'Keeffe, Georgia, 118
O'Neill, Eugene, 116
Observer, The 222–3
Office of Strategic Studies (US), 184–5;
  see also Central Intelligence Agency (CIA)
Ondegardo, Juan Polo de, 23
Ong, Walter, 94
opium 62, 71, 83, 95, 106, 107, 119, 131,
  143, 144, 161, 163, 192, 211; Opium
  Law (Germany, 1929) 163
Ordo Templi Orientis, 176
Osmond, Humphry, 3, 4, 193–8, 202–3,
  205, 206, 208, 215, 216–17, 219,
  221–2, 242; attends NAC meeting 208;
  experiment with adrenochrome 196–7;
  experiment with Aldous Huxley 3, 201–3;
  M-substance theory 194–7, 216–17;
  mescaline experience 193–4; schizophrenia
  research 4, 193–7; switches to LSD 206
Overhoser, Winfred, 184
Owsley, *see* Stanley, Augustus Owsley III

Paderewski, Ignacy Jan, 156
Paiute people, 57
Panpeyotl (pharmaceutical extract), 144–5,
  152, 153; *see also* Alexandre Rouhier
Parke, Davis & Co. (pharmacists), 59, 62–6,
  67, 85, 103, 108–9, 142; Aleister
  Crowley visits 108–9; Detroit headquar-
  ters 66, 108–9; Louis Lewin visits 66;
  'tincture of anhalonium' 67, 85, 108, 142
Parker, Cynthia Ann, 69
Parker, Quanah (Comanche), 69–75, 79,
  85–6, 249, 251, 256; chief of the
  Comanches 70; his grandfather peyote
  button 72, 249, 250; and James Mooney
  73–5; peyote roadman 71–3; rejects
  Ghost Dance 70
Parsons, Elsie Clews, 120
Parsons, Jack, 176
Pawnee people, 71
PCP (phencyclidine), 239
Pedro, Linda, 228–9
pellotine, 84, 98
Penrose, Lionel, 180
Penrose, Roland, 180
Peruvian Torch, 258n2; *see also* San Pedro
  cactus
Peta Nocona (Comanche), 69
peyote bird, 121–2
peyote cactus, 15, 33–49, 53–68, 70–5,
  79–100, 105–28, 138, 142–5, 152–5,
  163–7, 171–7, 206–9, 227–34, 236, 245,

249–56; alkaloid content 257n17, 18, 34;
  art inspired by 47–9, 96, 152–4; Antonin
  Artaud experiences 166–7; bad experiences with 62, 81, 82, 83, 90–1, 193–4;
  beatnik scene 227–8; John R. Briggs
  experiment 62; Carlos Castaneda and
  231–4; conservation issues 252–3;
  Aleister Crowley experiments 107–9;
  Mabel Dodge salon 114–16; Havelock
  Ellis experiments 93–4, 96; Erwin Ewell
  experiment 83; Arthur Heffter experiments 98–100; hippies 'up the cactus
  trail' 228–30; in Huichol culture 43–9;
  William James experiment 90–1; Carl
  Jung on 219; Carl Lumholtz experiments
  42–3; mail order suppliers 5, 113, 209,
  227–8, 236; Mexican ceremonies 38–41;
  Silas Weir Mitchell experiment 87–8;
  James Mooney reports on 54–5, 59–61;
  in Nahua culture 8, 35, 40; Native
  American ceremony, 4, 28, 54–5, 59–61,
  68, 70–5, 84, 173–5, 177, 206–9,
  249–50, 254–6; natural habitat 33, 45,
  252; pharmaceutical preparations 8, 67,
  85, 103, 106–9, 144–5, 153; Prentiss and
  Morgan experiments 79–83, 85;
  prohibition by League of Nations 145;
  prohibition in Mexico 39–40, 165;
  prohibition in USA 39, 95, 105, 112,
  119, 122, 127–8, 207, 227; remedy for
  alcoholism 60, 155, 208; Alexandre
  Rouhier on 142–5; as sacrament 36, 37,
  42, 45, 54, 71–5, 105, 107, 111–12, 115,
  127, 255; Arthur Symons experiment
  97–8; in Tarahumara culture 42–3, 47;
  taxonomy 34, 65, 66, 262n13, 100;
  Virgil Thomson experiments 113; as
  threat to public health 39, 60, 71, 95–6,
  105, 119–20, 208; as traditional medicine
  42, 55, 64, 71, 74, 121–2, 124, 143–5,
  208, 209, 252–5; visions induced by 35,
  36, 45–6, 62, 79, 81, 87–8, 89–90,
  93–100, 110, 113, 175, 219, 229; as
  western medicine 59–61, 67, 82–3, 103,
  143–4; Stanisław Witkiewicz experiments
  152–5; W.B. Yeats experiment 97
peyote gardens (Texas), 61, 68, 75, 112,
  122, 175, 252
peyoteros, 61, 62, 122, 227, 228, 229, 236,
  252
'Peyotyl R.D.' (pharmaceutical extract), 145
Pharmaceutische Zeitung, 85
phenethylamines, 19–20, 131, 193, 243–6

phenomenology 8, 146, 158–60, 187, 203, 211
Pliny (the Elder), 37
Plötner, Kurt, 185
Poco, Marcus (Comanche), 126
Ponca people, 71, 127
Post Oak Jim (Comanche), 125
Potter & Clarke (pharmacists), 91–2; 'Potter's Asthma Cure' 92
Powell, John Wesley, 56
Powick Hospital (Worcestershire), 215
Pratt, General R.H., 124–5
Prentiss, Daniel Webster, 79–83, 85, 86, 90, 93, 98, 103, 112, 133, 138, 142; mescaline experiments 79, 81–3
Progressive Association, 92
Progressive Era, 105, 110, 175, 201
Psalmodia christiana (1583), 35
psilocybin, 19, 187, 217, 235, 238; discovery 4, 235; mushrooms 4, 19, 33, 35, 235, 236–7; pharmaceutical (Indocybin) 235, 237
'psychedelic' (origin and use of term), 3, 94, 187
psychoanalysis, 132, 149, 172
psychosis, 133, 136–7, 141, 149, 157, 180, 182, 191–2, 194–7, 203, 216–17, 235, 238; 'mescal psychosis' 136–7, 141, 142, 143, 217, 238; *see also* schizophrenia
psychotomimetic theories 7, 136–7, 183–4, 191–2, 217, 235, 238
Pueblo Revolt (1680), 41
Puiwat (Comanche), 74–5
Pure Food and Drug Act (1906), 80
Purkinje, Jan, 139

Quahada (Comanche band), 69

Radcliffe, Raymond, 106
Rakoczi, Basil, *see* Beaumont, Basil
Ramón y Cajal, Santiago, 141
'Red Atlantis', 119
Red River War (1874–75), 69
Reed, John, 114, 117
Reiniger, Lotte, 29
Review of Reviews, 95
roadman (Native American peyote ceremony), 54–5, 72–5, 209, 249, 254–6
Rockefeller Foundation, 178, 190, 196, 216; funds mescaline research 178, 196
Roosevelt, President Franklin D., 118, 171–2
Roosevelt, President Theodore, 70

Ross, Jane, 4–5
Rouhier, Alexandre, 142–5, 149, 152, 153, 193, 243; on clairvoyance and indigenous medicine 143–4; Panpeyotl extract 144–5
Royal Bethlem Hospital (London), 179
Runke, Walter, 122
Rusby, Henry Hurd, 63, 67

Sahagún, Bernardino de, 34–8; describes peyote 34–5
Sainte-Anne Hospital (Paris), 191
St George's Hospital (London), 193, 195
Saints Herald, 110
St Thomas' Hospital (London), 103
Salm-Dyck, Prince Joseph de, 65
Salpêtrière Hospital (Paris), 155
Sandoz Pharmaceuticals, 188, 191, 206, 236, 237, 238
Sapir, Edward, 172
San Pedro cactus, 10, 15–29, 143, 234, 245, 251, 253–4; alkaloid content 10–11, 18–20, 257n17, 259n18; in art and archaeology 17, 24, 25; author's experiences with 28–9; biochemistry and metabolism 18–20; clairvoyance 26–7, 143–4; *Crystal Fairy and the Magical Cactus* 254; natural habitat 17–18, 20–1, 29; number of ribs 21; preparation 26, 27–8; as rooting and grafting stock 21; taxonomy 20–1, 258n2; traditional and contemporary use 25–7, 253–4; use in pre-Hispanic cultures 15, 23–5
Sandison, Ronald, 215
Sartre, Jean-Paul, 8, 157–60, 162, 220, 221; mescaline experiment 158–60
Saskatchewan Hospital, 195–6, 206
Sass, Louis, 203
Savoy Magazine, 96
Scalia, Antonin, 128
schizophrenia, 3, 133, 137, 142, 168, 179, 183–4, 190, 191–2, 194, 216–17, 223, 235; 'M-substance' theory of 4, 184, 194–7, 216–17; symptoms compared to mescaline intoxication 179, 183–4, 190, 194, 217, 235; *see also* psychosis
Schultes, Richard Evans, 174–5
Schumann, Karl, 85
scopolamine, 21
Sells, Cato, 128
serotonin (5-HT), 19, 258n7
Sertürner, Friedrich, 18, 131
Setkopti, Paul (Kiowa), 60, 144
shamans, shamanism, 15, 24, 25, 40, 42,

46, 47, 68, 72, 176, 231–4, 253–4; and Carlos Castaneda 231–4; *curanderismo* in Peru 25–7, 40, 253–4; Huichol *mara'akame* 44–5, 48

Sharon, Douglas, 234

Shulgin, Alexander, 243–6; mescaline trip 243; synthesises MDMA 244–5

Shumla caves (Texas), 34

Sia (Comanche Nation Ethno-Ornithological Initiative), 249, 261n46

Sigma-Aldrich, *see* Aldrich

Silva, Ramón Maria (Huichol), 44–5, 233; Castaneda's model for Don Juan 233; on peyote hunt 44–5

Simpsons, The, 243

Sitting Bull (Lakota), 57

Slade art school, 5

Slotkin, James Sydney, 4, 207; fieldwork 207; trustee of NAC 207

Slotta, Karl Heinrich, 178–9

Smith, Alfred Leo, 127

Smith, Frederick Madison, 110–13, 128, 243; and Native American peyote religion 111–12; peyote experiences 110; and 'second wind' 111

Smith, Joseph, 110

Smith, Kline & French (pharmaceutical company), 191

Smith, Ruth, 112

Smithsonian Institution, Bureau of Ethnology 53, 56, 59, 67, 80, 124, 128; founding by John Wesley Powell 56; publications 68, 124–5; recall of James Mooney from Oklahoma 128

Smurzło, Prosper, 152

Smythies, John R., 4, 5, 193–8, 201, 202–3, 205, 216–17, 219, 200, 242; gives mescaline to R.C. Zaehner 220; interest in the paranormal 5, 197; 'M-substance' theory 194–7; schizophrenia research 4, 193–7; visits Carl Jung 219

Smythies, Vanna, 193

Snyder, Gary, 176, 211

Society of American Indians, 123

Solís, Ruth Shady, 16

Southern, Terry, 228

Späth, Ernst, 131–2, 179, 239; first laboratory synthesis of mescaline (1919) 131–2

Stanley, Augustus Owsley III, 236, 244

Stein, Gertrude, 114, 117

Stephen, Karin, 182–3

Sterne, Maurice, 117, 118

Stockings, G. Tayleur, 183–4, 205

STP (phenethylamine), *see* DOM

strychnine, 67, 104

Supreme Court (US), 127–8

Surrealist movement, 150–1, 156, 157, 163, 180, 183

Symonds, John Addington, 92

Symons, Arthur, 92, 96–8, 107; hashish poetry 96; peyote experiment 97–8

Szuman, Stefan, 153, 155

Taíno people, 22

Tarahumara people, 42–3, 47, 48, 53, 68, 93, 143, 164–7, 173; visited by Antonin Artaud 165–7; visited by Carl Lumholtz 42–3

Takes Gun, Frank (Crow), 207–8

telepathy, *see* clairvoyance

Tello, Julio, 15–16, 23

Texas Rangers, 65

Texas–Mexico railroad, 8, 61, 70

Therapeutic Gazette, 59, 66, 82

Thomson, Virgil, 113

Thompson, Hunter S., 240–3; on Carlos Castaneda 240–1; *Fear and Loathing in Las Vegas* 240, 242; *First Trip with Mescalito* 241; mescaline trip

Time (magazine), 4, 205

Tiwanaku culture, 25

tobacco, 21–2, 27, 33, 38, 73, 155, 174–5, 209, 249, 250; Bull Durham brand 174–5

Tonarcy (Comanche, wife of Quanah Parker), 75

transmethylation hypothesis, 195–7

Trevelyan, Julian, 180–1; mescaline experiment 180–1

Trichocereus pachanoi/peruvianus, 15, 20–1; *see also* San Pedro cactus

tryptamines, 19

Tsao, Makepeace Uho, 239–40; mescaline synthesis 239

Tso, Andrew, 251

tuki (Huichol temples), 43, 46

Tzara, Tristan, 156

United Nations Convention on Psychotropic Substances (1971), 239

United Nations Narcotics Division, 250

United Nations Single Convention on Drugs (1961), 39

universities and medical schools: Berlin 65, 138; Berkeley 176, 243; Bucharest 155; Cambridge 103; Chicago 138, 145; Colorado 228; Columbian (now George

Washington) 79–80; Duke 227; Fordham 132; Freiburg 238–9; Hamburg 138; Harvard 89, 112–13; 174, 238; Heidelberg 135–7, 142, 146, 178; Jagellonian (Kraków) 153; Johns Hopkins 110, 178; King's College London 103; Minnesota 138; Oxford 219; Pennsylvania 142; Texas 229; UCLA 44, 233–4; Vienna 131; Yale 172; Zurich 132

vilca (DMT-containing snuff), 22–4, 25
Viracocha (Inca deity) 16
virola (DMT-containing bark), 22

Waddell, Leila, 106
Wain, Louis, 179–80
Waldo, James (Comanche), 126
Wallas, Graham, 149
'War on Drugs', 39
Wari culture, 25
Wasson, Gordon, 4
Waters, Frank, 176–7, 211, 228–9, 230; *Book of the Hopi* 177, 230; *The Man Who Killed the Deer* 177, 228–9; in Taos 177
Watson, Sereno, 65, 80
Watts, Alan, 237
Weber, Max, 104–5
Weil, Andrew, 237–8; mescaline experiences 238
Weiland, Eugene, 106
Wesley, John, 58
Whineray, Edward, 108
'whisky-root', 65; *see also* peyote cactus

White, Edmund, 103
Wichita Mountains, 54, 67, 75, 249
Wichita people, 53
Wiley, Harvey, 80, 83, 123, 124
Williams, William Carlos, 210
Wilson, Colin, 220–1; mescaline experiment 221
Wilson, Jack, *see* Wovoka
Wilson, John (Caddo roadman), 73
Wilson, Robert Anton, 272n20
Wirikuta (Huichol sacred land), 44–6, 252–3
Witkiewicz, Stanisław (father of Witkacy), 151
Witkiewicz, Stanisław Ignacy (Witkacy), 151–5, 158, 210, 243; art on peyote and mescaline 153–5; career 151–2; *Narcotics* (1932) 151–5
Wolfe, Jane, 176
Wolfe, Tom, 237
Woodcock, John, 205
Wordsworth, William, 7, 210
Wounded Knee massacre, 56–7
Wovoka (Paiute Ghost Dance prophet), 57–8, 69, 70; meets James Mooney 57–8
Wundt, Wilhelm, 132, 133
Wynter, Bryan, 5–6

yagé, see ayahuasca
Yeats, W.B., 92, 96–7, 107; peyote experiment 97

Zaehner, R.C., 219–20, 221; mescaline experiment 220
Zingg, Robert, 48–9

INDEX

Printed and bound by CPI Group (UK) Ltd, Croydon, CR0 4YY

20/12/2024

14615780-0001